主审　武阳丰

主编　胡继宏

编委　靳利梅　陈丽

流行病学

EPIDEMIOLOGY

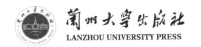

兰州大学出版社

LANZHOU UNIVERSITY PRESS

图书在版编目（ＣＩＰ）数据

　　流行病学 ＝ Epidemiology ： 汉文、英文 ／ 胡继宏
主编. －－ 兰州 ： 兰州大学出版社，2023.8
　　ISBN 978-7-311-06500-3

　　Ⅰ．①流… Ⅱ．①胡… Ⅲ．①流行病学－汉、英
Ⅳ．①R18

　　中国国家版本馆 CIP 数据核字(2023)第 111270 号

责任编辑　　陈红升　　牛涵波
封面设计　　琥珀视觉

书　　名　流行病学(Epidemiology)
作　　者　胡继宏　主编
出版发行　兰州大学出版社　（地址:兰州市天水南路 222 号　730000）
电　　话　0931-8912613(总编办公室)　0931-8617156(营销中心)
网　　址　http://press.lzu.edu.cn
电子信箱　press@lzu.edu.cn
印　　刷　西安日报社印务中心
开　　本　880 mm×1230 mm　1/16
印　　张　18.25
字　　数　499 千
版　　次　2023 年 8 月第 1 版
印　　次　2023 年 8 月第 1 次印刷
书　　号　ISBN 978-7-311-06500-3
定　　价　58.00元

序

流行病学是人类与疾病斗争过程中逐渐发展起来的一门学科，它的思想萌芽发端于 2000 多年前。流行病学以人群为对象，研究健康与疾病现象及决定因素，在疾病防治和健康促进方面发挥着巨大作用。流行病学作为预防医学的基础，也是预防医学的骨干学科、核心主干课程和执业医师考试的必考科目。流行病学研究方法作为医学界唯一研究群体的方法学，其提高人群健康水平的目标，也是医学与其他学科的重要内容。随着流行病学研究方法的不断完善和应用领域的不断扩展，它逐渐成为现代医学的基础学科，在医学教育、医学研究和医疗服务这三个领域中发挥着十分重要的作用，成为医学研究与实践中不可或缺的重要基础学科，是广大医学工作者从事防治工作必须要掌握的预防医学知识。

当前，不断涌现出很多新型传染病，如传染性非典型肺炎（SARS）、新型冠状病毒肺炎（COVID-19）、儿童不明原因肝炎等，这些传染病的暴发、流行，甚至大流行，给人民健康和社会经济带来巨大危害，彻底有效的防制需要明确其病因，消灭其源头。慢性非传染性疾病作为主要疾病负担，随着人口老龄化、环境污染等问题，其防制也任重道远。流行病学可以判断两个及两个以上事件是否有关联，以及关联性质和关联程度，从而确定其病因及作用大小，为疾病防控提供依据。

本书参考了美国耶鲁大学、印度 SRM 大学 *Epidemiology* 教材和美国著名流行病学家 Mark Woodward 编写的 *Epidemiology – Study Design and Data Analysis (Second Edition)*。本书采用中英文双语模式，内容主要包括绪论、疾病的分布、描述性研究、病例对照研究、队列研究、实验流行病学、病因和病因推断、筛检与诊断试验、疾病的预防和控制等九个章节内容，重点阐述流行病学原理和方法。本书适合医学专业的本科生和研究生使用，尤其适合预防医学专业的学生使用。

考虑到研究生教学和本科生考研的需要，我们经过不断查询资料、充分讨论后达成共识，最终完成该书的编写工作。在此，首先衷心感谢北京大学临床医学研究所武阳丰教授、中国医学科学院协和医学院阜外医院王增武教授、宁夏医科大学公共卫生学院张毓洪教授等给予的指导和帮助，还要感谢甘肃中医药大学公共卫生学院陈丽副教授（参与第9章的编写）、靳利梅讲师（参与第2章的编写）和曹良佳同学（参与格式编排和校对）的帮助。

鉴于主编水平有限，本书难免有不尽如人意的地方和疏漏之处，诚恳希望各位读者提出宝贵意见。

胡继宏

2023年5月

目　录

Chapter 1 Introduction to Epidemiology

Epidemiology is the basic science of preventive and social medicine. Its ramifications cover not only study of disease distribution and causation (and thereby prevention), but also health and health - related events occurring in human population. Modern epidemiology has entered the most exciting phase of its evolution. By identifying risk factors of chronic disease, evaluating treatment modalities and health services, it has provided new opportunities for prevention, treatment, planning and improving the effectiveness and efficiency of health services. The current interest of medical sciences in epidemiology has given rise to newer off-shoot such as infectious disease epidemiology, chronic disease epidemiology, clinical epidemiology, serological epidemiology, cancer epidemiology, malaria epidemiology, neuro epidemiology, genetic epidemiology, occupational epidemiology, psychosocial epidemiology, and so on. This trend is bound to increase in view of the increasing importance given to the pursuit of epidemiological studies. That these studies have added substantially to the advancement of medical knowledge is indisputable.

1.1 History of Epidemiology

Although epidemiologic thinking has been traced from Hippocrates (circa 400 B. C.) through Graunt (1662), Farr, Snow (both mid-1800's), and others, the discipline did not blossom until the end of the Second World War.

第 1 章 绪论

流行病学是预防医学和社会医学的基础学科，是研究人群中疾病和健康相关事件的分布及其影响因素，进一步开展疾病预防和健康促进的科学。现代流行病学已经进入到了重要的发展阶段。慢性病风险因素的识别、治疗模式及健康服务的评估，为疾病的预防、治疗、规划和卫生服务的效果和效率的提升提供了新的机遇。医学发展促使流行病学催生了很多新的分支，如传染病流行病学、慢性病流行病学、临床流行病学、血清流行病学、癌症流行病学、疟疾流行病学、神经流行病学、遗传流行病学、职业流行病学、心理社会流行病学等，这有利于提高流行病学研究的重要性，同时也大力促进了医学的发展。

1.1 流行病学简史

流行病学的思想最早可以追溯到希波克拉底（公元前 400 年左右），随后的 Graunt（1662 年）、Farr 和 Snow（19 世纪中期）等流行病学家相继出现，但直到第二次世界大战（以下简称"二战"）结束，流行病学都没有得到充分发展。

Hippocrates attempted to explain disease occurrence from a rational instead of a supernatural viewpoint. In his book entitled On *Airs, Waters, and Places*, Hippocrates suggested that environment and host factors such as behaviors might influence the development of disease.

Another early contributor to epidemiology was John Graunt, a London haberdasher who published his landmark analysis of mortality data in 1662. He was the first to quantify patterns of birth, death, and disease occurrence, noting male‑female disparities, high infant mortality, urban rural differences, and seasonal variations. No one built upon Graunt's work until the mid-800's, when William Farr began to systematically collect and analyze Britain's mortality statistics. Farr, considered the father of modern vital statistics and surveillance, developed many of the basic practices used today in vital statistics and disease classification. He extended the epidemiologic analysis of morbidity and mortality data, looking at the effects of marital status, occupation, and altitude. He also developed many epidemiologic concepts and techniques still in use today.

Meanwhile, an anesthesiologist named John Snow was conducting a series of investigations in London that later earned him the title "the father of modern epidemiology". Twenty years before the development of the microscope, Snow conducted studies of cholera outbreaks both to discover the cause of disease and to prevent its recurrence. His work classically illustrates the sequence from descriptive epidemiology to hypothesis generation to hypothesis testing (analytic epidemiology) to application. Snow conducted his classic study in 1854 when an epidemic of cholera developed in the Golden Square of London. He began his investigation by determining where in this area persons with cholera

希波克拉底曾试图摒弃超自然观点，科学地解释疾病的发生。在他的著作《空气、水和土壤》中，希波克拉底提出环境和宿主的行为等因素可能会影响疾病的发展。

另一个对早期流行病学有巨大贡献的是 John Graunt。他在1662年发表了具有里程碑意义的死亡数据的分析方法。他是第一个将出生、死亡和疾病进行定量分析的专家。通过分析，他发现死亡率存在性别差异、城乡差别、季节性变化及婴儿高死亡率等现象。Graunt 的工作并没有得到进一步的发展。直到19世纪80年代中期，William Farr 开始系统地收集和分析英国的死亡数据，扩展了发病率和死亡率的流行病学分析方法，探索分析了婚姻状况、职业和海拔对发病和死亡的影响，还开发了许多至今还在使用的流行病学概念和方法。Farr 是公认的现代统计分析和疾病监测的鼻祖，之后的科学家在他的研究基础上发展和实践了目前仍在使用的数据统计方法和疾病分类方法。

同时，John Snow 在伦敦对霍乱开展的系列研究为他赢得了"现代流行病学之父"的称号。在显微镜出现前20年，Snow 就发现了霍乱暴发的原因，并进行了复发的预防。1854年，伦敦黄金广场附近暴发了霍乱。Snow 为了调查引起霍乱暴发的原因，首先调查了这一区域所有患者居住和生活的地址，然后利用这些信息绘制了病例分布的散点地图。最后，他发现霍乱病例的分布可能和水井有关，故而推测宽街的水井作为黄金广场的主要水源，可能是导致霍乱的原因。封闭该水源后，病例数逐渐减少、消失，进一步验证了他关于病因的推测。这一经典研究，全面诠释了从描述性流行病学建立假设到分析流行病学检验假设

lived and worked. He then used this information to map the distribution of cases on what epidemiologists call a spot map. Lastly, he found a relationship between the distribution of cholera case households and the location of pumps. He thought that the Broad Street pump was probably the primary source of water for most persons with cholera in the Golden Square area.

In the mid-18th and late-18th, many others in Europe and the United States began to apply epidemiologic methods to investigate disease occurrence. At that time, most investigators focused on acute infectious diseases. In the 1900's, epidemiologists extended their methods to non-infectious diseases. The period since the Second World War has seen an explosion in the development of research methods and the theoretical underpinnings of epidemiology, and in the application of epidemiology to the entire range of health-related outcomes, behaviors, and even knowledge and attitudes. The studies by Doll and Hill linking smoking to lung cancer and the study of cardiovascular disease among residents of Framingham, Massachusetts, are the two examples of how pioneering researchers have applied epidemiologic methods to chronic disease since World War Ⅱ. Finally, during the lately 1960's and early 1970's health workers applied epidemiologic methods to eradicate smallpox worldwide. This was an achievement in applied epidemiology of unprecedented proportions. Today, Epidemiology is often practiced or used by non-epidemiologists to characterize the health of their communities and to solve day-to-day problems. This landmark in the evolution of the discipline is less dramatic than the eradication of smallpox, but it is no less important in improving the health of people everywhere.

的流行病学方法的应用过程。

19 世纪中晚期,欧美许多学者开始应用流行病学方法调查疾病的发生,该方法主要应用于调查急性传染病,20 世纪扩展到调查非传染病。二战以后,流行病学原理和方法得到了突飞猛进的发展,流行病学家们将流行病学方法的应用范围扩展到了与健康相关的所有问题上,甚至知识、态度和行为方面。Doll 和 Hill 关于吸烟与肺癌的研究及在弗明汉和马萨诸塞州进行的心血管疾病研究是二战以来将流行病学方法应用到慢性病的两个经典案例。20 世纪 60 年代末到 70 年代初,流行病学方法被用于在全球根除了天花,这是流行病学应用的又一重大成功。目前,流行病学方法还常被用于社区健康和日常问题的解决。

Definitions of epidemiology is listed as following, ranging from Hippocrates to those of the present.

① That branch of medical science which treatment epidemics (Parkin, 1873).

② The science of the mass phenomena of infectious diseases (Frost, 1927).

③ The study of disease, any disease, as a phenomenon (Greenwood, 1934).

④ The study of the distribution and determinants and disease frequency in man (MacMahon, 1960).

1.2　Definition of Epidemiology

The word "epidemiology" comes from the Greek words, "epi", meaning "on or upon", "demos", meaning "people", and "logos", meaning "the study of". Epidemiology has been defined by John M. Last. Epidemiology is the study of the distribution and determinants of health - related states or events in specified populations, and the application of this study to the control of health problems. This definition of epidemiology includes several terms which reflect some of the important principles of the discipline. As you study this definition, refer to the description of these terms below:

1.2.1　Study

Epidemiology is a basic course of public health and a basic method of scientific research.

1.2.2　Distribution

Epidemiology is concerned with the frequency and pattern of health events in a population. Frequency includes not only the number of such events in a population, but also the rate or risk of disease in the

流行病学的定义最早可以追溯到希波克拉底，到目前为止已有的流行病学相关定义简单列举如下：

①研究疫病治疗的医学分支学科（Parkin，1873）。

②研究传染病人群现象的学科（Frost，1927）。

③研究疾病及疾病现象的学科（Greenwood，1934）。

④研究人群中疾病分布、频率和决定因素的学科（MacMahon，1960）。

1.2　流行病学的定义

流行病学"epidemiology"一词源于希腊词汇，epi，意为"在……之上"；demos，意为"人群"；logos，意为"……研究"。John M. Last 将流行病学定义为研究人群中的健康相关状态或事件的分布及其影响因素，并用于健康问题防控的一门学科。这一定义包含了反映流行病学原理的几个重要术语，这几个术语可以解释如下：

1.2.1　学科

流行病学是一门公共卫生基础课程，也是科学研究的基本方法。

1.2.2　分布

流行病学关注人群中健康相关事件的频率和分布。频率不仅指人群中事件发生的数量，还包括人群中疾病的发生率或风险。发生率（事件发生人数与总人数相比）可以用来进行不同人群间

population. The rate (number of events divided by size of the population) is critical to epidemiologists because it allows valid comparisons across different populations.

Pattern refers to the occurrence of health-related events by time, place, and personal characteristics.

① Time characteristics include annual occurrence, seasonal occurrence, and daily or even hourly occurrence during an epidemic.

② Place characteristics include geographic variation, urban-rural differences, and location of worksites or schools.

③ Personal characteristics include demographic factors such as age, race, sex, marital status, and socioeconomic status, as well as behaviors and environmental exposures.

This characterization of the distribution of health-related states or events is one broad aspect of epidemiology called descriptive epidemiology. Descriptive epidemiology provides the What, Who, When, and Where of health-related events.

1.2.3 Determinants

Epidemiology is also used to search for causes and other factors that influence the occurrence of health-related events. Analytic epidemiology attempts to provide the why and how of such events by comparing groups with different rates of disease occurrence and with differences in demographic characteristics, genetic or immunologic make-up, behaviors, environmental exposures, and other so-called potential risk factors. Under ideal circumstances, epidemiologic findings provide sufficient evidence to direct swift and effective public health control and prevention measures.

的比较，所以在流行病学中十分重要。

分布指健康相关事件在时间、空间和人间上的分布特点：

①时间分布，包括年度变化、季节变化和流行期间每天甚至每小时的变化。

②空间分布，包括地理位置差异、城乡差异、工作或学习场所差异。

③人间分布，包括人口学因素，如年龄、民族、性别、婚姻状态、社会经济状况，也包括行为因素和环境暴露因素。

健康相关状态或事件的时间、空间和人间的"三间"分布特征是描述流行病学主要的研究内容。

1.2.3 影响因素

流行病学也用于探索健康相关事件的病因和其他影响因素。分析流行病学通过比较组间发病率的差异、人口学特点的差异、基因或免疫修饰的差异、行为因素的差异、环境暴露的差异和其他潜在危险因素的差异来回答这些健康相关事件为什么会发生、是如何发生的。理想情况下，流行病学研究结果为制定有效的公共卫生预防和控制措施提供了充分的证据。

1.2.4　Health-related states or events

Originally, epidemiology was concerned with epidemics of communicable diseases. Then epidemiology was extended to endemic communicable diseases and non-communicable infectious diseases. More recently, epidemiologic methods have been applied to chronic diseases, injuries, birth defects, maternal - child health, occupational health, and environmental health. Now, even behaviors related to health and well - being (amount of exercise, seat - belt use, etc.) are recognized as valid subjects for applying epidemiologic methods.

1.2.5　Specified populations

Although epidemiologists and physicians in clinical practice are both concerned with disease and the control of disease, they differ greatly in how they view "the patient". Clinicians are concerned with the health of an individual; epidemiologists are concerned with the collective health of the people in a community or other area. When faced with a patient with diarrheal disease, for example, the clinician and the epidemiologist have different responsibilities. Although both are interested in establishing the correct diagnosis, the clinician usually focuses on treating and caring for the individual. The epidemiologist focuses on the exposure (action or source that caused the illness), the number of other persons who may have been similarly exposed, the potential for further spread in the community, and interventions to prevent additional cases or recurrences.

1.2.4　健康相关状态或事件

流行病学最初研究的是传染病，后来逐渐扩展到地方病和非传染病。目前，流行病学方法已经应用到慢性病、意外伤害、出生缺陷、妇幼保健、职业卫生、环境卫生等领域，甚至涉及健康相关行为和生活质量（如体育锻炼、安全带的使用等）。

1.2.5　特定人群

虽然流行病学和临床医学都关注疾病及其控制，但它们的研究对象并不相同。临床医学的研究对象是病人个体，提倡个体化治疗；流行病学的研究对象是人群，关注的是人群的健康问题。例如，当霍乱发生时，临床医生在准确诊断的基础上，采用个体化的治疗和护理；流行病学家则关注的是引起疾病发生的暴露因素（病因）、相同暴露下的发病人数、疾病的传染力、预防疾病传播和复发的措施等。

1.2.6   Application

Epidemiology is more than "a discipline". As a discipline within public health, epidemiology provides data for directing public health action. However, using epidemiologic data is an art as well as a science. Consider again the medical model used above: To treat a patient, a clinician must call upon experience and creativity as well as scientific knowledge.

Similarly, epidemiologist also need personal experience and medical knowledge when applying descriptive and analytical epidemiological methods to community diagnosis and disease prevention and control.

1.3   Epidemiological Approach

1.3.1   The epidemiological approach to problems of health and disease is based on two major foundations

1. Asking questions

Epidemiology has been defined as "a means of learn to asking questions.... and getting answers that lead to find questions". For example, the following questions will be asked:

（1）Related to health events

① What is event?（the problem）

② What is its magnitude?

③ Where did it happen?

④ When did it happen?

⑤ Who are affected?

⑥ Why did it happen?

（2）Related to health action

① What can reduce the problem and its consequences?

1.2.6   应用

流行病学不单纯是一门学科，作为公共卫生的基础课程，它还为指导公共卫生实践提供了证据支持。流行病学数据的应用是一门艺术，也是一门科学。临床医生治疗患者时不仅需要依靠个人经验，还需结合医学模式，应用流行病学的科学知识。

同样，流行病学家应用描述性和分析性流行病学方法进行社区诊断和疾病防控时，也需要个人经验和医学知识。

1.3   流行病学方法

1.3.1   研究健康和疾病相关问题的流行病学方法主要基于两个方面

1.提出问题

流行病学研究方法的定义为"学习如何提出问题和寻找解决问题的方法"。例如，会提出以下的问题：

（1）与健康事件相关的问题

①是什么健康相关事件？（问题）

②事件发生的频率为多少？

③在哪里发生的？

④什么时候发生的？

⑤对哪些人有影响？

⑥为什么会发生？

（2）与采取的措施相关的问题

①什么可以减少这一健康相关事件的发生并减轻其后果？

② How can it be prevented in the future?

③ What action should be taken by the community? What health services should be provided? Which departments are involved? By other sectors? Where and for whom these activities be carried out?

④ What resources are required? How are the activities to be organized?

⑤ What difficulties may arise? and how might they be overcome?

Answer to the above questions may provide clues to disease aetiology, and help the epidemiologist to guide planning and evaluation.

2. Making comparison

The basic approach in epidemiology is to make comparisons and draw inferences. This may be comparison of two groups (or more groups)— one group having the disease (or exposed to risk factor) and the other group(s) not having the disease (or not exposed to risk factor), or comparison between individuals. By making comparisons, the epidemiologist tries to find out the crucial differences in the host and environmental factors between those affected and not affected. In the short, the epidemiologist weights, balances and contrasts. Clues to aetiology come from such comparison.

One of the first considerations before making comparisons is to ensure what is known as "comparability" between the study and control groups. In other words, both the groups should be similar so that "like can be compared with like". For facts to be comparable, they must be accurate, and they must be gathered in a uniform way. For example, the study and control groups should be similar with regard to their age and sex composition, and similar other pertinent variables. The best method of ensuring comparability, in such

②今后该如何预防？

③社区该采取什么措施？该提供什么健康服务？由哪些部门参与？提供健康服务的地点是哪里？对象是谁？

④健康服务需要哪些资源？如何组织？

⑤可能会出现哪些困难及如何解决？

以上问题的答案有助于提供病因线索，帮助流行病学家进行规划和评价。

2. 比较

流行病学的核心是通过比较进行推论。比较至少需要两组人群，一组病例组（或暴露组），一组对照组（或非暴露组）。通过比较，流行病学家可以发现两组在宿主和环境因素方面的差异，从而判断它们是否与疾病有关。简而言之，比较是流行病学的核心，病因的线索来源于比较。

通过比较确定病因线索前，要明确哪些因素在比较的组间具有可比性，即比较的组间在哪些方面是相似的，这样才能均衡混杂因素，从而控制混杂偏倚对结果真实性的影响。例如，试验组和对照组年龄、性别和其他非干预因素应该均衡可比。随机化分组是保证可比性、控制混杂偏倚的最好方法之一，但是在病例对照研究和队列研究中无法进行随机化分组，这时可以采用匹配的方法来减少混杂因素对结果的影响，或者采用标准化的方法或者分层分析的方法等减少年龄、性

cases, is by randomization or random allocation. Where random allocation is not possible (as in case control and cohort studies) what is known as "matching" is done for selected characteristics that might confound the interpretation of results. Another alternative is standardization which usually has a limited application to a few characteristics such as age, sex and parity.

1.3.2　Classification of epidemiological studies

Epidemiological studies can be classified as observational studies and experimental studies with further subdivisions:

1.Observational studies

（1）Descriptive studies

① Ecological or correlative, with populations as unit of study.

② Cross - sectional or prevalence, with individuals as unit of study.

（2）Analytical studies

① Case - control or case - reference, with individuals unit of study.

② Cohort or follow - up, with individuals unit of study.

2. Experimental studies or intervention studies

① Randomized controlled trials or clinical trials, with patients as unit of study.

② Field trials, with healthy people as unit of study.

③ Community trials, with communities as unit of study.

别、经济状况等混杂因素对结果的影响。

1.3.2　流行病学研究方法的分类

流行病学研究方法可以分为观察法和实验法。具体分类如下：

1. 观察法

（1）描述性研究

①生态学研究或相关性研究，以人群为研究单位。

②横断面研究或患病率研究，以个体为研究单位。

（2）分析性研究

①病例对照研究或病例参照研究，以个体为研究单位。

②队列研究或随访研究，以个体为研究单位。

2. 实验法或干预研究

①随机对照试验或临床试验，以病人为研究单位，目的是治疗疾病。

②现场试验，以健康高危个体为研究单位，目的是预防疾病。

③社区试验，以社区为研究单位，目的是预防疾病。

1.4　Using of Epidemiology

1.4.1　Three main aims of epidemiology study

According to the International Epidemiology Association (IEA), epidemiology has three main aims:

① To describe the distribution and magnitude of health and disease problems in human populations.

② To identify aetiological factors (risk factors) in the pathogenesis of disease.

③ To provide the data essential to the planning, implementation and evaluation of services for the prevention, control and treatment of disease and to the setting up of priorities among those services.

In order to fulfill these aims, three rather different classes of epidemiological studies may be mentioned: descriptive studies, analytical studies, and experimental or intervention studies.

1.4.2　The ultimate aim of epidemiology

The ultimate aim of epidemiology is lead to effective action:

① To eliminate or reduce the health problem or its consequences.

② To promote the health and well-being of society as a whole.

1.4.3　The uses of epidemiology

These uses are categorized and described below:

1. Population or community health assessment

To set policy and plan programs, public health of-

1.4　流行病学的用途

1.4.1　流行病学研究的三个主要目标

国际流行病学会总结了流行病学研究的三个主要目标：

①描述人群中疾病和健康问题的分布。

②确定疾病的病因（危险因素）。

③为疾病防治措施的确定、健康促进、卫生服务评价及卫生资源优先配置等提供科学依据。

为了实现以上三个目标，至少需要三种不同类型的流行病学研究方法：描述性研究、分析性研究、实验（或干预）性研究。

1.4.2　流行病学研究的最终目的

流行病学研究的最终目的是采取有效的措施，达到以下目的：

①消除或减少健康问题或其后果。

②促进健康，提高全人类的生活质量。

1.4.3　流行病学的用途

1. 人群或社区健康评价

制定疾病预防策略和措施时，要考虑这些措

ficials must assess the health of the population or community they serve and must determine whether health services are available, accessible, effective, and efficient. To do this, they must find answers to many questions: What are the actual and potential health problems in the community? Where are they? Who is at risk? Which problems are declining over time? Which ones are increasing or have the potential to increase? How do these patterns relate to the level and distribution of services available? The methods of descriptive and analytic epidemiology provide ways to answer these and other questions. With answers provided through the application of epidemiology, the officials can make informed decisions that will lead to improved health for the population they serve.

2. Individual decisions

People may not realized that they use epidemiologic information in their daily decisions. When they decide to stop smoking, take the stairs instead of the elevator, order a salad instead of a cheeseburger with French fries, or choose one method of contraception instead of another, they may be influenced, consciously or unconsciously, by epidemiologists' assessment of risk. Since World War Ⅱ, epidemiologists have provided information related to all those decisions. In the 1950's, epidemiologists documented the increased risk of lung cancer among smokers; in the 1960's and 1970's, epidemiologists noted a variety of benefits and risks associated with different methods of birth control; in the mid-1980's, epidemiologists identified the increased risk of human immunodeficiency virus（HIV）infection associated with certain sexual and drug-related behaviors; and, more positively, epidemiologists continue to document the role of exercise and proper diet in reducing the risk of heart disease. These

施在人群和社区中实施的可行性、科学性、效果和效益。为了达到这些目的，首先要找到以下问题的答案：社区主要和潜在的健康问题是什么？这些健康问题主要在哪里发生？谁是高危人群？哪些健康问题随着时间的变化频率减少？哪些健康问题的频率可能增加？如何采取措施影响健康问题的频率和分布？描述流行病学和分析流行病学为解决这些问题提供了方法。政府部门可以根据流行病学的研究结果进行政策决策，从而提高人群健康水平。

2. 个人决策

在日常生活的决策中，很多人没有意识到自己实际上也应用了流行病学的信息。比如决定采用戒烟、走楼梯替代乘坐电梯、吃色拉替代吃汉堡等健康的生活方式时，可能潜意识受到了流行病学关于疾病危险因素的影响。二战以来，大量流行病学研究提供了很多决策信息。例如，20世纪50年代，吸烟与肺癌关系的研究；20世纪60年代到70年代，不同避孕方法的益处和害处的研究；20世纪80年代中期，性行为与吸毒增加HIV感染风险的研究。这些流行病学研究结果直接影响了人们的日常决策，也将影响人们的终身健康。

and hundreds of other epidemiologic findings are directly relevant to the choices that people make every day, choices that affect their health over a lifetime.

3. Completing the clinical picture

When studying a disease outbreak, epidemiologists depend on clinical physicians and laboratory scientists for the proper diagnosis of individual patients. But epidemiologists also contribute to physicians' understanding of the clinical picture and natural history of disease. For example, in late 1989 three patients in New Mexico were diagnosed as having myalgias (severe muscle pains in chest or abdomen) and unexplained eosinophilia (an increase in the number of one type of white blood cell). Their physician could not identify the cause of their symptoms, or put a name to the disorder. Epidemiologists began looking for other cases with similar symptoms, and within weeks had found enough additional cases of eosinophilia-myalgia syndrome to describe the illness, its complications, and its rate of mortality. Similarly, epidemiologists have documented the course of HIV infection, from the initial exposure to the development of a wide variety of clinical syndromes that include acquired immunodeficiency syndrome (AIDS). They have also documented the numerous conditions that are associated with cigarette smoking — from pulmonary and heart disease to lung and cervical cancer.

4. Search for causes

Much of epidemiologic research is devoted to a search for causes, factors which influence one's risk of disease. Sometimes this is an academic pursuit, but more often the goal is to identify a cause so that appropriate public health action might be taken. Nevertheless, epidemiology often provides enough information

3.临床规划

当疾病暴发时，流行病学家能够依靠临床医生和实验室检测做出正确的疾病诊断。同时，流行病学也会帮助临床医生了解疾病自然史和做出临床规划。例如，1989年末，新墨西哥州有3名患者被发现患有肌痛（胸腹部的严重肌痛）和不明原因的嗜酸粒细胞增多（白细胞系中的一种细胞数目增多）。当时，临床医生不能判断引起这些症状的原因，也无法给予相应的诊断。于是流行病学家开始寻找其他相似的病例，几周内发现了足够数量的嗜酸粒细胞增多症-肌痛综合征病例，流行病学家通过描述疾病特征、并发症和死亡率，分析比较病例与对照的差异，阐明了HIV的感染过程。类似地，流行病学家还描述了从HIV暴露到AIDS临床症状的疾病自然变化过程。流行病学研究还阐明了吸烟与肺心病、肺癌和宫颈癌等疾病的关系，得出的结论是戒烟可以降低多个疾病的发生风险。

4.病因探索

流行病学作为预防医学的主干课程，就是为了帮助人们明确疾病的病因，这样人们才能提出有针对性的、有效的防治措施，如John Snow消毒水源预防霍乱的措施、禁售某牌子卫生棉条防控中毒休克综合征的措施等。需要注意的是，通常需要流行病学调查和实验室检验共同为病因的确

to support effective action. Examples include John Snow's removal of the pump handle and the withdrawal of a specific brand of tampon that was linked by epidemiologists to toxic shock syndrome. Just as often, epidemiology and laboratory science converge to provide the evidence needed to establish causation. For example, a team of epidemiologists were able to identify a variety of risk factors during an outbreak of pneumonia among persons attending the American Legion Convention in Philadelphia in 1976. However, the outbreak was not "solved" until the Legionnaires' bacillus was identified in the laboratory almost 6 months later.

1.5 Epidemiology and Clinical Medicine

The basic difference between epidemiology and clinical medicine is that in epidemiology, the unit of study is "defined population" or "population at risk"; in clinical medicine, the unit of study is a "case" or "cases". In clinical medicine, the physician is concerned with disease in individual patient, whereas the epidemiologist is concerned with disease patterns in the entire population. Epidemiologist is thus concerned with both sick and healthy. It has stated that clinicians are interested in cases with the diseases and the statistician with the population from which the cases are derived and the epidemiologist is interested in the relationship between cases and the population in the form of a rate.

In clinical medicine, the physician seeks a diagnosis which he derive a prognosis and prescribes specific treatment. In epidemiology, an analogous situation exists in epidemiologist is confronted with relevant data derived from particular epidemiological study. He seeks to identify the particular source of in-

定提供证据。例如，1976年参加费城退伍军人联谊会的老兵暴发急性肺炎，直到6个月后，实验室检测出军团菌才确定了疾病的病因。

1.5 流行病学和临床医学

流行病学和临床医学的基本区别在于，在流行病学中，研究单位是"特定人群"或"高危人群"；在临床医学中，研究单位是"病例个体"或"系列病例"。在临床医学中，医生关注患病个体，而在流行病学中，流行病学家关注人群的疾病模式。因此，流行病学既关心疾病，也关心健康。临床医学对患病病例感兴趣，统计学对病例来源的人群感兴趣，而流行病学对病例与人群之间以比率形式存在的关系感兴趣。

临床医学中，临床医生首先要明确诊断，才能给予相应的治疗和预后的判断；流行病学中，需要根据流行病学研究获得的数据进行逻辑推断。为了确定疾病流行的趋势和控制措施，流行病学家需要确定传染源和传播途径。流行病学还可以用来评价预防和治疗措施的效果，为政府管理部

fection, a mode of spread of aetiological factor in order to determine a future trend recommend specific control measures. The epidemiologist also evaluates the outcome of preventive and therapy measures instituted which provides the necessary guide and feed - back to the health care administrator for effective management of public health programmes.

In clinical medicine, the patient comes to the doctor. In the epidemiology, the investigator goes out into the community find persons who have the disease or experience suspected causal factor in question. Clinical medicine is on biomedical concepts with an ever - increasing concerning refining the technique of diagnosis and treatment an individual level. The subject matter of clinical medicine easily "perceived" by such techniques as clinical laboratory examinations including post - mortem report on contract, the subject matter of epidemiology is "concept" and can only be symbolized in the form of tables.

Finally, it may be stated that clinical medicine but epidemiology are not antagonistic. Both are closely relative co - existent and mutually helpful. Most epidemiologist enquiries could never be established without approach, clinical consideration as to how the disease in question of identified among individuals comprising the group of scrutiny. Likewise, knowledge of prevalence, aetiology, and prognosis derived from epidemiological research is important to clinician for the diagnosis and management in individual patients and their families.

门制定有效的公共卫生服务方案提供必要的指导和反馈。

临床医学是病人找医生看病，流行病学是研究人员深入社区，寻找患有该疾病或具有可疑病因的人。临床医学以生物医学概念为基础，考虑个体化的治疗方案，很大程度上受到临床实验室检查（包括检查后的分析报告）等技术的影响。

临床医学和流行病学不是对立的，二者密切相关，相互促进。大多数流行病学调查都离不开临床知识，如疾病的诊断。同样，流行病学研究的患病率、病因和预后知识对临床医生诊断和治疗患者及与其家属沟通都非常重要。

Chapter 2 Distribution of Disease

Distribution of disease refers to how a disease occurs in a population and addresses questions, such as who develop the disease and where and when the disease occurs. To answer these questions, it involves comparisons among population in different geographic areas, different subgroups within a population, or the same population over different periods of time. A disease normally exhibits a unique pattern of distribution. This distribution is determined by factors such as the characteristics of the population and the natural and socio-economic environment where the population lives. Thus, it may change over time. Knowledge of distributions by people, time and place (commonly known as three-dimension distribution in epidemiology) is usually the starting point of epidemiological investigations. It is also essential for formulating hypotheses concerning possible causal or preventive factors and for planning healthcare services and making public health policy decisions.

2.1 Measure or Index of Disease Frequency

Inherent in the definition of epidemiology is measurement frequency of disease, disability or death, and summarizing information in the form of rates and ratios (e. g., prevalence, incidence rate, death rate, etc.). Thus the basic measure disease frequency is rate or ratio. These rates are essential comparing disease frequency in different population subgroups of the same population in relation to suspect causal factors. Such

第2章 疾病的分布

疾病的分布是指疾病在什么人群中、什么时间点和什么地区发生，死亡及患病水平的频率变化及其分布特征为病因探求提供了线索。为了回答这些问题，需要对疾病在不同地区、不同人群、不同时间内的情况进行比较。不同疾病的分布通常有所不同，疾病的分布由人口特征以及人口所处的自然和社会经济环境等因素决定。因此，疾病的分布可能会随着时间而变化。疾病的分布（在流行病学中通常称为"三间分布"）是流行病学调查的起点。它不仅为形成病因假设及探索病因提供了线索，也为临床医学和卫生服务需求提供了重要信息，进而为制定和评价防治疾病及促进健康的策略和措施提供了科学依据。

2.1 疾病频率的测量指标

传统的流行病学定义是以比和率来测量疾病、伤残和死亡的频率（比如患病率、发病率、死亡率等）的。因此，比和率是测量疾病的基本频率指标。通过对不同亚组人群疾病频率的比较，可以建立病因假设，这也是制定预防和控制健康问题策略的重要一步。

comparisons may yield important clinical disease aetiology. This is a step in the development strategies for prevention or control of health problems.

Equally, epidemiology is also concerned with the measurement of health-related events and states in the community (e. g., health needs, demands, activities, tasks, health care utilization) and variables such as blood pressure, serum cholesterol, height, weight, etc. In this respect, epidemiology has the features of a quantitative science. Much of the subject matter of measurement of disease and health - related events falls in the domain of biostatistics, which is a basic tool of epidemiology. Epidemiologist needs a definition:

① That is acceptable and applicable to its use in large populations.

② That is precise and valid, to enable him to identify those who have the disease from those who do not. Clear definitions help to minimize errors in classification of data. Standardized methods of observation and recording are therefore essential before commencing any epidemiological study.

2.1.1 Tools of measurement

The epidemiologist usually expresses disease magnitude with a rate or proportion. A clear understanding of the tool is required for proper interpretation of epidemiological features. The basic tools of measurement in epidemiology are:

1.Rate

When we say there 500 deaths from vehicle accidents in City A during 1985, it is just nothing more counting deaths in that city during that particular year. Such statement might be sufficient for the municipal

流行病学也同样关注社区人群的健康相关事件和状态（例如，健康需要、需求、任务和卫生保健利用），以及血压、血清胆固醇、身高、体重等健康影响因素。流行病学需要定量测量健康相关事件及其影响因素，还需要利用生物统计学对测量的信息进行分析。定量分析前，需要确定健康相关事件及其影响因素的定义，这些相关定义必须具备以下特点：

①在大样本人群中使用，必须可接受且可行。

②必须精确且合理，能够准确区分有病（暴露）或无病（非暴露），减少错分偏倚。另外，在流行病学调查过程中采用统一的、标准化的方法收集信息也是十分必要的。

2.1.1 测量工具

频率测量是定量研究疾病分布特征的有效方法，流行病学通常用率或比表示疾病的强度。只有正确理解测量工具，才能合理解释疾病的流行病学特点。流行病学中基本的测量工具有：

1.率

当我们说1985年A城市有500人死于车祸时，绝对死亡人数不具有任何意义，因此单纯依靠该数据促使市政当局提供必要卫生服务的可能性极小。流行病学家通过比较A、B城市的事故发生

administration to provide necessary health services. But it conveys meaning to an epidemiologist who is interested in comparing the frequency of accidents in City A with City B allow such comparisons, the frequency must be expressed to rate.

A rate measure the occurrence of some particular effect（development of disease or the occurrence of death）in a population during a given time period. It is statement of the risk of developing a condition. It indicates the change in some event that takes place in a population over a period of time. An example of a typical rate is the death rate. It is written as below：

$$Death\ rate = \frac{Number\ of\ deaths\ in\ one\ year}{Mid\text{-}year\ population} \times 1\ 000‰$$

$$(2\text{-}1)$$

A rate comprises the following element - numerator, denominator, time specification and multiplier. The time dimension is usually a calendar year. The rate is expressed per 1 000 or some other round figure（10 000；100 000）selected according to convenience or convention to avoid fractions.

The various categories of rates as follows：

（1）Crude rates

These are the actual observed rates such as the birth and death rates. Crude rates are also known as unstandardized rates.

（2）Specific rates

These are the actual observed rates due to specific cause（e.g., tuberculosis）；or occurring in specific groups（e.g., age - sex groups）or during specific time periods（e.g., annual, monthly or weekly rates）.

（3）Standardized rates

These are obtained by direct or indirect method of standardization or adjustment, such as age and sex standardized rates, were primarily used for the compari-

率，方能为卫生服务决策提供科学依据。

率表示某一特定时期内，人群中某一特定事件（疾病或死亡）的发生频率，体现了事物发展过程中的风险。它可以显示一段时间内某一事件在人群中的变化。死亡率是率的典型示例，公式如下：

$$死亡率 = \frac{某人群某年总死亡人数}{该人群同年平均人数} \times 1\ 000‰$$

$$(2\text{-}1)$$

率包括分子、分母，时间维度和系数。时间维度通常以年为单位。根据惯例，为避免使用分数，率通常以每1 000或其他整数（如10 000、100 000）表示。

率的分类如下：

（1）粗率

通常是实际观察到的比率，如出生率和死亡率。粗率也称为非标准化率。

（2）专率

通常是具体病因的实际观察率（如肺结核死亡率）或发生在特定的群体中（如年龄、性别死亡率）或在特定的时间段内的专率（如年度、月度或每周死亡率）。

（3）标准化率

通过直接或间接的标准化法获得的，如年龄和性别标准化率，主要用于人口特征构成不同的人群间率的比较，以控制混杂偏倚。

son of rates between populations with different demographic characteristics to control for confounding bias.

2. Ratio

Another measure of disease frequency is a ratio. It expresses a relation in size between two random quantities. The numerator is not a component of the denominator. The numerator and denominator may involve an interval of time or may be instantaneous in time. Broadly, ratio is result of dividing one quantity by another. It is expressed in the form of ratio:

$$x : y \quad \text{or} \quad \frac{x}{y} \quad\quad (2\text{-}2)$$

Example 1 :

The ratio of white blood cells relative to red cells is $1 : 600$ or $1/600$, meaning that for each white cell, there are 600 red cells.

Example 2:

$$\frac{\text{The number of children with scabies at a certain time}}{\text{The number of children with malnutrition at a certain time}}$$

Other examples include sex-ratio, doctor-population ratio, child-woman ratio, etc.

3.Proportion

A proportion is a ratio which indicates relation in magnitude of a part of the whole. The numerator is always included in the denominator. A proportion is usually expressed as a percentage.

Example:

$$\frac{\text{The number of children with scabies at a certain time}}{\text{The total number of children in the village at the same time}} \times 100\%$$

4.Concept of numerator and denominator

（1）Numerator

Numerator refers to the number of times an event (e.g., sickness, birth, death, episodes of sickness) has

2. 比

比是疾病频率的另一个测量指标。它表示两个相关指标的比值。分子不是分母的一个组成部分。分子和分母可能是一个时间间隔或某一瞬间的数值。广义上，比是一个数除以另一个数的结果，可以表示为以下形式：

$$x : y \quad \text{或} \quad \frac{x}{y} \quad\quad (2\text{-}2)$$

示例1：

白细胞计数与红细胞的比是 $1 : 600$ 或 $1/600$，意味着每一个白细胞对应600个红细胞。

示例2：

$$\frac{\text{某一确定时间内患疥疮的儿童数}}{\text{某一特定时间内营养不良的儿童数}}$$

其他实例包括性别比、医患比、儿童妇女比等。

3. 构成比

构成比表示构成整体的各个组成部分所占的比例。分子是分母的一部分。构成比通常用百分数表示。

示例：

$$\frac{\text{某一确定的时间内村里患疥疮的儿童数}}{\text{同时期村里儿童的总数}} \times 100\%$$

4.分子和分母的概念

（1）分子

分子是在特定时间内，某一事件（疾病、生育、死亡）在人群中发生的次数。计算率时，分

occurred in a population, during a specified time-period. The numerator is a component of the denominator in calculating a rate, but not in a ratio.

（2）Denominator

Numerator has little meaning unless it is related to denominator, the epidemiologist has to choose appropriate denominator while calculating a rate. It may related to the population, or related to the total events.

1）Related to the population

The denominators related to the population comprise following:

① Mad-year population: Because population size changes daily due to births, deaths, migration, the mid-year population is commonly chosen denominator. The mid-point refers to the population estimated as on the first of July of a year.

② Population at risk: This is an important concept in epidemiology because it focuses on groups at risk of disease rather than individuals. The term is applied to all those to whom could have happened whether it did or not. For example, what are determining the rate of accidents for a town population at risk is all the people in the town. But some term it may be necessary to exclude people because they are not in risk, as for example, in food poisoning, only those who ate food are at of becoming ill. Similarly in calculating "general fertility rate", the denominator is restricted to who of child-bearing age (i.e., 15-49 years),older women and little girls are excluded because they are not "at risk" becoming pregnant. In short, "population at risk" is restricted solely to those who are capable of having or acquiring disease or condition in question.

③ Person-time: In epidemiological studies (e.g., cohort studies), persons enter the study at different time. Consequently, the under observation is for vary-

子是分母的一部分；计算相对比时，则不是。

（2）分母

只有与分母相关的分子才有意义。流行病学中必须选择合适的分母来计算率，其可能与人群总数相关或与事件总数相关。

1）与人群相关的概念
与人群相关的分母包括以下几种：

①年中人口数：由于出生、死亡、迁徙等原因，人口数量每天都在发生变化，因此分母通常选择年中人口数。年中人口数是指每年七月一日的人口估计数，或者年初与年终人口数的平均人口数。

②高危人群：这是流行病学中的一个重要概念，它聚焦高危群体而不是个体，是指所有可能发生疾病风险的人。例如，决定一个城镇居民发生事故的概率的是该城镇的所有居民。有时需要把那些不具备发病风险的人排除，例如，在食物中毒中，只有那些吃食物的人才可能生病。同样，在计算总生育率时，分母应限定在生育年龄内（即 15～49 岁），年龄较大的妇女和小女孩应该被排除在外，因为她们没有怀孕的"可能性"。简而言之，"高危人群"仅限于那些可能患有某种疾病或可能存在某种暴露的人。

③人时：在流行病学研究（如队列研究）中，人们在不同的时间进入研究，观察的时间不同。在这种情况下，分母是人与时间的结合。经常使

ing time periods. In such case denominator is a combination of persons and time. The frequently used person-time is persons-years. Sometimes may be person-months, person-weeks or man-hours. For example, if 10 persons remain in the study for 10 years, they are said to be 100 person-years of observation. The figure would be derived if 100 persons were observation per one year. These denominators have advantage of summarizing the experience of persons within different durations of observation or exposure. The figure would be derived if 100 persons were observation per one year. These denominators have advantage of summarizing the experience of persons within different durations of observation or exposure.

④ Sub - group of population: The denominator may be subgroups population, e.g., age, sex, occupation, social class, etc.

2)Related to total events

In some instances, the denominator may be related to events instead of the total population, as in the case of mortality rate and case fatality rate. In the case of accident, the number of accidents "per 1 000 vehicles" or "per motor kilometers" will be a useful denominator than total population, many of them may not be using vehicle.

2.1.2　Measure or index of disease frequency

1. Incidence rate

Incidence rate is a measurement of the occurrence of new cases in a defined population size and in a certain period of time.

（1）It requires the definition of two important units

用的人时是人年，有时可能是人月、人周或人时。例如，如果10人的研究开展了10年，那就是观察了100人年；如果对100人观察了一年，同样会得到100人年。人时作为分母，具有综合研究对象观察时间或暴露期限的优点。

④亚组人群：分母可以是亚组人群，如不同年龄组、性别组、职业组和社会阶层等。

2）与事件相关的概念

在某些情况下，分母可能是相关事件数，而不是总人数，如病例死亡率和病死率。计算事故发生率时，以"每1 000辆汽车"或"每辆机动车行驶公里数"作为分母比总人数更有意义，因为许多人可能不使用车辆。

2.1.2　疾病频率测量指标

1.发病率

发病率是衡量一定期间内、一定人群中新病例发生的频率指标。

（1）计算发病率时需要注意的两个重要概念

①A unit of place: A defined geographical place that would be common to the two statistics used in the computation. Any incidence rate would normally correspond to a geographically defined population.

②A unit of time: Because the rate will be equivalent to a measurement of speed, it should be defined according to a unit of time.

（2）It requires the gathering of two statistics

①The number of cases, which is the numerator, with cases defined as number of individuals with a specific health condition.

②The underlying population of origin, which is the denominator. This population is the number of persons living in the region of origin of cases.

With these two statistics, one can calculate the incidence rate such as:

$$R = \frac{N}{P} \qquad (2-3)$$

Where N is the new cases were occurring during a defined period. The numerator (N) should include only new cases of the disease that occurred during the specified period, and should not include cases that occurred or were diagnosed earlier. This is very important when working with chronic infectious diseases such as tuberculosis, malaria and HIV.

The denominator (P) is the population at risk. This means that the people included in the denominator should be able to develop the disease in question during the time period covered. In practice, we usually use census data for the denominator. The denominator should also represent the population from which the cases in the numerator arose. The population may be defined by geographic area (e.g., XX City) or by membership in a specific group (e.g., employee of company X, student at school Y). If we are studying a specific

①地域：计算发病率时，分子和分母都应该是特定区域内的人群。发病率通常是特定区域内人群的发病率，不同地区人群的发病率会不同。

②时间：因为率是类似于速率的测量值，所以应该根据时间单位来定义，不同时间的发病率会不同。

（2）计算发病率时需要的两个数据

①新发病例数：即分子。病例数定义为特定时间内具有特定健康状况的数量，而不是人数，因为流感、腹泻等疾病一年中可多次患病。

②可能发病的人数：即分母，是与病例同一区域的病例来源的人群，对已经患病而观察期内不可能发病成为新病例的人，不应计入分母。

利用以上两个数据可以计算发病率，例如：

$$R = \frac{N}{P} \qquad (2-3)$$

式中，N 是在特定时期内的新发病例数。分子（N）应仅包括指定时期内的新发病例，而不应包括旧病例或早期诊断的病例，尤其在计算慢性传染性疾病（如结核、疟疾和 HIV 感染）的发病率时。

分母（P）是处于风险中的人数。这意味着分母是那些在特定时期内可能发生该疾病的人。在实践中，通常使用普查数据作为分母。分母还应代表分子中新发病例来源的人群，可根据地理区域（如 XX 市）或特定群体的成员（如 X 公司员工、Y 学校学生）来确定。如果正在研究某一特定群体，比如学校的学生或护理机构的长期居民，应该使用该人群的人口普查数据作为分母。

group such as students in a school or residents in a long term care facility, we should use a census of that population for an exact denominator.

2. Attack rate

In epidemiology, an attack rate is the cumulative incidence of infection in a group of people observed over a period of time during an epidemic, usually in relation to foodborne illness. Quantitatively, it is the number of exposed people who develop the disease divided by the total number of exposed people.

3. Prevalence rate

Prevalence, sometimes referred to as prevalence rate, is the proportion of persons in a population who have a particular disease or attribute at a specified point in time or over a specified period of time. Prevalence differs from incidence in that prevalence includes all cases, both new and pre-existing, in the population at the specified time, whereas incidence is limited to new cases only.

Method for calculating prevalence of disease:

Prevalence rate=

$$\frac{\text{All new and pre-existing cases during a given time period}}{\text{Population during the same time period}} \times K$$

$$(2-4)$$

The value of K might be 100%, 1 000‰, or even 100 000/100 000 for rare attributes and for most diseases.

Differences between incidence and prevalence as follows:

①Prevalence and incidence are frequently confused. Prevalence refers to proportion of persons who have a condition at or during a particular time period, whereas incidence refers to the proportion or rate of persons who develop a condition during a particular time period. So prevalence and incidence are similar,

2. 罹患率

在流行病学中，罹患率是疾病流行期间短时间局限范围内的发病率，主要用于食物中毒、职业中毒或传染病暴发及流行中。它是暴露后患上该病的人数除以同期暴露人数的数值。

3. 患病率

患病率，有时称为现患率，是指在特定时间点或特定时间段内患有特定疾病的人数（新旧病例数）所占的比例。患病率与发病率的不同之处在于，患病率的分子包括特定时间人群中所有新发病例和先前存在的旧病例，而发病率的分子仅限于新病例；患病率的分母为总人数，发病率的分母为暴露人数（即可能发病的人口数）。

患病率计算公式：

患病率=

$$\frac{\text{特定时期内某人群中某病新旧病例数}}{\text{同期观察人数}} \times K$$

$$(2-4)$$

根据疾病的属性是罕见病还是常见病，K 的值可能是 100%、1 000‰，甚至 100 000/10 万。

发病率与患病率的区别如下：

①患病率和发病率经常被混淆。患病率是指在某一特定时间段内患病的人数（包括新旧病例）所占的比例，而发病率是指在某一特定时间段内新发病例数所占的比例或发生的频率。因此，患病率和发病率是相似的，但患病率包括新的和先前存在的旧病例，而发病率仅包括新病例，它们

but prevalence includes new and pre - existing cases whereas incidence includes new cases only. The key difference is in their numerators.

Numerator of incidence = new cases that occurred during a given time period

Numerator of prevalence = all cases present during a given time period

② The denominator of an incidence proportion or rate is the underlying population of origin. This population is the number of persons living in the region of origin of cases. The denominator of a prevalence rate is the total people in the region.

③ Prevalence is based on both incidence and duration of illness.

Prevalence = incidence×duration

High prevalence of a disease within a population might reflect high incidence or prolonged survival without cure or both. Conversely, a low prevalence might indicate low incidence, a rapidly fatal process, or rapid recovery.

④ Prevalence rather than incidence is often measured for chronic diseases such as diabetes or osteoarthritis which have long duration and dates of onset that are difficult to pinpoint.

4.Infection rate

The infection rate is widely used in epidemiology and is usually to measure the proportion of infected persons in a given time range.

Infection rate is often used to study the infection status, popular trend and the effect of the prevention and treatment of infectious or parasitic diseases. Infection rate can also to provide evidence for planning prevention and control measures.

的重要区别在于分子不同。

发病率分子=特定时间段内新发病例数

患病率分子=特定时间段内出现的所有病例数

②发病率的分母是病例来源的人群，即暴露于疾病风险可能发病的人数；患病率的分母是特定地区观察的所有人的数量。

③患病率与发病率及病程有关。当某病的发病率和病程在一段时间内保持相对稳定时：
患病率=发病率×病程
高患病率可能与高发病率、寿命延长而疾病久治不愈等有关。相反，低患病率可能意味着低发病率、快速病死或快速治愈等。

④对于慢性病（如糖尿病或骨关节炎），通常计算其患病率而不是发病率，因为这些疾病病程长，难以确定其发病日期。

4.感染率

感染率在流行病学工作中应用较为广泛，通常用于衡量在特定时间范围内被检人群中现有感染者所占的比例。

感染率通常用于研究传染病或寄生虫病的感染状况、流行趋势和防治效果。感染率也可为制定预防控制措施提供依据。

5. Secondary attack rate

The secondary attack rate is defined as the probability that infection occurs among susceptible persons within a reasonable incubation period following known contact with an infectious person or an infectious source. It is a key epidemiologic parameter in infectious diseases that are transmitted by contact. A secondary attack rate is sometimes calculated to document the difference between community transmission of illness versus transmission of illness in a household, barracks, or other closed population. It is calculated as:

$$\text{Secondary attack rate} = \frac{\text{Number of cases among contacts of primary cases}}{\text{Total number of contacts}} \times K \quad (2\text{-}5)$$

Often, the total number of contacts in the denominator is calculated as the total population in the households of the primary cases, minus the number of primary cases. For a secondary attack rate, K usually is 100%.

6.Mortality rate

A mortality rate is a measure of the frequency of occurrence of death in a defined population during a specified interval. Morbidity and mortality measures are often the same mathematically; it's just a matter of what you choose to measure, illness or death. The formula for the mortality of a defined population, over a specified period of time, is:

$$\text{Mortality rate} = \frac{\text{Deaths occurring during a given time period}}{\text{Size of the population among which the deaths occurred}} \times K \quad (2\text{-}6)$$

When mortality rates are based on vital statistics (e.g., counts of death certificates), the denominator most commonly used is the size of the population at the middle

5.续发率

续发率是指在潜伏期内，易感者接触传染源后在最短潜伏期到最长潜伏期之间发生感染的概率。它是评价传染病传播的一个重要的流行病学指标，用于比较传染病传染力的强弱。有时计算续发率是为了记录社区疾病传播与家庭、军营或其他封闭人群疾病传播之间的差异。公式如下：

$$续发率 = \frac{潜伏期内易感接触者中发病人数}{易感接触者总人数} \times K \quad (2\text{-}5)$$

续发率的分子和分母都应该减去原发病例数，且分母中的接触者为可能发病的易感者。续发率计算公式中的 K 通常为100%。

6.死亡率

死亡率是在特定时间内特定人群死亡发生的频率指标。患病率和死亡率是相似的测量指标，选择什么来衡量疾病或死亡是一个重要的问题。死亡率是测量人群死亡危险最常用的指标。特定时期内特定人群的死亡率计算公式为：

$$死亡率 = \frac{某人群某年总死亡人数}{该人群同年平均人数} \times K \quad (2\text{-}6)$$

当死亡率基于生命统计数据（如死亡证明计数）时，分母通常是时间段中点的人数。大多数疾病死亡率计算公式中的 K 使用1 000‰或100 000/10万。

of the time period. Values of 1 000‰ and 100 000/100 000 are both used for K for most types of mortality rates.

The crude mortality rate is the mortality rate from all causes of death for a population.

The cause-specific mortality rate is the mortality rate from a specified cause for a population. The numerator is the number of deaths attributed to a specific cause. The denominator remains the size of the population at the midpoint of the time period. An age-specific mortality rate is a mortality rate limited to a particular age group. The numerator is the number of deaths in that age group; the denominator is the number of persons in that age group in the population.

The infant mortality rate is perhaps the most commonly used measure for comparing health status among nations. The infant mortality rate is generally calculated on an annual basis. It is a widely used measure of health status because it reflects the health of the mother and infant during pregnancy and the year thereafter. The health of the mother and infant, in turn, reflects a wide variety of factors, including access to prenatal care, prevalence of prenatal maternal health behaviors (such as alcohol or tobacco use and proper nutrition during pregnancy, etc.), postnatal care and behaviors (including childhood immunizations and proper nutrition), sanitation, and infection control.

$$\text{Infant mortality} = \frac{\text{Deaths occuring during a given time period}}{\text{Number of livings}} \times 1\,000‰$$

$$(2-7)$$

7. Fatality rate

The fatality rate is the proportion of persons with a particular condition (cases) who die from that condition. It is a measure of the severity of the condition. The formula is:

粗死亡率是指某人群中所有死因的死亡率。

死因别死亡率是指人群中特定原因的死亡率。分子是归因于特定原因的死亡人数，分母仍然是时间段中点的人数。年龄别死亡率是指仅限于特定年龄组的死亡率，分子是该年龄组的死亡人数，分母是人群中该年龄组的人数。

婴儿死亡率可能是比较不同国家健康状况最广泛使用的指标，因为它反映了产妇和婴儿在孕期及产后一年的健康状况。婴儿死亡率一般每年计算一次，反映一周岁以内婴儿的死亡水平。产妇和婴儿的健康反映了多种因素，包括获得产前护理的机会、产前母亲健康行为（如孕期饮酒、吸烟和合理营养等）、产后护理和行为（包括儿童免疫接种和适当营养）、医疗卫生条件、社会经济实力、感染控制等，是衡量人口素质的重要依据之一。公式如下：

$$婴儿死亡率 = \frac{某年婴儿死亡总数}{同期活产总数} \times 1\,000‰$$

$$(2-7)$$

7. 病死率

病死率是指患有特定疾病的人（病例）中死于该病的病例所占的比例。它可以衡量疾病的严重程度。公式如下：

Fatality rate=

$$\frac{\text{Number of cause-specific deaths among}}{\text{Number of incident cases}} \times 100\%$$

（2-8）

The fatality rate is a proportion, so the numerator is restricted to deaths among people included in the denominator. The time periods for the numerator and the denominator do not need to be the same; the denominator could be cases of HIV/AIDS diagnosed during the calendar year 1990, and the numerator, deaths among those diagnosed with HIV in 1990, could be from 1990 to the present.

8.Survival rate

Survival rate is a part of survival analysis, indicating the percentage of people in a study or treatment group who are alive for a given period of time after diagnosis. Survival rates are important for prognosis, but because this rate is based on the population as a whole, an individual prognosis may be different depending on newer treatments since the last statistical analysis as well as the overall general health of the patient.

$$\text{Survival rate}=\frac{\text{Total number of patients alive after 5 years}}{\text{Total number of patients digagosed or treated}} \times 100\%$$

（2-9）

9. Potential years of life lost

Potential years of life lost (PYLL) is one measure of the impact of premature mortality on a population. Additional measures incorporate disability and other measures of quality of life. PYLL is calculated as the sum of the differences between a predetermined end point and the ages of death for those who died before that end point. The two most commonly used end points are age 65 years and average life expectancy.

$$病死率=\frac{\text{一定时期内因某病死亡的人数}}{\text{同期确诊的某病病例数}} \times 100\%$$

（2-8）

病死率本质上是一个构成比，其分子限于分母中患病人群中因该病死亡的人数。分子和分母的时间段不需要相同，分母可以是1990年诊断的HIV感染/艾滋病病例数，分子（即1990年诊断出的HIV感染者中的死亡人数）的时间段可以是1990年到现在。

8. 生存率

生存率是生存分析的一部分，表示接受某种治疗的病人中或患某病的病人中，经过 n 年随访后，存活的病人所占的比例。生存率对预后很重要，反映了疾病对生命的危害程度，可用于评价某些慢性病的远期疗效。但由于其基于整个人群，因此个体预后可能会因上次统计分析以来的新疗法以及患者的总体健康状况而有所不同。公式如下：

$$生存率=\frac{\text{5年后尚存活的病人数}}{\text{被诊断或治疗的病人总数}} \times 100\%$$

（2-9）

9. 潜在减寿年数

潜在减寿年数（PYLL）是衡量过早死亡对人群健康影响的一个指标，是人群疾病负担测量的一个直接指标。其他衡量指标还包括残疾和其他生活质量。PYLL是某病某年龄组人群死亡者的预期寿命与实际死亡年龄的差值之和。最常用的预期寿命是65岁和平均预期寿命。

The use of PYLL is affected by this calculation, which implies a value system in which more weight is given to a death when it occurs at an earlier age. Thus, deaths at older ages are "devalued". However, the PYLL before age 65 (PYLL$_{65}$) places much more emphasis on deaths at early ages than does PYLL based on remaining life expectancy (PYLLLE). In 2000, the remaining life expectancy was 21.6 years for a 60-year-old, 11.3 years for a 70-year-old, and 8.6 for an 80-year-old. PYLL$_{65}$ is based on the fewer than 30% of deaths that occur among persons younger than 65. In contrast, PYLL for remaining life expectancy (PYLLLE) is based on deaths among persons of all ages, so it more closely resembles crude mortality rates.

10. Disability adjusted life year

The disability-adjusted life year (DALY) is a measure of overall disease burden, expressed as the number of years lost due to ill - health, disability or early death. Traditionally, health liabilities were expressed using one measure: (expected or average number of) "Years of Life Lost" (YLL). This measure does not take the impact of disability into account, which can be expressed by: "Years Lived with Disability" (YLD). DALYs are calculated by taking the sum of these two components. In a formula: DALY = YLL+YLD. The DA-LY relies on an acceptance that the most appropriate measure of the effects of chronic illness is time, both time lost due to premature death and time spent disabled by disease. One DALY, therefore, is equal to one year of healthy life lost.

2.2 Epidemic Strength of Disease

The common terms of epidemic strength include sporadic, outbreak and epidemic.

PYLL的使用体现了一种价值体系，在这种体系中，当死亡发生在生命早期时，会给予更多的权重。因此，高龄死亡被"贬值"。然而，与基于剩余预期寿命的PYLL（PYLLLE）相比，65岁之前的PYLL（PYLL$_{65}$）受到早期死亡的影响更大。2000年，60岁的剩余预期寿命为21.6岁，70岁的为11.3岁，80岁的为8.6岁。PYLL$_{65}$根据65岁以下人群中不到30%的死亡率计算。相比之下，基于剩余预期寿命的PYLL（PYLLLE）是根据所有年龄段的死亡计算得到的，因此更接近粗死亡率。

10.伤残调整寿命年

伤残调整寿命年（DALY）是一种衡量总体疾病负担的指标，指从发病到死亡所损失的全部健康寿命年，包括残疾或过早死亡。传统上，疾病负担是用一个指标来表示的：（预期或平均）"寿命损失年数"（YLL）。YLL没有考虑到残疾的影响，需要用"残疾生活年限"（YLD）来表示。伤残调整寿命年是通过计算这两部分的总和来计算的，公式为：DALY=YLL+YLD。DALY是反映疾病对人群寿命损失影响的综合指标，包括因过早死亡而造成的寿命损失和因疾病致残而造成的健康寿命损失。因此，一个伤残调整寿命年等于失去健康生命的一年。

2.2 疾病流行的强度

疾病流行的强度通常包括散发、暴发和流行。

2.2.1 Sporadic

Occurring upon occasion or in a scattered, isolated, or seemingly random way; occurring occasionally, singly, or in irregular or random instances. It means that there is no significant relationship between cases.

2.2.2 Outbreak

Outbreak is a term used in epidemiology to describe the sudden rise in the incidence of a disease at a particular time and place, it affect a small and localized group in a short time. E.g. food poisoning on a collective canteen, measles outbreak in kindergarten units.

2.2.3 Epidemic

In epidemiology, an epidemic occurs when new cases of a certain disease, in a given human population, and during a given period, substantially exceed what is expected based on recent experience. Epidemiologists often consider the term outbreak to be synonymous to epidemic, but the general public typically perceives outbreaks to be more local and less serious than epidemics. An epidemic may be restricted to one location; however, if it spreads to other countries or continents and affects a substantial number of people, it may be termed a pandemic.

2.3　The Distribution of the Disease

2.3.1　Person

Because personal characteristics may affect ill-

2.2.1　散发

散发即偶然发生或以分散、孤立或看似随机的方式发生。发病率呈历年一般水平，病例间没有明显的关系，即表现为散发。确定散发时，多与当地近三年该病的发病率比较，如果没有明显超过既往平均水平，即为散发。

2.2.2　暴发

暴发是流行病学中的一个术语，用于描述在特定时间和地点发病率的突然上升，它指短时间小范围内的影响。病例往往有相同的传染源或传播途径，大多数病例出现在最短和最长潜伏期之间。例如，食堂食物中毒，幼儿园麻疹暴发。

2.2.3　流行

在流行病学中，当特定人群和特定时期内某病的发病率显著超过以往水平时，就会发生流行。相对于散发，流行出现时各病例呈现明显的时间和空间联系；相对于流行，暴发涉及的范围更局限。疾病流行后迅速蔓延，如果传播到其他国家或大陆，并影响到相当数量的人，则可称为大流行。

2.3　疾病的分布

2.3.1　人间分布

人群的一些固有特征或社会特征可能会影响

ness, organization and analysis of data by "person" may use inherent characteristics of people (for example, age, sex, race), biologic characteristics (immune status), acquired characteristics (marital status), activities (occupation, leisure activities, use of medications/tobacco/drugs), or the conditions under which they live (socioeconomic status, access to medical care). Age and sex are included in almost all data sets and are the two most commonly analyzed "person" characteristics. However, depending on the disease and the data available, analyses of other person variables are usually necessary. Usually epidemiologists begin the analysis of person data by looking at each variable separately. Sometimes, two variables such as age and sex can be examined simultaneously. Person data are usually displayed in tables or graphs.

1. Age

Age is probably the single most important "person" attribute, because almost every health - related event varies with age. A number of factors that also vary with age include: susceptibility, opportunity for exposure, latency or incubation period of the disease, and physiologic response (which affects, among other things, disease development).

When analyzing data by age, epidemiologists try to use age groups that are narrow enough to detect any age-related patterns that may be present in the data. For some diseases, particularly chronic diseases, 10-year age groups may be adequate. For other diseases, 10-year and even 5-year age groups conceal important variations in disease occurrence by age. Consider the graph of pertussis occurrence by standard 5-year age groups shown in Figure 2-1a. The highest rate is clearly among children 4 years old and younger. But is the rate equally high in all children within that age group,

疾病分布，这些特征包括遗传特征（年龄、性别、种族）、生物特征（免疫状态）、获得特征（婚姻状况）、活动（职业、休闲活动、烟草/药物的使用）或者生活的条件（社会经济地位、获得医疗服务的机会）等。其中，年龄和性别是最常被分析的两个人间分布特征。通常也会根据研究目的对其他人间分布特征进行分析，尤其在研究初期会对所有特征都进行分析。人间分布结果通常以统计表或图的形式展现。

1. 年龄

年龄可能是最重要的人间分布特征，因为几乎所有与健康相关的事件都随年龄而变化，许多因素也随年龄而变化，包括：易感性、接触机会、疾病的潜伏期及生理反应（这些都会影响疾病的发展）。

当按年龄分析数据时，可以通过不同年龄组的疾病情况判断疾病与年龄的相关性。对于某些疾病，特别是慢性病，通常按10岁划分年龄组。对于其他一些疾病，10岁年龄组甚至5岁年龄组可能掩盖了不同年龄段疾病发生的重要差异。图2-1a表示按5岁年龄组划分的百日咳发生情况。显然，4岁及以下儿童的发病率最高。但是，是这个年龄组的所有儿童的发病率都同样高，还是有些年龄儿童的发病率高于其他儿童？要回答这个问题，需要观察更小的年龄分组。图2-1b显示了利用相同数据，1岁以下儿童的百日咳发病率明显

or do some children have higher rates than others? To answer this question, different age groups are needed. Examine Figure 2-1b, which shows the same data but displays the rate of pertussis for children less than 1 year of age separately. Clearly, infants account for most of the high rate among 0-4 year olds. Public health efforts should thus be focused on children less than1 year of age, rather than on the entire 5-year age group.

高于其他年龄段。显然，婴儿时期是0~4岁儿童中高发病率的重要年龄段。因此，公共卫生工作的重点应该是1岁以下的儿童，而不是整个5岁年龄组。

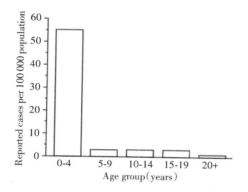

Figure 2-1a　Pertussis by 5-year age groups

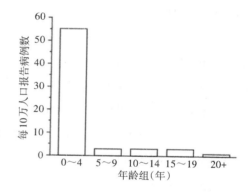

图2-1a　按5岁年龄组划分的百日咳发病情况

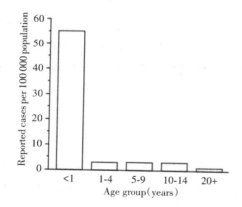

Figure 2-1b　Pertussis by <1, 4-year, then 5-year age groups

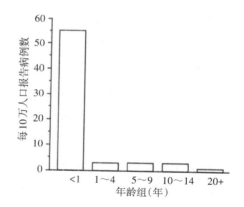

图2-1b　按<1岁、4岁和5岁年龄组划分的百日咳发病情况

Figure 2-1　Pertussis infection situation of different age groups

图2-1　不同年龄组的百日咳发病情况

Methods of studying the age distribution of diseases as follows:

（1）Cross section analysis

Cross section analysis mainly analyzes the differences of different age groups within the same year or

研究疾病年龄分布的方法如下：

（1）横断面分析

横断面分析主要分析同一年代（断面）或不同年代（断面）各年龄组的发病率、患病率或死

changes of the same age group in the different years on prevalence or mortality (seen in Figure 2-2). However, it can't present the accurate relation of risk factors and age.

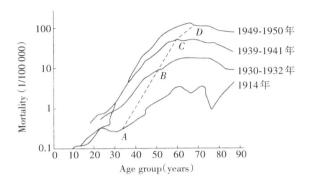

Figure 2-2　Age mortality rates of lung cancer in men from 1914 to 1950

(MacMahon and Pugh, 1970)

（2）Birth cohort analysis

A birth cohort is a group of individuals born during a given calendar time period within a specified geographical region.For example, the U.S. 1950 annual birth cohort refers to the group of people born in the United States during the calendar year 1950, and the 1950 to 1952 birth cohort identifies those born during the period covering the three consecutive calendar years 1950, 1951, and 1952. Birth cohort analysis is an observational cohort analysis of an entire birth cohort or of a selected sample of the birth cohort which will be followed up to observe the incidence or mortality (seen in Figure 2-3), and can show the relation of risk factors and age.

亡率等的不同或变化（图2-2所示）。结果可以显示年龄与疾病的关系，但不能显示致病因素与年龄的关系。

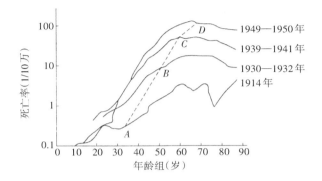

图2-2　1914—1950年不同年龄男性肺癌死亡率

（MacMahon and Pugh, 1970）

（2）出生队列分析

出生队列是指在特定地理区域内同一时期出生的一群人。例如，美国1950年的出生队列指的是1950年间在美国出生的人群，而1950年至1952年的出生队列指的是连续三年，即1950年、1951年和1952年间出生的人群。出生队列分析是对整个出生队列或出生队列的选定样本进行的观察性队列分析，是对同一时期出生的一组人随访若干年，观察其发病或死亡情况（图2-3所示），该分析方法的结果可以呈现出致病因子与年龄的关系。

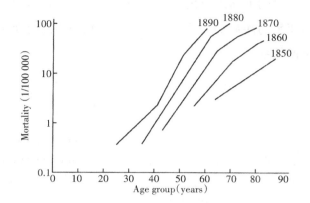

Figure 2-3　Age mortality rates of lung cancer among men born between 1850 and 1890

（MacMahon and Pugh, 1970）

2.Sex

Males have higher rates of illness and death than do females for many diseases. For some diseases, this sex-related difference is because of genetic, hormonal, anatomic, or other inherent differences between the sexes. These inherent differences affect susceptibility or physiologic responses. For example, premenopausal women have a lower risk of heart disease than men of the same age. This difference has been attributed to higher estrogen levels in women. On the other hand, the sex-related differences in the occurrence of many diseases reflect differences in opportunity or levels of exposure. For example, Figure 2-4 shows the differences in lung cancer death rates over time among men and women. The difference noted in earlier years has been attributed to the higher prevalence of smoking among men in the past. Unfortunately, prevalence of smoking among women now equals that among men, and lung cancer death rates in women have been climbing as a result.

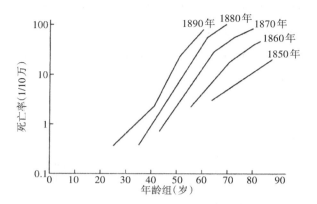

图2-3　1850—1890年出生队列中不同年龄男性肺癌死亡率

（MacMahon 和Pugh, 1970）

2.性别

绝大多数疾病都呈现出男性的患病率和死亡率高于女性的特点。这些疾病的性别差异与遗传特征、内分泌代谢、生理解剖特点及致病因子暴露机会差异有关，这些差异影响易感性或生理反应。例如，绝经前的女性患心脏病的风险比同龄男性低。这种差异归因于女性雌激素水平较高，而雌激素具有一定的保护作用。另一方面，许多疾病发生的性别差异反映了接触机会或接触水平的差异。例如，图2-4显示了男性和女性肺癌死亡率随时间的差异。其中，早期的差异是过去男性吸烟率较高造成的。不幸的是，现在女性吸烟率与男性持平，因此女性肺癌死亡率一直在攀升。

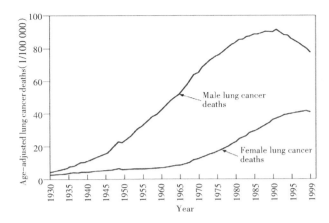

Figure 2-4　Lung Cancer Rates in the United States,
1930-1999

Data Source: American Cancer Society [Internet]. Atlanta: The American Cancer Society, Inc. Available from: http://www. cancer. org/docroot/PRO/content/PRO_1_1_ Cancer_ Statistics_ 2005_Presentation.asp.

3.Occupation

Different occupation exposed to various physical factors, chemical factors, biological factors and occupational stress, and all this could be lead to the different of disease distribution.

4.Ethnic and racial groups

Sometimes epidemiologists are interested in analyzing person data by biologic, cultural or social groupings such as race, nationality, religion, or social groups such as tribes and other geographically or socially isolated groups. Differences in racial, ethnic, or other group variables may reflect differences in susceptibility or exposure, or differences in other factors that influence the risk of disease, such as socioeconomic status and access to health care. Figure 2-5 shows the infant mortality rates by different races and ethnic groups of the mother in 2002.

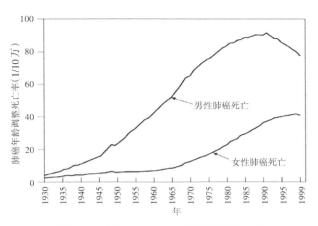

图2-4　1930—1999年美国肺癌死亡率

数据来源：American Cancer Society [Internet]. Atlanta：The American Cancer Society, Inc. Available from：http：//www. cancer. org/docroot/PRO/content/PRO_1_1_ Cancer_ Statistics_2005_Presentation.asp.

3.职业

不同职业暴露于各种不同的物理因素、化学因素、生物因素和职业压力，可导致疾病分布的职业差异。

4.种族和民族

种族和民族是长期共同生活并具有共同生物学和社会学特征的相对稳定的群体。根据生物、文化或社会群体（如种族、国籍、宗教、部落）和其他地理位置的不同分析数据，不同种族和民族由于长期受一定自然环境、社会环境和遗传背景的影响，疾病的分布差异可能反映了易感性或暴露的差异，或具有影响疾病风险的其他因素的差异，如社会经济地位和获得医疗保健的机会。图2-5显示了2002年不同民族和种族的母亲所生婴儿的死亡率。

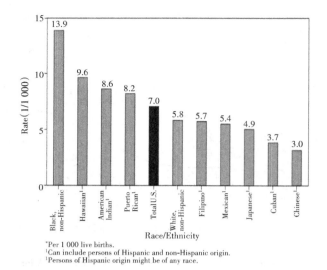

*Per 1 000 live births.
¹Can include persons of Hispanic and non-Hispanic origin.
¹Persons of Hispanic origin might be of any race.

Figure 2-5　Infant Mortality Rates for 2002, by Race and Ethnicity of Mother

Source: Centers for Disease Control and Prevention. Quick-Stats: Infant mortality rates, by selected racial/ethnic populations—United States, 2002, MMWR,2005, 54(5):126.

5. Religion

6. Marriage and Family

7. Floating population

2.3.2　Time

The occurrence of disease changes over time. Some of these changes occur regularly, while others are unpredictable. Two diseases that occur during the same season each year include influenza (winter) and West Nile virus infection (August - September). In contrast, diseases such as hepatitis B and salmonellosis can occur at any time. For diseases that occur seasonally, health officials can anticipate their occurrence and implement control and prevention measures, such as an influenza vaccination campaign or mosquito spraying. For diseases that occur sporadically, investigators can conduct studies to identify the causes and modes of spread, and then develop appropriately targeted actions to control or prevent further occurrence of the disease.

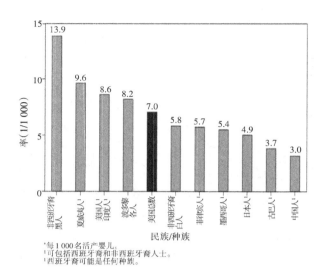

*每1 000名活产婴儿。
¹可包括西班牙裔和非西班牙裔人士。
¹西班牙裔可能是任何种族。

图2-5　2002年按母亲民族和种族分列的婴儿死亡率

数据来源：Centers for Disease Control and Prevention. QuickStats：Infant mortality rates, by selected racial/ethnic populations—United States, 2002, MMWR ,2005, 54 (5)：126.

5. 宗教信仰

6. 婚姻和家庭

7. 流动人口

2.3.2　时间分布

疾病的发生随时间而变化。其中一些变化是规律发生的，而另一些变化是不可预测的。例如，流感（冬季）和西尼罗河病毒感染（8月至9月）的发生呈季节性规律；而乙型肝炎和沙门氏菌病等疾病可以随时发生，不具有季节规律。对于季节性发生的疾病，可以通过预测其流行规律，实施预防和控制措施，如流感疫苗接种或喷洒灭蚊剂。对于偶尔发生的疾病，可以通过调查确定病因和传播方式，然后制定适当的、有针对性的措施，以控制或防止疾病的进一步扩散。

In either situation, displaying the patterns of disease occurrence by time is critical for monitoring disease occurrence in the community and for assessing whether the public health interventions made a difference. The patterns of disease by time usually include rapid fluctuation, and seasonal variation, and cyclic change and secular trends to describe the distribution and variation of disease.

1. Rapid fluctuation

Rapid fluctuation is also called outbreak, it describes the sudden rise in the incidence of a disease at a short time in a collectivity or a fixed crowd.

2. Seasonal variation

Disease occurrence can be graphed by week or month over the course of a year or more to show its seasonal pattern, if any. Some diseases such as influenza and West Nile infection are known to have characteristic seasonal distributions. Seasonal patterns may suggest hypotheses about how the infection is transmitted, what behavioral factors increase risk, and other possible contributors to the disease or condition. Figure 2-6 shows the seasonal patterns of rubella, influenza, and rotavirus. All three diseases display consistent seasonal distributions, but each disease peaks in different months—rubella in March to June, influenza in November to March, and rotavirus in February to April. The rubella graph is striking for the epidemic that occurred in 1964 (rubella vaccine was not available until 1969), but this epidemic nonetheless followed the seasonal pattern.

按时间显示疾病发生的模式，对监测社区疾病的发生和评估公共卫生干预措施至关重要。疾病的时间分布及变化规律往往从短期波动、季节性变化、周期性变化和长期趋势等方面进行描述。

1. 短期波动

短期波动也称为暴发，它描述了一种疾病在短时间内在集体或固定群体中发病率的突然上升。

2. 季节性变化

疾病的发生可以周或月为单位绘制成一年或更长时间的变化图表，以显示其季节性模式（如果有的话）。季节性可以有两种表现形式，即严格的季节性和季节性升高。例如，虫媒传播的传染病有严格的季节性（如乙型脑炎与蚊虫的繁殖季节有关，仅在某些季节出现），而一些疾病一年四季均发病，但在一定月份呈现季节性发病率升高的特点，比如肠道传染病和呼吸道传染病。根据季节性模式，可以提出以下假设：感染如何传播，哪些行为因素增加了风险，以及其他可能导致疾病或状况发生的因素。图2-6显示了风疹、流感和轮状病毒的季节性模式。这三种疾病的季节分布都是一致的，但出现高峰的月份不同——风疹在3月至6月，流感在11月至次年3月，轮状病毒感染在2月至4月。风疹曲线图显示1964年风疹曾出现流行高峰（直到1969年风疹疫苗才开始使用），但这种流行目前仍然遵循季节性模式。

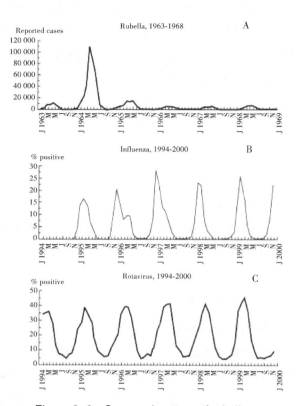

Figure 2-6   Seasonal pattern of rubella,
influenza and rotavirus

Source: DOWELL S F. Seasonal variation in host susceptibility and cycles of certain infectious diseases. Emerg Infect
Dis. 2001, 7(3):369-374.

3.Cyclic change or periodicity

Cyclic change means that the disease frequency
presents a regular changes status after a fairly regular
interval. Common causes and necessary condition of
periodicity are follows:

① Prevalently in the cities of densely populated
and traffic congestion.

② Mechanism of transmission of disease is easy
to implement.

③ After an epidemic of a disease, the incidence
rate could fall rapidly.

④ The occurrence of periodicity also depends on
the speed of the accumulation of susceptible people
and the speed of the pathogens variation.

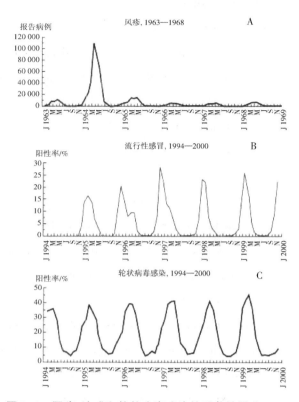

图2-6   风疹、流感和轮状病毒感染的季节性模式

数据来源：DOWELL S F. Seasonal variation in host susceptibility and cycles of certain infectious diseases. Emerg Infect Dis，2001，7（3）：369-374.

3.周期性变化或周期性

周期性变化是指疾病频率按照一定的时间间
隔，有规律地起伏波动，每隔一段时间出现一个
流行高峰的现象。周期性变化的常见原因和必要
条件如下：

①普遍存在于人口密集和交通拥挤的城市。

②疾病的传播机制很容易实现。

③疾病流行后，发病率可能会迅速下降。

④周期性的发生还取决于易感人群的积累速
度和病原体的变化速度。

4. Secular trends or secular change

Graphing the annual cases or rate of a disease over a period of years shows long - term or secular trends in the occurrence of the disease. Health officials use these graphs to assess the prevailing direction of disease occurrence (increasing, decreasing, or essentially flat), help them evaluate programs or make policy decisions, infer what caused an increase or decrease in the occurrence of a disease (particularly if the graph indicates when related events took place), and use past trends as a predictor of future incidence of disease.

2.3.3　Place

Describing the occurrence of disease by place provides insight into the geographic extent of the problem and its geographic variation.

Characterization by place refers not only to place of residence but to any geographic location relevant to disease occurrence. Such locations include place of diagnosis or report, birthplace, site of employment, school district, hospital unit, or recent travel destinations. The unit may be as large as a continent or country or as small as a street address, hospital wing, or operating room. Sometimes place refers not to a specific location at all but to a place category such as urban or rural, domestic or foreign, and institutional or non - institutional.

Analyzing data by place can identify communities at increased risk of disease. Even if the data cannot reveal why these people have an increased risk , it can help generate hypotheses to test with additional studies. For example, is a community at increased risk because of characteristics of the people in the community such as genetic susceptibility, lack of immunity, risky behaviors, or exposure to local toxins or contaminated food?

4.长期趋势或长期变化

将疾病在一段比较长的时间内（通常为几年或几十年）的年度病例数或发病率绘制成图表，可以看出疾病发生的长期变化或长期趋势。利用长期趋势变化可以评估疾病流行的主要方向（增加、减少或不变），有助于做出决策，推断出导致疾病发生的增加或减少（尤其是图表中所显示的相关事件随时间的变化）的原因，还可利用过去的趋势预测疾病未来的发生情况。

2.3.3　空间分布

通过描述疾病的空间分布，可以深入了解疾病涉及的地理范围及在不同地区间的差异。

疾病的空间分布特征不仅指居住地点，还指与疾病发生相关的任何地理区域。这些区域包括诊断或报告地点、出生地、工作地点、学区、医院单位或最近的旅行目的地。区域可能与国家或大陆一样大，也可能与街道地址、校医院或手术室一样小。有时，区域根本不是指一个特定的地点，而是指地区类别，如城市或农村、国内或国外、机构或非机构。

根据空间分布数据可以确定高危地区。即使不能揭示风险增加的原因，也有助于建立病因假设。例如，疾病高发地区可能由于遗传易感性、缺乏免疫力、危险行为、暴露于当地毒素或受污染的食物、恶劣的自然环境等而增加风险。

1. Endemic disease

An endemic disease refers a pathological condition entrenched and perpetuated within a population group, a country or continent without any external influences.

2. Exotic diseases

Exotic diseases are infectious diseases that normally do not occur in the region either because they have never been present there or because they were eradicated and then kept out by government control measures. Exotic diseases are usually contracted by people traveling to Third World nations. Other times people purchase rare animals that may have come from a foreign country and may be infected with an unusual parasite or virus. Some exotic diseases are relatively harmless while others may prove fatal.

3. The judgment criterions of endemic diseases

① All kinds of resident and nationality in the region have a high incidence rate.

② The similar people in other region all have a low incidence rate, or even don't develop the disease.

③ The incidence rate of immigration in the region is similar to the local residents after a period of time.

④ The incidence rate of people who move away from the region become low, or the patient's symptoms will alleviate to heal.

⑤ In addition to the local people, susceptible animals may occur to the same disease.

1.地方病

地方病是指在没有任何外部影响的情况下，在某些特定区域内相对稳定、持续存在的一类疾病。

2.外来性疾病(输入性疾病)

凡本国或本地区不存在或已消灭的传染病，从国外或其他地区传入时，均称为外来性疾病。外来性疾病通常因为前往第三世界国家旅行而感染，有时也会因为购买感染了不常见寄生虫或病毒的外国珍稀动物而感染。一些外来性疾病相对无害，而另一些则可能致命。

3.地方病的判定标准

①该地区居民发病率高。

②其他地区的类似人群发病率低，甚至不发病。

③迁入该地区一段时间后，迁入人群的发病率与当地居民的相似。

④迁出该地区后，迁出人群的发病率下降，患病症状减轻或自愈。

⑤除了当地居民之外，当地易感动物也可发生同样的疾病。

4. The disease distribution in domestic or foreign, in urban or rural

There are significant differences in the distribution of certain diseases in different countries, in different parts of the same country, in urban and rural areas.

2.3.4 Migrant epidemiology

Large scale migration of human populations from one country to another provides a unique opportunity to evaluate the role of the possible genetic and environmental factors in the occurrence of disease in a population. Supposing there are marked geographic differences in the occurrence of a disease in two areas—area "A" and area "B". Let us assume that the environments in these two places are very different. The question arises whether the environmental differences in the two areas account for the variations in the occurrence of the disease in question.

Ideally, samples of population in area "A" should be sent to area "B", and vice versa to study change in incidence of disease. In human populations this is hardly possible, so we restrict our study to observation of changes in disease frequency among migrants.

Migrant studies can be carried out in two ways:

1.Comparison of disease and death rates for migrants with those of their kin who have stayed at home

The study need to genetic similarity, life in a different environment or exposed population. If the disease and death rates in migrants are similar to country of adoption over a period of time, the likely explanation would be change in the environment. A special

4.国内外和城乡疾病分布情况

某些疾病在不同国家、同一国家的不同地区、城市和农村的分布存在明显差异。

2.3.4 移民流行病学

从一个国家到另一个国家的大规模人口迁移，为评估遗传和环境因素在人群中发病的可能作用提供了一个独特的机会。假设两个地区（A 和 B）的疾病发生有明显的地区差异，如果两地环境因素有明显差异，是否就可以得出环境因素差异决定了移民发病率的变化。

理想情况下，A 地区的人群到 B 地区后，发病率会发生变化，反之亦然。通过研究移民疾病发生率的变化，可以判断其是否与环境因素差异有关，但在一般人群中研究不太可能得到这样的结论。因此，有必要在移民中观察疾病发生率的变化，通过比较移民、移居地居民和原居住地居民的发病率或死亡率的差异，判断环境因素或遗传的作用。

移民研究可以从以下两方面开展：

1.移民与原居住地人群的发病率或死亡率进行比较

需要遗传相似、生活或暴露在不同环境中的人群。如果经过一段时期，移民的发病率和死亡率与移居地人群的相似，与原居住地人群的不同，那么发病率或死亡率的变化主要由环境因素解释。有一个特殊案例是利用暴露在不同迁移环境中的

case is the use of twins who have been exposed to different environments of migration.

2. Comparison of disease and death rates for migrants with local population of the host country

The study required different genetic groups living in similar environments. If the migration rates of disease and death are similar to the country of origin, the likely explanation would be the genetic factors.

Migrant studies have shown that men of Japanese ancestry living in USA experience a higher rate of coronary heart disease than do the Japanese in Japan. Taking another example, Japan has a higher rate for stomach cancer and a lower rate for colon cancer than the United States has. However, third - generation descendants of Japanese immigrants to USA have rates of stomach and colon cancer like those of the total US population. These studies suggest that as the Japanese were probably adopting the American way of life their susceptibility to coronary heart disease gastric and colonic cancer was moving in the direction of that found in the Americans. Further, migrant studies may also indicate the duration of residence necessary to acquire susceptibility to the disease in question by comparing groups that left home at different ages. Studies of this kind provide a basis for further studies of specific environmental factors to which the migrants may have been exposed or of changes in their habits of life that may be of aetiological importance.

Migrant studies suffer from the usual defects of observational studies, deriving from lack of random assignment to the groups under observation. Migrants may be self - selected in that fit, vigorous and perhaps the temperamentally unstable are more likely to mi-

双胞胎的发病率进行比较。

2. 移民与移居地人群的发病率或死亡率进行比较

需要生活在相似环境中的不同遗传群体。如果移民的发病率或死亡率与原住地人群的相似，与移居地人群的不同，那么发病率或死亡率的差异就可能是遗传因素引起的。

移民研究表明，居住在美国的日本后裔男子冠心病发病率比在日本本土的日本人高；日本人的胃癌发病率高于美国，而结肠癌发病率低于美国。然而，美籍日裔第三代移民的胃癌和结肠癌发病率与美国人的类似。这些结果提示，日本移民可能适应了美国的生活方式后，他们对冠心病和胃肠癌的易感性正朝着接近美国人的方向发展。此外，移民研究还表明，通过对不同时代移民的比较，可获知对该病易感所必需的移居时间。这类研究为进一步研究环境暴露或生活习惯的变化等环境因素可能为移民的重要病因提供了基础。由此可见，移民流行病学是进行疾病人间、空间、时间分布综合描述的典型。

由于缺乏对观察群体的随机分配，移民研究通常存在观察性研究的缺陷。人群迁移可能是自我选择的，也可能是情绪所致。环境因素可能只在某一临界点或某一特定年龄起作用。如果这种疾病的潜伏期很长，那么可能经过很多年移民都

grate. The environmental factors may only act at a certain critical point or at a certain specific age. If the incubation period of the disease is very long, migrants may not show any increased incidence or mortality of the disease for many years.

2.4　Adjusted or Standardized Rates

If we want to compare the death rates of two populations with different age-composition, the crude death rate is not the right yardstick. This is because, rates are only comparable if the populations upon which they are based are comparable. And it is cumbersome to use a series of age specific death rates. The answer is "age adjustment" or "age standardization", which removes the confounding effect of different age structures and yields a single standardized or adjusted rate, by which the mortality experience can be compared directly. The adjustment can be made not only for age but also sex, race, parity, etc. Thus one can generate age-sex, and race-adjusted rates.

Standardization is carried out by either one of two methods - direct or indirect standardization. Both the methods begin by choosing a "standard population", not the age-structures of the populations.

2.4.1　Direct standardization

Two examples of direct standardization are given. In the first, a "standard population" is selected. A standard population is defined as one for which the numbers in the age and sex group are known. A frequently used standard age-composition is shown in Table 2-1. The standard population may also be "created" by combining populations, this is shown in the second example.

表现不出发病率或死亡率的升高。

2.4　调整率或标准化率

当比较两个人群的死亡率时，如果其年龄构成不同，那么粗死亡率并不是正确的评价指标，因为不同年龄的死亡率不同。只有比较的两组人群年龄构成具有可比性时，才可以直接使用粗死亡率进行比较。通过进行"年龄调整"或"年龄标准化"，可以消除年龄构成差异的混杂效应，得到的年龄标准化率或调整率可以直接用于进行比较。这种方法不仅可以用于年龄，还可以用于性别、种族、胎次等的调整或标准化，由此可以得到年龄、性别或种族的调整率。

标准化法有直接标准化或间接标准化两种方法。这两种方法都是从选择"标准人群"开始的，而不是从人群的年龄构成开始的。

2.4.1　直接标准化

以下将通过两个直接标准化法的例子进行阐述。第一步，选择"标准人群"。标准人群中不同年龄和性别组的人数是已知的。表2-1是常用的标准人群年龄构成显示方法。标准人群也可以是通过人群合并获得的，如例2所示。

The next step is to apply to the standard population age-specific rates of the population whose crude death rate to be adjusted or standardized. As a result for each group, an "expected" number of deaths (or events) in standard population is obtained; these are added together all the age groups, to give the total expected deaths. The operation is to divide the "expected" total number of deaths by the total of the standard population, which yields standardized or age-adjusted rate.

【Example 1】

Example 1 shows: the computation of age-specific death rates per 1 000 population for City X (Table 2-1); and application of these rates to a standard population to obtain "expected deaths" and the standardized or age-adjusted deaths rate(Table 2-2).

Table 2-1　Calculation of the standardized death rate for City X

Age	Standard population	Age-specific death rates per 1 000/‰	Expected deaths
0	2 400	15.0	36
1-4	9 600	4.4	42.24
5-14	19 000	3.0	57
15-19	9 000	3.0	27
20-24	8 000	4.0	32
25-34	14 000	3.1	43.4
35-44	12 000	5.3	63.6
45-54	11 000	12.5	137.5
55-64	8 000	21.4	171.2
Total	93 000		609.94

Note: Standardized death rate per 1 000‰ $= \dfrac{609.94}{93\,000} \times 1\,000‰ = 6.56‰$

第二步，将要比较人群的年龄别粗死亡率应用到标准人群中进行调整或标准化。这样，每个年龄组的标准人群都可以得到预期死亡数（或阳性事件数）；所有年龄组加在一起，可以得到预期死亡总数；然后将预期的死亡总数除以标准人群总人数，就可以得到标准化率或年龄调整率。

【例1】

已知X市每1 000人年龄别死亡率（表2-1），将这些率应用于标准人群，可获得"预期死亡"和标准化或年龄调整死亡率（表2-2）。

表 2-1　X市标准化死亡率的计算

年龄	标准人口	每1 000人年龄别死亡率/‰	预期死亡人数
0	2 400	15.0	36
1～4	9 600	4.4	42.24
5～14	19 000	3.0	57
15～19	9 000	3.0	27
20～24	8 000	4.0	32
25～34	14 000	3.1	43.4
35～44	12 000	5.3	63.6
45～54	11 000	12.5	137.5
55～64	8 000	21.4	171.2
合计	93 000		609.94

注：每1 000人中人均标准化死亡率 $= \dfrac{609.94}{93\,000} \times 1\,000‰ = 6.56‰$

Table 2-2   Calculation of age-specific death rates for City X

Age	Mid-year population	Deaths in the year	Age-specific death rates per 1 000/‰
0	4 000	60	15.0
1-4	4 500	20	4.4
5-14	4 000	12	3.0
15-19	5 000	15	3.0
20-24	4 000	16	4.0
25-34	8 000	25	3.1
35-44	9 000	48	5.3
45-54	8 000	100	12.5
55-64	7 000	150	21.4
Total	53 500	446	

Note:Crude death rate per 1 000=8‰

表 2-2　X市特定年龄死亡率的计算

年龄	年中人数	年内死亡人数	每1 000人年龄别死亡率/‰
0	4 000	60	15.0
1～4	4 500	20	4.4
5～14	4 000	12	3.0
15～19	5 000	15	3.0
20～24	4 000	16	4.0
25～34	8 000	25	3.1
35～44	9 000	48	5.3
45～54	8 000	100	12.5
55～64	7 000	150	21.4
合计	53 500	446	

注：每1 000人粗死亡率=8‰

It can be seen from Tables 2-1 and 2-2 that standardizing for age distribution has reduced the crude death rate from 8.3‰ to 6.56‰. The choice of the standard population is, to some extent, arbitrary. Clearly, use of a different standard population will given rise to a different value for the standardized death rate, but it must be remembered that these compared between themselves - they have no intrinsic meaning other than for this purpose.

It is usual to use the national population as standard when inter - regional comparisons between cities within a range are made. In order that comparisons can be made over a period of years' a "standard population" can be maintained for that period. The standard population used in Table 2-2 is given by WHO in its publication " Health for All" Series No 4.

【Example 2】

Table 2-3 shows that in a study of lung cancer and smoking, 42 percent of cases and 18 percent of controls were heavy smokers.

从表2-1和表2-2看出，根据标准人群的年龄分布调整，粗死亡率由8.3‰降低到标准化率6.56‰。在某种程度上标准人口是任意选择的。显然，使用不同的标准人口会得到不同的标准化率。必须记住，标准化率的意义仅在于比较。

在一定范围内的城市间进行比较时，通常使用国家人口作为标准人口。为了能够在一段时间内进行比较，"标准人口"可以一直使用。表2-2中使用的标准人口出自世界卫生组织（WHO）颁布的"全民健康"系列4号文件。

【例2】

表2-3显示,在一项肺癌和吸烟的研究中,42%的病例和18%的对照是重度吸烟者。

Table 2-3　Population of heavy smokers in cases and controls (lung cancer)

Age	Total subjects	Cases			Controls		
		No.	Heavy smokers	%	No.	Heavy smokers	%
40-49	500	400	200	50	100	50	50
50-59	500	100	10	10	400	40	10
Total	1 000	500	210	42	500	90	18

Age adjustments were carried out: First, by combining the number of subjects in both the age groups (500+500=1 000) to create a standard population; Second, applying the observed age-specific proportions of heavy smokers (i. e, 50% and 10% in both cases and controls) to the same standard population. The results or "expected" values are shown in Table 2-4, which shows that the age adjusted proportions of heavy smokers are identical (30%) for cases and controls. The previously observed difference is explained entirely by the difference in age composition.

Table 2-4　Age-adjusted proportions

Age	Subject	Expected number of heavy smokers	
		Cases	Controls
40-49	500	$\frac{500 \times 50}{100} = 250$	$\frac{500 \times 50}{100} = 250$
50-59	500	$\frac{500 \times 10}{100} = 50$	$\frac{500 \times 10}{100} = 50$
Total	1 000	300	300
Standardized rates		$\frac{300}{1 000} \times 100\% = 30\%$	$\frac{300}{1 000} \times 100\% = 30\%$

The direct method of standardization is feasible only if the actual specific rates in subgroups of the observed population are available, along with the number of individuals in each subgroup.

2.4.2　Indirect age standardization

1. Standardized mortality ratio (SMR)

The simplest and most useful form of indirect

表 2-3　病例组和对照组重度吸烟人群(肺癌)

年龄	总人数	病例组			对照组		
		人数	重度吸烟人数	占比/%	人数	重度吸烟人数	占比/%
40～49	500	400	200	50	100	50	50
50～59	500	100	10	10	400	40	10
总数	1 000	500	210	42	500	90	18

进行年龄调整：首先，通过合并两个年龄组研究对象的数量（500 + 500 = 1000）创建一个标准人口；其次，将观察到的重度吸烟者年龄比例（即病例组和对照组的50%和10%）应用到相同的标准人口中。表2-4的结果显示了两组重度吸烟者的期望值，表明病例组和对照组重度吸烟者的年龄调整肺癌发病率均是30%。说明以前观察到的肺癌发病率差异完全是由年龄构成的差异造成的。

表 2-4　年龄调整比例

年龄	人数	预期重度吸烟人数	
		病例组	对照组
40～49	500	$\frac{500 \times 50}{100} = 250$	$\frac{500 \times 50}{100} = 250$
50～59	500	$\frac{500 \times 10}{100} = 50$	$\frac{500 \times 10}{100} = 50$
总数	1 000	300	300
标准化率		$\frac{300}{1 000} \times 100\% = 30\%$	$\frac{300}{1 000} \times 100\% = 30\%$

只有已知观察人群的亚组的实际率，以及每个亚组的具体人数时，直接标准化法才可以使用。

2.4.2　间接年龄标准化

1.标准化死亡比(SMR)

最简单和最实用的间接标准化指标是标准化

standardization is the Standardized Mortality Ratio (SMR) in England, it is the basis for the allocation of govern money to the health regions of the country. The concerns are that the regions with higher mortality also have the higher morbidity, and should therefore receive proportion higher funding to combat ill health.

Standard mortality ratio is a ratio (usually expressed by the percentage) of the total number of deaths that occur in study group to the number of deaths that would have expected to occur if that study group had experienced death rates of a standard population (or other reference population). In other words. SMR compares the mortality study group (e.g, an occupational group) with the mortality that the occupational group would have had if they had experienced national mortality rates. In this method, the stable rates of the larger population are applied to the study group. It gives a measure of the likely excess mortality due to the occupation.

$$SMR = \frac{Observed \quad deaths}{Expected \quad deaths} \times 100\% \qquad (2-10)$$

If the ratio had value greater than 100, then the occupational would appear to carry a greater mortality risk than that the whole population. If the ratio had value less than 100, then the occupation risks of mortality would seem the proportionately less than that for the whole population.

Table 2-5 shows that the mortality experience of coal worker was 129 percent, which meant that their mortality was 29 percent more than that experienced by the national population. Values over 100 percent represent an unfavourable mortality experience and those below 100 percent relatively favourable mortality experience. Table 2-5 display the calculations.

The SMR has the advantage over the direct meth-

死亡比（SMR）。在英国，国家卫生资源分配以SMR为基础。死亡率高的地区也有较高的发病率，因此这些地区应该获得更多的经费用来防治疾病。

SMR是一个比值（通常用百分比表示），是研究人群中实际观察到的死亡人数与通过标准人口计算得到的预期死亡人数的比值。可以通过SMR进行职业人群死亡率的比较。当人口数较大时，死亡率相对稳定。而当研究对象数目较少，结局时间的发生率比较低时，不宜直接计算率，常用SMR评价发病或死亡的风险。SMR在职业流行病学中常用，可以用来测量职业所导致的超额死亡。

$$SMR = \frac{实际死亡数}{预期死亡数} \times 100\% \qquad (2-10)$$

如果SMR大于1，那么职业人群的死亡风险比一般人群高。如果SMR小于1，那么职业人群的死亡风险比一般人群低。

表2-5显示煤炭工人的SMR为129%，表明煤炭工人的死亡率比全国人口的死亡率高29%。超过100%代表了增加死亡风险，低于100%代表了降低死亡风险。

SMR相对于直接标准化法的优势在于，由于

od adjustment in that it permits adjustment for age and other factors where age specific rates are not available and unstable because of small numbers. One needs to know the number of persons in each age group in the population and the age specific rates of the nature population (or other reference population). It is possible use SMR if the event of interest is occurrence of diseases than death.

死亡例数少，它不需要像直接标准化法那样对年龄和其他因素进行调整或得到年龄别死亡率。直接标准化法需要知道人群中每个年龄组的人数和标准人口（或其他参考人口）的年龄别率。SMR不仅可以用于评价死亡风险，也可以用于评价发病风险。

Table 2-5　Calculation of the SMR for coal workers

Age	National population death rates per 1 000/‰	Coal workers population	Observed deaths	Expected deaths
25-34	3.0	300	*	*
35-44	5.0	400	*	*
45-54	8.0	200	*	*
55-64	25.0	100	*	*
Total		1 000	9	7

Note：*It is not necessary to known these values；only the total for the whole age-range is required.

表 2-5　煤矿工人SMR的计算

年龄	全国人口每1 000人死亡率/‰	煤矿工人人数	观察到的死亡人数	预期死亡人数
25～34	3.0	300	*	*
35～44	5.0	400	*	*
45～54	8.0	200	*	*
55～64	25.0	100	*	*
总计		1 000	9	7

注：*没有必要知道这些值；只需要整个年龄段的总数。

2. Other standardization techniques

① A more complicated method of in direct adjusted, which yields absolute age adjusted rate, involved calculation of an index death rate and a standardizing rate for each population of interest. The reader is referred to A.B. Hill's *Principles of Medical Statistics.*

② Life table：An age-adjusted summary of current all-causes mortality.

③ Regression techniques：These are an efficient means of standardization.

④ Multivariate analysis：A computer, using regression or similar methods, can standardize for many variables simultaneously.

2.其他标准化技术

①一种可以获得绝对年龄调整率的更复杂的直接调整方法，涉及研究人群的死亡率指数和标准化率的计算。读者可以参考 A.B.Hill 的《医学统计原则》。

②生命表：全死因死亡率年龄调整的汇总表。

③回归技术：一种有效的控制混杂因素的标准化方法。

④多因素分析：使用回归或类似的方法，可以同时对多个变量进行调整。

Chapter 3 Descriptive Studies

Descriptive epidemiologic studies describe the distribution of disease, health status and exposure in different populations by factors such as age, gender and race, and estimate the pattern and trends in disease occurrence over time or in different geographic areas. These studies are mainly used to generate hypotheses for further study and cannot testify the causal relation between disease and exposure or ascertain the degree of exposure. Descriptive studies mainly include case report, disease surveillance, cross - sectional study, ecological study and screening. The cross - sectional study measures disease and exposure status simultaneously in a population, in which the frequency and characteristics of a disease in the population at a particular point in time can be described. This type of data may be useful for assessing the prevalence of acute or chronic conditions but can not tell whether the exposure proceeded or followed the disease. Ecologic study, also known as correlation study, relates the frequency of a disease to an exposure at population or group level. Thus, the observational unit in ecological studies is groups or populations rather than individuals. Descriptive studies are mainly used for estimating the prevalence of disease or health status, probing into the natural history of disease, ascertaining high - risk individuals and providing clues for further studies.

Such studies basically ask the questions:

①When is the disease occurring?—time distribution

②Where is it occurring?—place distribution

第3章 描述性研究

描述性流行病学研究通过描述疾病、健康状况和暴露因素的"三间"分布情况，提出病因假设，为进一步调查研究提供病因线索。描述性研究不能检验暴露或暴露水平与疾病的因果关系。描述性流行病学研究主要包括个案调查、疾病监测、横断面研究、生态学研究和筛查。横断面研究同时测量人群中疾病和暴露的情况，描述疾病在特定时间的频率和特征，可用于评估急性、慢性疾病的流行情况，但不能确定暴露在疾病发生之前还是之后。生态学研究又称相关性研究，研究的是群体暴露状况或群体暴露水平与疾病频率的关系。因此，生态学研究的观察单位是群体，而不是个体。描述性研究主要用于估计疾病或健康状况的流行情况，探索疾病的自然史，确定高危人群，并为进一步进行病因研究提供线索，是分析性研究的基础。

这类研究要问的基本问题：

①疾病什么时候发生？——时间分布

②疾病在哪里发生？——空间分布

③ Who is getting the disease?—person distribution

③什么样的人患了疾病？——人间分布

3.1 Cross-sectional Study

3.1 横断面研究

3.1.1 Conception

A cross-sectional study is a descriptive study in which disease and exposure status both are measured simultaneously in a given population. Cross-sectional studies can be thought of as providing a "snapshot" of the frequency and characteristics of a disease in a population at a particular point in time. This type of data can be used to assess the prevalence of acute or chronic conditions in a population. For example, in a study of hypertension, we can also collect data during the survey about age, sex, physical exercise, body weight, salt intake and other variables of interest. Then we can determine how prevention of hypertension is related to certain variables simultaneously measured. Such a study tells us about the distribution of a disease in population rather than its aetiology.

The most common reason that epidemiologist examines the inter-relationships between a disease, or one of its precursors, and other variables is to attempt to establish a causal chain and so give lead to possible ways of preventing that disease. However, since exposure and disease status are measured at the same point in time, it may not be possible to distinguish whether the exposure preceded or followed the disease, and thus cause and effect relationships are not certain. Although a cross-sectional study provides information about disease prevalence, it provides very little information about the natural history of disease or about the rate of occurrence of new cases (incidence).Cross-

3.1.1 概念

横断面研究是一种描述性研究，是在特定时期和特定人群中同时测量疾病和相关暴露因素的研究。横断面研究被形象地比喻为提供特定时间、特定人群中疾病频率和特征的"快照"，可用于评估人群中急性或慢性疾病的患病率。例如，在一项高血压研究中，调查期间可以收集年龄、性别、体育锻炼、体重、盐摄入量等高血压相关因素的数据。横断面研究可以描述疾病在人群中的分布情况，但不能确定病因。

流行病学通过研究疾病或其临床先兆与影响因素之间的相互关系，尝试建立因果链，从而提出预防疾病的可能措施。然而，由于横断面研究同时测量暴露和疾病状态，无法区分暴露与疾病的先后顺序，因此无法确定二者的因果关系。虽然横断面研究提供了关于疾病流行的信息，但无法提供关于疾病的自然史或新发病例（发病率）的信息。横断面研究也称为横断面分析、现况研究、现患率研究。

sectional studies also known as cross - sectional analyses, transversal studies, prevalence study.

3.1.2 Purpose and application scope

① To know the distribution of the disease or health in the target groups.

② To provide clues for disease etiology research.

③ To confirm the high risk group.

④ To evaluate the effect of disease surveillance and vaccination.

3.1.3 Characteristics and types of cross-sectional studies

1. Characteristics of cross-sectional studies

① At the beginning of the cross - sectional studies do not have a control group.

② The special time of cross - sectional studies.

Cross - sectional studies focus on the connection between exposure and disease in a population in a special time - point or a specific period.

③ Cross - sectional studies are limited in determining the causal association.

④ If the exposed factor does not change, the cross-sectional study could prompt the causal association.

2. Types of cross-sectional studies

（1）Census

Census is complete survey. A survey that measures the entire target population is called a census. It is a survey that all population in a special time - point or period in a particular range are objects of study. The special time - point should be short. The particular range is an area or population with a characteristic, such as children's physique survey.

3.1.2 研究目的与应用范围

①了解疾病或健康状况在目标人群中的分布。

②提供病因线索。

③确定高危人群。

④评价疾病监测、预防接种的效果。

3.1.3 研究特点与研究类型

1. 现况研究的特点

①现况研究设计阶段不设对照组。

②现况研究有特定时间。现况研究侧重于特定时间点或特定时期人群中暴露与疾病之间的关系。

③现况研究不能确定暴露与疾病的因果联系。

④对研究对象固有的暴露因素，可以提示其与疾病的因果联系。

2. 现况研究的类型

（1）普查

普查即全面调查，指在特定时间或时期内对整个目标人群进行调查。普查是在研究目标下，以特定时间或范围内的所有人为研究对象。特定时间可以是时间点或时间段，但不宜太长，应该相对较短。特定范围是某个地区或具有某种特征的人群。

The objectives of census: ①Early discovery, early diagnosis and early treatment; ②To know the prevalence of chronic disease and the epidemics distribution of acute infectious diseases; ③To know the health conditions of local residents, such as nutrition surveys; ④To know the range of normal value of all kinds of physiological and biochemical refers to the human body.

Advantage of census: ①The objects of study are the all target population, so there is no sampling error; ②Could survey the distribution of a variety of disease or health at the same time; ③Could discover all cases of target population.

Disadvantage of census: ①Cross - sectional studies do not suitable for the rare disease; ②Exist failing to report unavoidably; ③Can't guarantee the quality of survey; ④Cross - sectional studies are often very expensive and time-consuming.

（2）Sampling survey

Survey sampling describes the process of selecting a sample of elements from a target population in order to conduct a survey. A survey may refer to many different types or techniques of observation, but in the context of survey sampling it most often involves a questionnaire used to measure the characteristics and/or attitudes of people. Different ways of contacting members of a sample once they have been selected is the subject of survey data collection. The purpose of sampling is to reduce the cost and/or the amount of work that it would take to survey the entire target population.

普查的目的：①早发现、早诊断、早治疗（即"三早"）；②了解慢性病的流行情况和急性传染病的流行分布情况；③了解当地居民的健康状况，如营养状况调查；④了解人体各种生理生化指标的正常值范围。

普查的优点：①调查对象为全体目标人群，不存在抽样误差；②可以同时调查目标人群中多种疾病或健康状况的分布情况；③可以发现目标人群中的全部病例，实现"三早"，达到二级预防。

普查的缺点：①现况研究不适用于罕见疾病；②不可避免地存在漏报现象；③工作量大，无法保证调查质量；④通常非常昂贵、耗时。

（2）抽查

抽查即抽样调查。抽样调查描述了从目标人群中选择样本以进行调查的过程。抽样调查包括不同类型或观察方法，通常利用调查表测量样本人群的特征和/或态度。一旦通过不同抽样方法确定样本，就需要进行数据的收集。抽样的目的是减少调查整个目标人群的成本和/或工作量。

3.1.4 Study design and implementation

1. Clear and definite the investigation purpose and types

2. Determine the objects of study

3. Determine the sample size and sampling methods

（1）Sample size

The influencing factors of sample size: ① Expected prevalence (p); ② The requirement of accuracy, if the allowable error (d) is bigger, and the sample size is smaller; ③ Level of significance (α), The higher requirements of significance level, the bigger the sample size requirements. The calculation formula of sample size as follows:

$$s_p = \sqrt{\frac{pq}{n}} \qquad (3-1)$$

After the transformation：

$$n = \frac{pq}{s_p^2} \qquad (3-2)$$

Made $s_p = \dfrac{d}{z_\alpha}$,

$$n = \frac{pq}{(\frac{d}{z_\alpha})^2} = \frac{z_\alpha^2 \times pq}{d^2} \qquad (3-3)$$

In the formula, p is expected prevalence, $q=1-p$, d is allowable error, z_α is summary statistic of significance testing, when $\alpha =0.05$, $z_\alpha =1.96$, and when $a=0.01$, $z_\alpha=2.58$. n is the sample size.

Assume that d is a fraction of p. Generally $d=0.1\times p$, and when $\alpha=0.05$, $z=1.96\approx2$.

So formula 3-3 could transform into the follow:

$$n = 400 \times \frac{q}{p} \qquad (3-4)$$

If $d=0.15p$, $n=178\times q/p$, similarly, when $d=0.2p$, $n=100\times q/p$, level of significance, $\alpha=0.05$. We could esti-

3.1.4 研究设计与实施

1. 明确调查目的与类型

2. 确定研究对象

3. 确定样本量和抽样方法

（1）样本量

样本量的影响因素：①预期现患率（p）；②对调查结果精确性的要求：容许误差（d）越大，所需样本量就越小；③显著性水平（α）：α 值越小，显著性水平要求越高，样本量要求越大。一般来讲，在做某病的现患率调查时，其样本量可用下式估计：

$$s_p = \sqrt{\frac{pq}{n}} \qquad (3-1)$$

经转换，可改写成下式：

$$n = \frac{pq}{s_p^2} \qquad (3-2)$$

令 $s_p = \dfrac{d}{z_\alpha}$，则有

$$n = \frac{pq}{(\frac{d}{z_\alpha})^2} = \frac{z_\alpha^2 \times pq}{d^2} \qquad (3-3)$$

式中，p 为预期的现患率；$q=1-p$；d 为容许误差；z_α 为显著性检验的统计量，$\alpha=0.05$ 时，$z_\alpha=1.96$，$\alpha=0.01$ 时，$z_\alpha=2.58$；n 为样本量。

设 d 为 p 的一个分数。一般采用 $d=0.1\times p$，并且当 $\alpha=0.05$ 时，$z=1.96\approx2$。

则式 3-3 可写成：

$$n = 400 \times \frac{q}{p} \qquad (3-4)$$

若容许误差 $d=0.15p$，则 $n=178\times q/p$；同理，$d=0.2p$ 时，$n=100\times q/p$，以上计算中显著性水平 α 均

mate the sample size according Table 3-1. When the prevalence or positive rate is smaller than 10% obviously, we could not use this table.

取0.05。据此，表3-1可作为估计调查样本量大小的参考（$\alpha=0.05$）。但当患病率或阳性率明显小于10%时，此表不适用。

Table 3-1　The required sample size of expected prevalence and allowable error

Expected prevalence	Allowable error		
	0.1p	0.15p	0.2p
0.050	7 600	3 382	1 900
0.075	4 933	2 193	1 328
0.100	3 600	1 602	900
0.150	2 264	1 009	566
0.200	1 600	712	400
0.250	1 200	533	300
0.300	930	415	233
0.350	743	330	186
0.400	600	267	150

表3-1　不同预期现患率和容许误差时所需的样本量大小

预期现患率	容许误差		
	0.1p	0.15p	0.2p
0.050	7 600	3 382	1 900
0.075	4 933	2 193	1 328
0.100	3 600	1 602	900
0.150	2 264	1 009	566
0.200	1 600	712	400
0.250	1 200	533	300
0.300	930	415	233
0.350	743	330	186
0.400	600	267	150

The formulas above apply only to the situation that $n \times p > 5$, if $n \times p \leq 5$, we could use the method of Poisson distribution to estimate the sample size. Table 3-2 is confidence limits table of expected values of Poisson distribution.

以上样本量估计公式仅适用于 $n \times p > 5$ 的情况，如果 $n \times p \leq 5$，则宜用 Poisson 分布的办法来估算样本量。表3-2为 Poisson 分布期望值的可信限简表。

Table 3-2　Confidence limits table of expected values of Poisson distribution

Expected numbers of cases	0.95		0.90	
	Lower limit	Upper limit	Lower limit	Upper limit
0	0.00	3.69	0.00	3.00
1	0.025 3	5.57	0.051 3	4.74
2	0.242	7.22	0.355	6.30
3	0.619	8.77	0.818	7.75
4	1.09	10.24	1.37	9.15
5	1.62	11.67	1.97	10.51
6	2.20	13.06	2.61	11.84
7	2.81	14.42	3.29	13.15
8	3.45	15.76	3.93	14.43

表3-2　Poisson 分布期望值的可信限简表

预期病例数	0.95		0.90	
	下限	上限	下限	上限
0	0.00	3.69	0.00	3.00
1	0.025 3	5.57	0.051 3	4.74
2	0.242	7.22	0.355	6.30
3	0.619	8.77	0.818	7.75
4	1.09	10.24	1.37	9.15
5	1.62	11.67	1.97	10.51
6	2.20	13.06	2.61	11.84
7	2.81	14.42	3.29	13.15
8	3.45	15.76	3.93	14.43

Expected numbers of cases	0.95		0.90	
	Lower limit	Upper limit	Lower limit	Upper limit
9	4.12	17.08	4.70	15.71
10	4.30	18.29	5.43	16.96
11	5.49	19.68	6.17	18.21
12	6.20	20.96	6.92	19.44
13	6.92	22.23	7.69	20.67
14	7.65	23.49	8.46	21.89
15	8.40	24.74	9.25	23.10
16	9.15	25.98	10.04	24.30
17	9.90	27.22	10.83	25.50
18	10.67	28.45	11.63	26.69
19	11.44	29.67	12.44	27.88
20	12.22	30.89	13.25	29.06
21	13.00	32.10	14.07	30.24
22	13.79	33.31	14.89	31.42
23	14.58	34.51	15.72	32.59
24	15.38	35.71	16.55	33.75
25	16.18	36.90	17.38	34.92
26	16.98	38.10	18.22	36.08
27	17.79	39.28	19.06	37.23
28	18.61	40.47	19.90	38.39
29	19.42	41.65	20.75	39.54
30	20.24	42.83	21.59	40.69
35	24.38	48.68	25.87	46.40
40	28.58	54.47	30.20	52.07
45	32.82	60.21	34.56	57.69
50	37.11	65.92	38.96	63.29

If the analysis index of sampling survey is measurement data, we should use formula 3-5 to calculate the sample size.

$$n = \frac{4s^2}{d^2} \tag{3-5}$$

预期病例数	0.95		0.90	
	下限	上限	下限	上限
9	4.12	17.08	4.70	15.71
10	4.30	18.29	5.43	16.96
11	5.49	19.68	6.17	18.21
12	6.20	20.96	6.92	19.44
13	6.92	22.23	7.69	20.67
14	7.65	23.49	8.46	21.89
15	8.40	24.74	9.25	23.10
16	9.15	25.98	10.04	24.30
17	9.90	27.22	10.83	25.50
18	10.67	28.45	11.63	26.69
19	11.44	29.67	12.44	27.88
20	12.22	30.89	13.25	29.06
21	13.00	32.10	14.07	30.24
22	13.79	33.31	14.89	31.42
23	14.58	34.51	15.72	32.59
24	15.38	35.71	16.55	33.75
25	16.18	36.90	17.38	34.92
26	16.98	38.10	18.22	36.08
27	17.79	39.28	19.06	37.23
28	18.61	40.47	19.90	38.39
29	19.42	41.65	20.75	39.54
30	20.24	42.83	21.59	40.69
35	24.38	48.68	25.87	46.40
40	28.58	54.47	30.20	52.07
45	32.82	60.21	34.56	57.69
50	37.11	65.92	38.96	63.29

若抽样调查的分析指标为计量资料，则应按计量资料的样本估计公式来计算，公式如下：

$$n = \frac{4s^2}{d^2} \tag{3-5}$$

n is the sample size, d is allowable error, s is estimated value of population standard deviation.

（2）Sampling methods

Common methods of random sampling are simple random sampling, systematic sampling, stratified sampling, cluster sampling, and multistage sampling.

1）Simple random sampling

A simple random sample is a subset of individuals (a sample) chosen from a larger set (a population). Each individual is chosen randomly and entirely by chance, such that each individual has the same probability of being chosen at any stage during the sampling process, and each subset of k individuals has the same probability of being chosen for the sample as any other subset of k individuals. This process and technique is known as simple random sampling, and should not be confused with systematic random sampling. A simple random sample is an unbiased surveying technique.

Simple random sampling is a basic type of sampling, since it can be a component of other more complex sampling methods. The principle of simple random sampling is that every object has the same probability of being chosen. For example, suppose N college students want to get a ticket for a basketball game, but there are only $X < N$ tickets for them, so they decide to have a fair way to see who gets to go. Then, everybody is given a number in the range from 0 to $N-1$, and random numbers are generated, either electronically or from a table of random numbers. Numbers outside the range from 0 to $N-1$ are ignored, as are any numbers previously selected. The first X numbers would identify the lucky ticket winners.

上式中，n 为样本量，d 为容许误差，s 为总体标准差的估计值。

（2）抽样方法

抽样方法可分为非随机抽样（如典型抽样和方便抽样）和随机抽样。常用的随机抽样方法有简单随机抽样、系统抽样、分层抽样、整群抽样和多级（多阶段）抽样。

1）简单随机抽样

简单随机样本是从更大的集合（总体）中选择的个体子集（样本）。总体中的每个个体在抽样过程中都有相同的概率或机会被抽中，成为样本中的成员。这一过程和技术被称为简单随机抽样，简单随机抽样不应与系统随机抽样相混淆。简单随机抽样是一种无偏调查技术。

简单随机抽样是最简单、最基本的抽样方法，它可以是其他更复杂抽样方法的组成部分。简单随机抽样的原理是，总体中的每个对象都有相同的概率被选择成为样本人群中的研究对象。例如，假设 N 名大学生想得到篮球比赛的票，但只有 X（$X<N$）张票，所以采用公平的方式来决定谁去。首先，给每个学生 0 到 $N-1$ 范围内的数字编码，然后利用软件或随机数表生成随机数字，随机数字也要求是 0 到 $N-1$ 范围内的数字，这样每个学生对应一个随机数字，之后再进行简单随机抽样。事先规定，前 X 个随机数字为幸运票的获得者。

The standard error of mean:

$$s_{\bar{x}} = \sqrt{\left(1 - \frac{n}{N}\right)\frac{s^2}{n}} \qquad (3\text{-}6)$$

The standard error of rate:

$$s_p = \sqrt{\left(1 - \frac{n}{N}\right)\frac{p(1-p)}{n-1}} \qquad (3\text{-}7)$$

s is the standard deviation of sample; p is sample rate; n/N is sampling fraction, if n/N is less than 5%, it could be ignore.

2）Systematic sampling

Systematic sampling is a statistical method involving the selection of elements from an ordered sampling frame.

The most common form of systematic sampling is an equal - probability method. In this approach, progression through the list is treated circularly, with a return to the top once the end of the list is passed. The sampling starts by selecting an element from the list at random and then every k^{th} element in the frame is selected, where k, the sampling interval (sometimes known as the skip), this is calculated as: $k=N/n$. Where n is the sample size, and N is the population size.

The advantages of systematic sampling: Samples can be performed without the number of overall units; the sample is extracted from the units of each part of the overall, and the distribution is relatively uniform and the representative is better.

The disadvantages of systematic sampling: If the distribution of the overall units has a periodic trend, the extraction interval is exactly in line with this cycle, the sample may produce bias.

3）Stratified sampling

In statistical surveys, when subpopulations within an overall population vary, it is advantageous to sam-

均数的标准误：

$$s_{\bar{x}} = \sqrt{\left(1 - \frac{n}{N}\right)\frac{s^2}{n}} \qquad (3\text{-}6)$$

率的标准误：

$$s_p = \sqrt{\left(1 - \frac{n}{N}\right)\frac{p(1-p)}{n-1}} \qquad (3\text{-}7)$$

式中：s 为样本标准差；p 为样本率；N 为总体含量；n 为样本量；n/N 为抽样比，若其小于5%，则可以忽略不计。

2）系统抽样

系统抽样又称机械抽样，是从一个有序总体中，机械地每隔若干单位抽取一个个体的抽样方法。

系统抽样最常见的形式是等概率法。在这种方法中，需要进行多次循环抽样。首先从总体中随机选择一个个体，然后每隔 k 个人选择一个个体作为样本中的研究对象，其中 k 为抽样间隔（有时称为跳过），计算公式为 $k=N/n$。其中，n 为样本大小，N 为总体大小。

系统抽样的优点：可以在不知道总体单位数的情况下进行抽样；样本是从总体内部各部分的单元中抽取的，分布比较均匀，代表性较好。

系统抽样的缺点：如果总体各单位的分布有周期性趋势，抽取的间隔恰好与此周期吻合，则样本可能产生偏倚。

3）分层抽样

调查中，当总体中的亚组人群间存在变异时，适合对亚组人群（阶层）分别进行独立抽样。分

ple each subpopulation （stratum） independently. Stratification is the process of strata should be mutually exclusive: Every element in population must be assigned to only one stratum. The dividing members of the population into homogeneous subgroups before sampling. The strata should also be collectively exhaustive: no population element can be excluded. Then simple random sampling or systematic sampling is applied within each stratum. This often improves the representativeness of the sample by reducing sampling error. It can produce a weighted mean that has less variability than the arithmetic mean of a simple random sample of the population.

Stratified sampling includes two types: Proportional allocation and optimum allocation. Proportional allocation uses a sampling fraction in each of the strata that is proportional to that of the total population. Optimum allocation—Each stratum is proportionate to the standard deviation of the distribution of the variable. Larger samples are taken in the strata with the greatest variability to generate the least possible sampling variance.

4）Cluster sampling

Cluster sampling is a sampling technique where the entire population is divided into groups, or clusters and a random sample of these clusters are selected. And cluster sampling includes simple cluster sampling and two stages sampling.

5）Multistage sampling

A multistage sample is one in which sampling is done sequentially across two or more hierarchical levels, such as first at the province level, second at the city level, third at the block level, fourth at the household level, and ultimately at the within-household level.

层是在抽样前，将总体划分为同质亚组的过程。层与层之间应该是相互排斥的，总体中的每个个体只能分配给某个层。分层也应该是全面的，分层应该涵盖分层因素的所有情况。然后，在每个层内采用简单随机抽样或系统抽样。分层抽样通过减少抽样误差来提高样本的代表性。分层抽样获得的加权均数比简单随机抽样的算术均数的变异度小，这样抽样误差也就小。总的来说，分层抽样就是将总体按某种特征分为若干层，然后在每层内进行简单随机抽样，组成样本。

分层抽样有两种方法：比例分配和最优分配。比例分配根据样本在总体中的比例（各层内抽样比例相同），在每层中随机选择样本。最优分配，即各层抽样比例不同，分层因素与变量分布的标准偏差成比例。内部变异小的层抽样比例小，内部变异大的层抽样比例大，以产生尽可能小的抽样误差。

4）整群抽样

整群抽样是将总体人群分成若干组或若干群，并从中随机抽取部分群组作为样本。整群抽样包括简单整群抽样和两阶段抽样。整群抽样的特点是易于组织实施和抽样误差较大。

5）多级抽样

多级抽样是指抽样过程分阶段进行，每个阶段的抽样方法往往不同。多级抽样在大型流行病学调查中常用。例如，首先在省级层面随机抽样，其次在市级层面随机抽样，再次在街区一级随机抽样，之后在家庭一级随机抽样，最终在家庭成员一级随机抽样，每个阶段可以将以上抽样方法结合使用。

4. Data collection

The methods of data collection include two types: One is determination or examination; another is using questionnaires to ask the objects.

5. Evaluating sources and data analysis

3.1.5　The common bias and its control

1. The common bias

Bias is system error from the various stages of research design, implementation and data processing and analyzing, bias also from the one-sideness of results explanation and inference, all those lead to a difference between research results and true value, also lead to a wrong connection between exposure and disease. The causes of bias as follows:

① Subjective select objects of study.

② Change the sampling method arbitrarily.

③ Non-respondent bias.

④ Survivor bias.

⑤ Recall bias.

⑥ Investigation bias.

⑦ Measurement bias.

2. Bias's control

① Strictly in accordance with the requirements of sampling method.

② Increase the compliance and examination rate of the research objects.

③ To select the measuring tools and testing methods correctly.

④ Investigators must be trained.

⑤ Completes the data review seriously.

⑥ Choose the correct statistical analysis technique.

4. 资料的收集

数据收集的方法有两种：一种是使用检测或检查；另一种是使用问卷调查。

5. 数据的整理和分析

3.1.5　常见偏倚及其控制

1. 常见的偏倚

偏倚是指从研究设计、实施、数据处理和分析的各个环节中产生的系统误差，引起结果解释、推论中的片面性，导致研究结果与真实值之间的差异，从而得到错误的暴露与疾病关系。现况研究中，偏倚产生的原因主要有：

①选择偏倚。

②任意变换抽样方法。

③无应答偏倚。

④幸存者偏倚。

⑤回忆偏倚。

⑥调查偏倚。

⑦测量偏倚。

2. 偏倚的控制

①严格遵循抽样方法的要求。

②提高研究对象的依从性和受检率。

③正确选择测量工具和检测方法。

④调查员接受培训。

⑤做好资料的复查、复核等工作。

⑥选择正确的统计分析方法。

3.1.6 Advantages and disadvantages

1. Advantages

①The research results of cross-sectional studies have stronger meaning of promotion.

②There have a concurrent control group formed naturally, so the results are comparable.

③A cross-sectional study could observe multi-factor simultaneously. It is one of the absolutely necessary basic works in exploration process of disease causes.

2. Disadvantages

①The cross-sectional studies are difficult to determine the information on the sequence ofhappenings.

②The cross-sectional studies could not get the data of incidence. The cross-sectional studies may underestimate the level of prevalence.

3.2 Ecological Study

All the study types described thus far share the characteristic that the observations made pertain to individuals. It is possible, and sometimes necessary, to conduct research in which the unit of observation is a group of people rather than an individual. Such studies are called ecologic or aggregate studies. The groups may be classes in a school, factories, cities, counties, or nations. The only requirement is that information on the populations studied is available to measure the exposure and disease distributions in each group. Incidence or mortality rates are commonly used to quantify disease occurrence in groups. Exposure is also measured by an overall index; for example, county

3.1.6　优点与局限性

1. 优点

①现况研究的结果具有较强的病因提示作用。

②在同一研究人群中自然形成的对照组，结果具有可比性。

③可以同时观察多个因素。现况研究是病因研究中必不可少的基础性工作之一。

2. 局限性

①现况研究无法确定时间的先后顺序，不能得到因果关系。

②现况研究无法获得发病率数据，可能低估患病率。

3.2　生态学研究

迄今为止，所有的研究方法都有一个共同的特点，即以个体为观察对象。开展以群体而非个体为观察对象的研究是可能的，有时也是必要的。这类研究被称为生态学或相关性研究。这些群体可以是学校的班级、工厂、城市、县或国家。生态学研究以群体为观察和分析单位，在群体水平上研究暴露因素与疾病之间的关系。发病率或死亡率通常用于量化群体中的疾病频率，暴露也通过一个整体指数来测量。例如，根据酒精纳税数据估算酒精消费量，可通过人口普查数据获得社会经济信息，还可获得当地或该区域的环境数据（温度、空气质量等）。这些环境数据只能在群体水平上收集，个体数据无法获得或收集不可行。

alcohol consumption may be estimated from alcohol tax data, information on socioeconomic status is available for census tracts from the decennial census, and environmental data (temperature, air quality, etc.) may be available locally or regionally. These environmental data are examples of exposures that are measured by necessity at the level of a group, because individual - level data are usually unavailable and impractical to gather. Thus, a bias is unavoidable in ecological study—ecological fallacy.

因此，生态学研究不可避免地存在偏倚——生态学谬误。

Chapter 4　Case-Control Studies

Case-control study is one of the most basic and important type of analytic epidemiology, and normally used to investigate the association between the occurrence of a disease and an exposure suspected of causing (or preventing) that disease. In particular, case-control studies start by identifying cases from those who had the disease of interest and controls from those who have not. In a well-designed case-control study, cases are selected from a clearly defined population, which is sometimes called the source population, and controls are selected from the same population that yielded the cases. The past exposure status in both cases and controls is then collected and compared to assess the relationship between the exposure and disease. For rare disease or harms, case-control studies can be only practical approach to identifying their possible cause. Thus, as compared with cohort studies, case-control study is relatively less expensive and less time consuming but provides less strong evidence for the temporal order of a causal relation. Case-control studies are commonly used to estimate the relative magnitude of risk of disease due to environmental factors, investigate the cause of adverse effects due to drugs, discovering factors that cause or prevent disease, and study the impact of a diagnosis on the prognosis of disease. More recently, case-control studies have also been used to study gene-disease associations.

Suppose you are a clinician and you have seen a few patients with a certain type of cancer, almost all of

第4章　病例对照研究

病例对照研究是分析性流行病学方法中最基本、最重要的研究方法之一，常用于调查疾病与可疑暴露之间的关系。病例对照研究首先根据研究对象是否患有所研究疾病，将其分为病例组和对照组。一个设计良好的病例对照研究中，病例是从特定人群中筛选出来的患病的人，该特定人群也被称为源人群，对照是从病例来源的源人群中筛选出来的未患病的人。然后收集并比较病例组和对照组的暴露状况，以评估暴露与疾病之间的统计学关联及关联程度。病例对照研究是研究罕见病或伤害的病因的唯一可行办法。与队列研究相比，病例对照研究的花费较少、不耗时，但因无法确定暴露与疾病的时间先后顺序，所以提供的因果关系证据力度较弱。病例对照研究常用于评估环境因素导致疾病的风险程度，以及研究药物不良反应的影响因素、探索疾病的致病因素或保护因素和研究疾病的预后因素等。近年来，病例对照研究也被用于研究基因与疾病的相关性。

假设作为一名临床大夫，你发现患有某种癌症的患者几乎都曾暴露于某种化学物，有人据此

whom report that they have been exposed to a particular chemical. You hypothesize that the exposure is related to the risk of developing this type of cancer. How would you go about confirming or refuting your hypothesis?

Consider two real-life examples:

A first example: In the early 1940's, Alton Ochsner, a surgeon in New Orleans, observed that virtually all of the patients on whom he was operating for lung cancer gave a history of cigarette smoking. Although this relationship is accepted and well recognized today, it was relatively new and controversial at the time that Ochsner made his observation. He hypothesized that cigarette smoking was linked to lung cancer. Based only on his observations in cases of lung cancer, was this conclusion valid?

A second example: Again in the 1940's, Sir Norman Gregg, an Australian ophthalmologist, observed a number of infants and young children in his ophthalmology practice who presented with an unusual form of cataract. Gregg noted that these children had been in utero during the time of a rubella (German measles) outbreak. He suggested that there was an association between prenatal rubella exposure and the development of the unusual cataracts. Keep in mind that at that time there was no knowledge that a virus could be teratogenic. Thus, he proposed his hypothesis solely on the basis of observational data, the equivalent of data from ambulatory or bedside practice today.

Let us suppose that Gregg had observed that 90% of these infants had been in utero during the rubella outbreak. Would he have been justified in concluding that rubella was associated with the cataracts? Clearly, the answer is no. For although such an observation would be interesting, it would be difficult to interpret

推测这种暴露可能与该癌症有关，那么下一步你该怎样证实或驳倒这一推测？

现列举生活中两个真实的例子：

第一个例子：20世纪40年代早期，新奥尔良的一名外科大夫 Alton Ochsner 发现，几乎所有经他手术的肺癌患者都有吸烟史。尽管目前吸烟与肺癌的关系已被大众承认，但在 Ochsner 发现这个现象时，吸烟与肺癌的关系是相对新的发现并存在争议。基于对肺癌患者的观察，提出吸烟与肺癌有关的假设，这种结论是否合理、正确？

第二个例子：同样在20世纪40年代，澳大利亚的一名眼科医生 Norman Gregg 发现，他的眼科病人中，许多婴幼儿都患有一种不常见类型的白内障。Gregg 注意到这些孩子在母亲子宫内时已经感染了风疹病毒，故认为产前风疹病毒暴露与白内障可能有关，而那个年代人们还没有认识到病毒可以致畸。因此，他仅仅基于观察数据（相当于根据现在的日间或床旁数据）提出了假设。

假设 Gregg 发现90%的白内障婴幼儿在母亲子宫内时就已感染了风疹病毒，是否就可以证明风疹病毒与白内障有关？很明显不能。尽管这些发现很有意义，但缺乏与未患白内障婴幼儿（对照组）的风疹感染数据的比较，因此无法确定二者关系。例如，一个社区在风疹暴发期间，90%的

without data for a comparison group of children cataracts. It is possible, for example, that 90% of all mothers in that community — both mothers of children with the cataracts and mothers of children with no cataracts — had been pregnant during the outbreak of rubella. In such a case, the exposure history would be no different for mothers of children with cataracts than for mothers of controls. The question was, therefore, whether the prevalence of rubella exposure (i.e., having been in utero during the outbreak) was greater in children with cataracts than in a group of children without cataracts.

To determine the significance of such observations in a group of cases, a comparison or control group is needed. Without such a comparison, Ochsner's or Gregg's observations would only constitute a case series. The observations would have been intriguing, but no conclusion is possible without comparative observations in a series of cases. Comparison is an essential component of epidemiologic investigation and is well exemplified by the case-control study design.

4.1　Basic Theory

To examine the possible relation of an exposure to a certain disease, we identify a group of individuals with that disease (called cases) and, for purposes of comparison, a group of people without that disease (called controls). We determine what proportion of the cases were exposed and what proportion were not. We also determine what proportion of the controls were exposed and what proportion were not. In the example of the children with cataracts, the cases would consist of children with cataracts and the controls would consist of children without cataracts. For each

母亲是孕妇，包括白内障患儿的母亲和未患白内障儿童的母亲。这种情况下，白内障患儿母亲的风疹暴露风险与对照组母亲的暴露风险无差异。因此，问题是，白内障患儿的风疹病毒暴露率（如风疹暴发期间的子宫内感染）是否高于未患白内障的儿童?

　　为了确定病例组观察数据的意义，必须设置对照组进行比较。没有对照组进行比较，Ochsner或Gregg的研究就仅是系列的病例观察，不能得出结论。比较是流行病学研究的核心，病例对照研究很好地体现了这一点。

4.1　基本原理

　　为了检验暴露与疾病的可能关系，以确诊患有研究疾病的一组人群为病例组，以不患有研究疾病但是具有可比性的一组人群为对照组，计算和比较病例组与对照组的暴露比（暴露人数与非暴露人数之比）。以前面的婴幼儿白内障为例，病例组由患有白内障的婴幼儿组成，对照组由未患白内障的婴幼儿组成，必须确定每个婴幼儿的母亲在其孕期是否曾暴露于风疹病毒。假设暴露于风疹病毒与白内障确实相关，那么病例组（白内障儿童）的风疹暴露率将高于对照组（无白内障儿童）的暴露率。因此，在病例对照研究中，如

child, it would then be necessary to ascertain whether or not the mother was exposed to rubella during her pregnancy with that child. We anticipate that if the exposure (rubella) is in fact related to the disease (cataracts), the prevalence of history of exposure among the cases — children with cataracts — will be greater than that among the controls — children with no cataracts. Thus, in a case-control study, if there is an association of an exposure with a disease, the prevalence of history of exposure should be higher in persons who have the disease (cases) than in those who do not (controls).The structural model shows in Figure 4-1.

果暴露与疾病有关，那么病例组的暴露率应该高于对照组的暴露率。病例对照研究的原理示意图见图4-1。

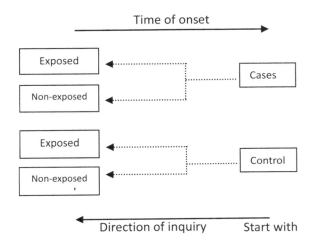

Figure 4-1　The schematic diagram of case control study

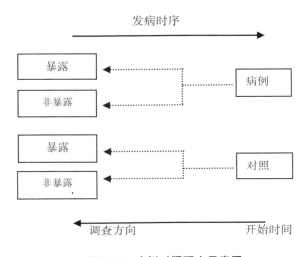

图 4-1　病例对照研究示意图

4.2　Types of Case-Control Studies

4.2.1　Cases does not match with the controls

Cases and controls were selected within a source population (according to the design), generally, the number of controls should be more than or equal to the number of cases. The choices of controls have no special provisions.

4.2　病例对照研究的类型

4.2.1　成组病例对照研究（病例与对照不匹配）

根据研究目的，在同一来源人群中分别选择病例组和对照组，一般对照组人数应多于或等于病例组人数。对照组的选择没有特殊规定。

4.2.2　Matching

A major concern in conducting a case - control study is that cases and controls may differ in characteristics or exposures other than the one that has been targeted for study. If more cases than controls are found to have been exposed, we may be left with the question of whether the observed association could be due to differences between the cases and controls in factors other than the exposure being studied. For example, if more cases than controls are found to have been exposed, and if most of the cases are poor and most of the controls are affluent, we would not know whether the factor determining development of disease is exposure to the factor being studied or another characteristic associated with being poor. To avoid such a situation, we would like to ensure that the distribution of the cases and controls by socioeconomic status is similar, so that a difference in exposure will likely constitute the critical difference, and the presence or absence of disease is not likely to be attributable to a difference in socioeconomic status.

One approach to dealing with this problem in the design and conduct of the study is to match the cases and controls for factors about which we may be concerned, such as income, as in the preceding example. Matching is defined as the process of selecting the controls so that they are similar to the cases in certain characteristics, such as age, race, sex, socioeconomic status, and occupation. Matching may be of two types: group matching and individual matching.

1. Group matching

Group matching (or frequency matching) consists of selecting the controls in such a manner that the

4.2.2　匹配病例对照研究

在进行病例对照研究时，主要关心的一个问题是非研究特征或暴露在病例组和对照组间是否存在差异。当病例组的暴露率高于对照组时，观察到的关联可能受到病例组和对照组非研究因素的差异影响。例如，病例组的暴露率高于对照组，同时大部分病例较贫穷，而对照组人群较富裕，则无法判断决定疾病发展的因素是所要研究的暴露因素还是与贫穷相关的特征。为了避免这种情况，就要确保病例组与对照组的社会经济状况可比，这时两组间主要的不同是暴露差异，疾病的发生就与社会经济状况无关。

处理这类问题的一种方法就是，在研究设计阶段和实施过程中将所担心的因素进行病例和对照的匹配，比如上例中的经济收入。匹配就是选择对照时，某些特征要与病例保持相似，例如，年龄、种族、性别、社会经济状况及职业。目的是两组进行比较时，可以排除匹配因素的干扰。匹配分为两种类型：成组匹配和个体匹配。

1.成组匹配

成组匹配（又称为频数匹配），即对照组在某一特征上的构成比例与病例组相似。例如，病例

proportion of controls with a certain characteristic is identical to the proportion of cases with the same characteristic. Thus, if 25% of cases are married, the controls will be selected so that 25% of that group is also married. This type of selection generally requires that all of the cases be selected first. After calculations are made of the proportions of certain characteristics in the group of cases, then a control group, in which the same characteristics occur in the same proportions, is selected.

2.Individual matching

A second type of matching is individual matching (or matched pairs). In this approach, for each case selected for the study, a control is selected who is similar to the case in terms of the specific variable or variables of concern. For example, if the first case enrolled in our study is a 45-year-old white woman, we will seek a 45-year-old white female control. If the second case is a 24-year-old black man, we will select a control who is also a 24-year-old black man. This type of control selection yields matched case-control pairs; that is, each case is individually matched to a control.

Continuous variables, such as age, are matched within a specified range. Sometimes this is done by grouping the variables; for example, age might be categorized into 5-year age groups and the control must be within the same 5-year age group as the case.

Individual matching is often used in case-control studies that use hospital controls. The reason for this is more practical than conceptual. Let us say that sex and age are considered important variables, and it is thought to be important that the cases and the controls be comparable in terms of these two characteristics. It is easier to identify a case and then to choose the next hospital admission that matches the case for sex and

组中有 25% 已婚，那么在选择对照组时已婚人士的占比也要控制在 25% 左右。这种类型的匹配通常要求先选择病例组。在计算好病例组某一特征的构成比例后，再按照该特征的比例选择对照组。

2. 个体匹配

个体匹配又称为配对。研究中每确定一个病例，即选择与病例在某些特征或变量上相似的对照。例如，如果第一个进入研究的病例是一位 45 岁的白人妇女，那么同样选择一位 45 岁的白人女性作为对照；如果第二个进入研究的病例是一位 24 岁的黑人男子，那么对照也要选择一位 24 岁的黑人男子。配对即病例和对照以个体为单位进行匹配，最终形成病例-对照的对子。

连续性变量（如年龄）要在特定范围内匹配，有时通过对变量进行分组来实现。例如，年龄按照每 5 岁为一个年龄段进行分组，那么对照必须和病例在同一个年龄段里面。

个体匹配在病例对照研究中较常使用，考虑到其可操作性（可行性），对照一般在医院中选择。通常，年龄和性别是重要的匹配变量，以保证两组间的可比性。首先确定病例，然后在入院患者中选择年龄、性别匹配的对照，这种操作相对简单。因此，以医院患者为基础来选择对照时，个体匹配是最可行的办法。

age. Thus individual matching is most expedient in studies using hospital controls.

（1）Advantage

①There is direct control of the confounders.

② Under certain conditions, matching improves the efficiency of the investigation.

（2）There are two issues to consider in matching

1）Practical problems with matching

If an attempt is made to match according to too many characteristics, it may prove difficult or impossible to identify an appropriate control. For example, suppose that it is decided to match each case for race, sex, age, marital status, number of children, zip code of residence, and occupation. If the case is a 48-year-old black woman who is married, has four children, lives in Zip code 21209, and works in a photo-processing plant, it may prove difficult or impossible to find a control who is similar to the case in all of these characteristics. Therefore, the more variables that we choose to match, the more difficult it will be to find a suitable control.

2）Conceptual problems with matching

Perhaps a more important problem is the conceptual one: Once we have matched controls to cases according to a given characteristic, we cannot study that characteristic. For example, suppose we are interested in studying marital status as a risk factor for breast cancer. If we match the cases（breast cancer）and the controls（no breast cancer）for marital status, we can no longer study whether or not marital status is a risk factor for breast cancer. Why not? Because in matching according to marital status we have artificially established an identical proportion in cases and controls. If 35% of the cases are married, and through matching we create a control group in which 35% are also mar-

（1）匹配的优点

①控制混杂因素。

②提高检验效能。

（2）匹配需要考虑的两个问题

1）可行性问题

如果匹配的因素过多，合适对照的选择就会很困难。例如，假设要对种族、性别、年龄、婚姻状况、子女人数、住宅邮编和职业等因素进行匹配。如果有一个病例是48岁的黑人、已婚妇女、有四个孩子、住宅邮编为21209、在相片处理厂工作，那么很难匹配同时符合以上特征或类似的对照。因此，匹配的因素越多，合适的对照就越不好找。也就是说，匹配因素过多，容易造成过度匹配。

2）理论性问题

理论性问题可能更重要，一旦设定某因素为匹配因素，就不能再研究它与疾病的关系。例如，假设婚姻状况是乳腺癌的危险因素，如果根据婚姻状况进行病例（乳腺癌患者）和对照（非乳腺癌患者）的匹配，就无法进一步研究婚姻状况是否为乳腺癌的一个危险因素。因为，匹配后病例组和对照组的婚姻状况构成比例无差异。如果病例组有35%的已婚人士，匹配人为地使已婚对象的比例在两组中是相同的，对照组同样有35%的已婚人士。通过匹配使病例和对照在某一因素上的相似性加强，确保了该因素的构成情况在病例组和对照组中的一致。很明显，该因素在病例组和对照组中的构成不可能存在差异。因此，在本

ried, we have artificially ensured that the proportion of married subjects will be identical in both groups. By using matching to impose comparability for a certain factor, we ensure the same prevalence of that factor in the cases and the controls. Clearly, we will not be able to ask whether cases differ from controls in the prevalence of that factor. We would therefore not want to match on the variable of marital status in this study. Indeed, we do not want to match on any variable that we may wish to explore in our study.

It is also important to recognize that unplanned matching may inadvertently occur in case - control studies. For example, if we use neighborhood controls, we are in effect matching for socioeconomic status as well as for cultural and other characteristics of a neighborhood. If we use best-friend controls, it is likely that the case and his or her best friend share many lifestyle characteristics, which in effect produces a match for these characteristics. For example, in a study of oral contraceptive use and cancer in which best-friend controls were considered, there was concern that if the case used oral contraceptives it might well be that her best friend would also be likely to be an oral contraceptive user. The result would be an unplanned matching on oral contraceptive use, so that this variable could no longer be investigated in this study.

In carrying out a case - control study, therefore, we only match on variables that we are convinced are risk factors for the disease, which we are therefore not interested in investigating in this study. Matching on variables other than these, in either a planned or inadvertent manner, is called overmatching. Common matching variables are age and sex.

研究中不应该匹配婚姻状况。也就是说，研究因素均不应该进行匹配。

没有计划的无意匹配在病例对照研究中也需要重视。当以邻居为对照时，也可能无意间对社会经济状况、文化以及其他特征进行了匹配；当以好友为对照时，因为病例和其好朋友很可能有很多类似的生活方式，所以实际上也对这些特征进行了匹配。例如，在研究口服避孕药与癌症的关系时，以病例的好朋友为对照，如果病例使用口服避孕药，她的好朋友也可能使用口服避孕药，这会导致口服避孕药使用的无意匹配，从而无法分析口服避孕药与癌症的关系。

因此，在病例对照研究中，应匹配那些已经确定的危险因素，且这些因素不是要研究的因素。超过此范围，不论是计划内的，还是无意的匹配，都称为过度匹配。常见的匹配因素为年龄和性别。

4.2.3　Variants of the case-control design

1. Nested case-control studies

Epidemiologists sometimes refer to specific case-control studies as nested case-control studies when the population within which the study is conducted a fully enumerated cohort, which allows formal random sampling of cases and controls to be carried out. The term is usually used in reference to a case-control study conducted within a cohort study, in which further information (perhaps from expensive tests) is obtained on most or all cases, but for economy is obtained from only a fraction of the remaining cohort members (the controls often matched to cases). Nonetheless, many population—based case-control studies can be thought of as nested within an enumerated source population. Simply, taking a cohort study that has run for some time, the cases are identified as those in the cohort study who have developed the disease of interest. For each case, a random selection of corresponding controls is drawn from amongst all these in the cohort who have not experienced the disease at the time when the case gets the disease. These controls may get the disease later and may also act as controls for other cases. The great advantage of a nested study, over a standard case-control design, is that cases and controls come from the same population, reducing the issues of selection bias and recall bias. Relative to the parent cohort study, and assuming the disease under study is rare, nested case-control studies save numbers and time, and expense.

2. Case-cohort studies

A case-cohort study is, like the nested case-control study, set within a parent cohort study both de-

4.2.3　衍生的病例对照研究类型

1. 巢式病例对照研究

巢式病例对照研究是一种特殊的病例对照研究，是在一个事先确定好的队列人群进行随访的基础上，随机选择病例和对照，即在队列研究中开展病例对照研究。大部分或全部患者作为病例组。从经济角度考虑，仅以小部分非患者为对照（通常要与病例匹配），然后进一步收集信息（包括实验室检测信息）。很多基于人群的病例对照研究都可被认为是嵌入源人群的研究。简单地讲，就是在一个已经随访了一段时间的队列中，以其中发生所研究疾病的人为病例组，从队列中随机选择与每个病例对应的未发生该病的人作为对照。这些对照未来可能发生该病，也可以作为其他疾病研究的对照。相对于传统的病例对照研究而言，巢氏病例对照研究最大的优势就是病例和对照来于同一人群，可以减少选择偏倚和回忆偏倚。相对于队列研究而言，巢氏病例对照研究在研究罕见病时所需的样本相对较小，也比较省时和节约经费。

2. 病例队列研究

病例队列研究与巢氏病例对照研究类似，都是在一个队列研究的基础上开展的研究。其设计

signs take the cases identified from the cohort study in the same way, but the case-cohort study, rather than adding matched controls, adds a random subset of the initial cohort, called the subcohort. No matching is involved. The case-cohort study is a case-control study in which the source population is a cohort and (within sampling or matching strata) every person in this cohort has an equal chance of being included in the study as a control, regardless of how much time that person has contributed to the person-time experience of the cohort or whether the person developed the study disease. As like is common in prenatal studies. An advantage of the case-cohort design is that it facilitates conduct of a set of case-control studies from a single cohort, all of which use the same control group. As a sample from the cohort at enrollment, the control group can be compared with any number of case groups. One disadvantage is that, because of the overlap of membership in the case and control groups (controls who are selected may also develop disease and enter the study as cases), one will need to select more controls in a case-cohort study than in an ordinary case-control study with the same number of cases, if one is to achieve the same amount of statistical precision. Extra controls are needed because the statistical precision of a study is strongly determined by the numbers of distinct cases and non-cases.

3.Case-only studies

There are a number of situations in which cases are the only subjects used to estimate or test hypotheses about effects. For example, it is sometimes possible to employ theoretical considerations to construct a prior distribution of exposure in the source population and use this distribution in place of an observed control series. Such situations arise naturally in genetic

和病例的确定与巢氏病例对照研究相同，不同的是，它不是通过匹配确定对照，而是在队列中随机选择一个亚队列作为对照，即病例对列研究的源人群是一个队列人群，该源人群中（抽样或匹配阶段）每名研究对象都有均等的机会进入对照组，无论研究对象进入队列的时间长或短，也无论其是否已经发展为目标疾病。也就是说，病例队列研究的基本设计是在队列的研究开始时，在队列中按一定比例随机抽样选出一个有代表性的样本（子队列）作为对照组，观察结束时，队列中出现的所有病例作为病例组。病例队列研究常用于围产期研究。病例队列研究的优点是，在一个队列研究中，一个随机对照可以同时和几个病例组比较。缺点是，因为病例和对照有一部分重叠（对照组研究对象也有可能发生目标疾病而进入病例组），所以对于相同数量的病例，病例队列研究需要比一般病例对照研究更多的对照才能获得相同的统计效率（因为统计效率由病例组和对照组的例数决定）。

3.病例—病例研究

在许多情况下，只使用病例估计或检验效应假设。例如，在患有某病的源人群中，根据某暴露因素的分布，部分有该暴露的患者为病例组，没有该暴露的为对照组。该方法常用于基因相关研究，也可以用于研究基因与环境的交互作用。

studies. It is also possible to study certain aspects of joint effects (interactions) of genetic and environmental factors without using control subjects.

4. Case-crossover studies

Sometimes the risk factor of interest is transient but repeatable. For such risk factors, a special type of matched study can be very useful—the case-crossover study, in which each case acts as her or his own control. The case-crossover study is a case-control analog of the crossover study (Maclure, 1991). For each case, one or more pre-disease or post-disease time periods are selected as matched "control" periods for the case. The exposure status of the case at the time of the disease onset is compared with the distribution of exposure status for that same person in the control periods. Such a comparison depends on the assumption that neither exposure nor confounders are changing over time in a systematic way.

4.3　Design and Implementation

4.3.1　General steps

① Put forward the hypothesis of etiology.
② Develop a plan of study.
③ Collect of data.
④ Sorting and analyzing the collected data.
⑤ Summarize and submit the report.

4.3.2　Specific implementation

1. Put forward the hypothesis

According to the understanding of the distribution of the disease and known related factors to put forward the hypothesis.

4.病例交叉研究

有时，要研究的危险因素是短暂暴露且可重复暴露。这种情况下，有一种特殊的配对研究有助于开展研究，即病例交叉研究，这是一种以病例自身为对照的研究。1991年，Maclure提出了这种模拟交叉研究的病例对照研究，即病例交叉研究。以每一病例病前或病后的一个或多个时期作为对照时期，将发病时的暴露状态与自身对照时期暴露的分布情况相比较，这种比较是基于暴露和混杂因素都不随着时间而变化的假设。

4.3　研究设计与实施

4.3.1　一般步骤

①提出病因假说。
②制定研究计划。
③收集数据。
④对收集的数据进行整理和分析。
⑤总结并提交报告。

4.3.2　具体实施

1.提出假设

根据对疾病分布和已知相关因素的了解提出假设。

2. Clear and definite the purposes of research

3. Selection of cases and controls

（1）Selection of cases

1）Definition

Before cases can be selected, a precise definition of disease to be studies must be formulated. If this is not precise, there will be a danger of misclassification of potential cases and controls. If the definition is too broad, then the case-control study may be futile. For instance, the definition "mental illness" will encompass a range of condition with very different aetiology. Even if certain clinical conditions are strongly associated with specific risk factors, the complete set of cases may have no, or only a minimal, excess of these risk factors compared with controls.

2）Diagnostic criteria

The diagnostic criteria of the disease and the stage of disease any（e. g, breast cancer Stage Ⅰ）to be included in the study must be specified before the study is undertaken. Supposing we are investigating cases of cancer, we should be quite clear that our cases group have the same histology. Once the diagnostic criteria are established, they should not be altered or changed till the study is over.

3）Inclusion and exclusion criteria

Sometimes subjects with the disease are considered eligible to be cases only if they satisfy certain inclusion and exclusion criteria. These may be chosen so as to improve the validity of the study—for example, when subjects with co-existing diseases or well-established risk factors are excluded. Some restrictions on time and place are, in any case, necessary for practical reasons in all case-control studies.

2. 明确研究目的

3. 选择病例和对照

（1）病例的选择

1）定义

在选择病例之前，所研究的疾病必须有精确的定义，否则病例和对照会出现错分。如果疾病定义太广，病例对照研究就可能是徒劳的。例如，"精神病"的定义包含一系列不同病因引起的健康状况。即使某些危险因素与某种临床状况相关性很强，但与对照组相比，病例组也可能没有或仅有很小的超额风险。

2）诊断标准

在研究开始之前，必须明确疾病的诊断标准和疾病分期（例如：乳腺癌Ⅰ期）。假设研究对象是癌症患者，那么这些病例在组织学上应该有相同表现。诊断标准一旦确定，在研究结束之前，就不应改变或变更诊断标准。

3）纳入和排除标准

有时，患有研究疾病的研究对象需要满足某些纳入和排除标准后才能被认为是合格的病例。这样的选择有利于提高研究的准确度。例如，排除有共存疾病或已知危险因素的研究对象。在病例对照研究中，从可行性角度对研究对象进行时间和空间的限制也是必要的。

Sometimes diseased people are excluded from the case series because they have no, or very little, chance of exposure to the risk factors. Thus, in a study of oral contraceptives as risk factors for breast cancer, we should exclude postmenopausal women; including them would be a waste of resources. Exclusions on grounds of efficiency often utilize age and sex criteria.

4）Incident or prevalent

Incident disease is a better criterion for case selection. Prevalent cases introduce a greater element of ambiguity in the time sequence. For instance, alcohol consumption may be associated with the absence of diabetes simply because many of those with diabetes have been told to stop drinking by their doctor.

The great advantage with prevalent cases is their ready availability in large numbers for certain conditions. This would represent a distinct saving in time and effort when studying a rare, but nonfatal, chronic condition. When prevalent cases are used, steps should be taken to minimize the chance of error; for example, lifetime histories of exposures might be sought.

5）Source

Cases are usually selected from medical information systems. The most common source is hospital admission records, but operating theatre or pathology department records, sickness absence forms and disease registers are other potential source.

（2）Selection of controls

The definition of the source population determines the population from which controls are sampled. Ideally, selection will involve direct sampling of controls from the source population.

1）Three basic rules for choosing controls

①Controls should be drawn from those who are free of the disease being studied. Usually, we should

有时患者因为没有或有非常少的机会暴露于危险因素而被从病例中排除。因此，在口服避孕药与乳腺癌关系的研究中，应该排除绝经妇女，否则是资源的浪费。为了提高研究效率，通常将年龄和性别作为排除标准中的选项，即育龄妇女是合适的研究对象。

4）新发病例还是现患病例的选择

选择病例时，新发病例是更好的选择，因为现患病例的暴露时间无法准确判断。例如，饮酒可能是糖尿病的保护因素，仅仅因为大部分糖尿病患者都被大夫告知要戒酒。

现患病例最大的优点是有大量的可用病例，在研究非致命性的、罕见的慢性病时，可以节省大量的时间和精力。当使用现患病例时，应该采取减少误差（回忆偏倚）的措施，例如，可以探寻既往暴露史。

5）病例来源

病例一般从医院信息系统中选取。最常用的资源是住院记录、手术室记录、病理科记录或疾病登记等其他潜在的资源。

（2）对照的选择

源人群的定义决定了抽取对照的人群，理想的对照应直接从源人群中抽取。

1）选择对照的三个基本原则

①对照应该从未患研究疾病的人群中选取。以前患有研究疾病现在已治愈者，通常也排除在

exempt anyone who, although disease free now, has had the disease in the past.

②Controls should be from the same population - the source population—that gives rise to the study cases. If this rule cannot be followed, there needs to be solid evidence that the population supplying controls has an exposure distribution identical to that of the population that is the source of cases, which is a very stringent demand that is rarely demonstrable.

③ Controls should have some potential for the disease. For instance, women who have had their womb removed should not be considered as controls in a study of endometrial cancer. If they were, some of those without a womb but with the risk factor would be expected to have become cases if they had retained their womb. Consequently, the comparison between cases and controls would underestimate the effect of the risk factor, assuming that no equal (for greater) bias is associated with the cases.

2）Sources for control series

The controls must be free from the disease under study. They must be as similar to the cases as possible, except for the absence of the disease under study. As a rule, comparison group is identified before a study is done comprising of persons who have not been exposed to the disease or some other factor whose influence is being studied. Difficulties may arise in the selection of controls the disease under investigation occurs in subclinical form whose diagnosis is difficult. Selection of an appropriate control group is therefore an important prerequisite, for it is against this, we make comparisons, draw inferences and make judgements about the outcome of the investigation.

① Hospitals controls. Hospitals are convenient and cheap source of controls, especially in situations

外。

②对照应当来自病例来源的人群，即与病例是同一个源人群。如果不能满足这个原则，则需要有确凿的证据证明产生对照的人群与病例来源的人群其暴露分布是相同的，以保证比较的两组具有可比性。这是十分必要的，但一般很难论证。

③对照应该有患病的可能。例如，子宫切除的妇女不能作为子宫内膜癌研究的对照人群。这些子宫切除而又有子宫内膜癌危险因素的妇女，如果不切除子宫，可能会成为病例。假设选择子宫切除的妇女作对照，那么其与病例存在不可比的偏倚，会导致子宫内膜癌危险因素的作用被低估。

2）对照的来源

对照组不得患有所研究的疾病。对照组除了不患有所研究的疾病外，其他特征应与病例相似。一般来说，在研究之前，首先将未患有所研究疾病的人群定义为对照组。如果研究的疾病处于亚临床阶段，其诊断困难，对照的选择也困难。因此，合适的对照是开展病例对照研究的重要前提，通过与病例组比较，进行推论，并对调查结果作出判断。

①医院来源的对照。医院是方便、廉价的对照来源，尤其在需要收集一些与疾病相关的血样

when a clinical procedure, such as a blood sample, is required to measure the risk factor. They have the advantage that their medical data are likely to be of comparable quality to those from the case and may have been collected prior to classification as controls (removing the possibility of observer bias). There is a good chance that their quality of recall will also be similar to that for cases (reducing the chance of anamnestic bias) because they are in the same environment. As with the cases, they are likely to be thinking about the antecedents of their illness and they are to be co-operative, especially because they have time to spare. One disadvantage is that the risk factor for the study disease may also be a risk factor for the condition that a particular control has, which is the cause of her or his hospitalization. To reduce such problems, it is best to choose controls from a range of conditions, exempting any disease that is likely to be related to exposure.

② Community controls. Controls drawn from the community have the great advantage of being drawn directly from the true population of those without the disease. The disadvantages with random community controls are that they are inconvenient to capture and their data are often of inferior quality. Locating and visiting a random selection of controls at home may be expensive and time consuming.

③ Other sources. Other sources for controls are medical systems other than hospitals and special groups in the community who have some relation to the cases (such as friends, neighbours and relatives).

4. Size of sample

(1) The influencing factors of sample size

① The exposure rate of study factor in controls (p_0).

② Relative risk (RR) or odds ratio (OR).

③ The significance level of test, the probability

检测指标时。医院来源的对照有一个优点，即与病例的医学数据质量相当，且在归类为对照前就已经收集了（避免观察者偏倚）。病例和对照在相同环境下，回忆信息的质量也相同（减少了歧视性偏倚）。医院来源的对照配合度较好，时间也相对充裕，愿意回忆患病的经历。缺点为所研究疾病的危险因素可能也是导致对照入院的原因。解决这个问题的方法就是，选择的对照不应该具有与暴露有关的任何疾病。

②社区来源的对照。社区来源的对照最大的优点是，对照直接来自未患目标疾病的全人群，选择偏倚较小；缺点是，随机选择的社区对照不易获取，且数据质量较低。若对随机抽样获得的对照进行入户调查，则要耗费较多财力和时间，且这些对照也不易配合。

③其他来源的对照。其他来源如除医院以外的其他医疗系统、社区中与病例相关的特殊群体（例如，朋友、邻居和亲戚等）。

4. 确定样本量

（1）影响样本量的因素

①对照组的暴露率p_0。

②相对危险度RR或暴露的比值比OR。

③显著性水平，即Ⅰ类错误的概率α。

of Error type Ⅰ in hypothesis testing (α).

④ The power of test ($1-\beta$), β is the probability of Error type Ⅱ in hypothesis testing.

（2）Method of estimation

Methods of calculate the sample size change with the way of matching, we could use the formulas, also use the ready-made tables. Pay attention:

① The estimated sample size is not absolutely precise value.

② We should correct errors in thinking that bigger sample size is better.

③ In the condition of the total sample size unchanged, the statistical efficiency is highest when the sample size of cases is equal to the controls.

（3）Non-matching design and the sample size of cases is equal to the controls

$$n = 2\bar{p}\bar{q}(z_\alpha + z_\beta)^2/(p_1 - p_0)^2 \qquad (4-1)$$

$$p_1 = \frac{p_0 RR}{1 + p_0(RR - 1)}, \ \bar{p} = 0.5 \times (p_1 + p_0),$$

$$\bar{q} = 1 - \bar{p}$$

In the formula, p_1 is the exposure rate in cases, p_0 is the exposure rate in controls, z_α and z_β could get by checking Table 4-1, or get by checking Table 4-2 directly.

Table 4-1　Quantile table of standard normal distribution

α or β	z_α (one-tailed test) z_β (one-tailed and two-tailed)	z_α (two-tailed test)
0.001	3.09	3.29
0.005	2.58	2.81
0.010	2.33	2.58
0.025	1.96	2.24
0.050	1.64	1.96
0.100	1.28	1.64
0.200	0.84	1.28
0.300	0.52	1.04

④把握度（$1-\beta$），β为Ⅱ类错误的概率。

（2）估算方法

根据是否匹配，样本量计算公式有所不同。另外，还可以利用查表法得到样本量。需要注意的是：

①所估计的样本量并非绝对精确的数值，因为样本量的估计是有条件的，而这些条件并非一成不变的。

②应当纠正样本量越大越好的这种错误看法。样本量过大，常会影响调查工作的质量，增加负担、费用。

③总的样本量相同的情况下，病例组和对照组样本量相等时统计学效率最高。

（3）病例数与对照数相等的非匹配设计

$$n = 2\bar{p}\bar{q}(z_\alpha + z_\beta)^2/(p_1 - p_0)^2 \qquad (4-1)$$

$$p_1 = \frac{p_0 RR}{1 + p_0(RR - 1)}, \ \bar{p} = 0.5 \times (p_1 + p_0),$$

$$\bar{q} = 1 - \bar{p}$$

式中，p_1为病例组的暴露率，p_0为对照组的暴露率，z_α和z_β可查表4-1得到，也可直接查表4-2得到。

表4-1　标准正态分布的分位数表

α 或 β	z_α（单侧检验） z_β（单侧和双侧）	z_α（双侧检验）
0.001	3.09	3.29
0.005	2.58	2.81
0.010	2.33	2.58
0.025	1.96	2.24
0.050	1.64	1.96
0.100	1.28	1.64
0.200	0.84	1.28
0.300	0.52	1.04

Table 4-2 Sample size of case-control study

(Non-matching, sample sizes are same in cases and controls)

[$\alpha=0.05$ (two-tailed), $\beta=0.10$]

RR	p_0						
	0.01	0.10	0.20	0.40	0.60	0.80	0.90
0.1	1 420	137	66	31	20	18	23
0.5	6 323	658	347	203	176	229	378
2.0	3 206	378	229	176	203	347	658
3.0	1 074	133	85	71	89	163	319
4.0	599	77	51	46	61	117	232
5.0	406	54	37	35	48	96	194
10.0	150	23	18	20	31	66	137
20.0	66	12	11	14	24	54	115

(Schlesselman, 1982)

(4) Non-matching design and the sample size of cases is not equal to the controls

Hypothesis number of cases: number of controls = $1:c$, so the number of case is n.

$$n = (1 + 1/c)\bar{p}\bar{q}(z_\alpha + z_\beta)^2/(p_1 - p_0)^2 \qquad (4-2)$$
$$\bar{p} = (p_1 + cp_0)/(1 + c)$$
$$\bar{q} = 1 - \bar{p}$$

In the formula, p_1 is same with formula 4-1, the number of controls = $c \times n$.

(5) 1:1 matched design

Pairs is meaningful for the analysis when the status of exposure in case is different with control.

Formula recommended by Schlesselman:

$$m = \left[z_\alpha/2 + z_\beta \sqrt{p(1-p)} \right]^2/(p - 1/2)^2 \qquad (4-3)$$
$$p = OR/(1 + OR) \approx RR/(1 + RR) \qquad (4-4)$$

m is the number of pairs that the status of exposure in case is different with control. So the total numbers of pairs are:

$$M \approx m/(p_0q_1 + p_1q_0) \qquad (4-5)$$

In the formula p_1 is the exposure rate in cases, p_0 is the exposure rate in controls.

表4-2 病例对照研究样本量(非匹配、两组人数相等)

[$\alpha=0.05$(双侧), $\beta=0.10$]

RR	p_0						
	0.01	0.10	0.20	0.40	0.60	0.80	0.90
0.1	1 420	137	66	31	20	18	23
0.5	6 323	658	347	203	176	229	378
2.0	3 206	378	229	176	203	347	658
3.0	1 074	133	85	71	89	163	319
4.0	599	77	51	46	61	117	232
5.0	406	54	37	35	48	96	194
10.0	150	23	18	20	31	66	137
20.0	66	12	11	14	24	54	115

(Schlesselman, 1982)

(4) 病例数与对照数不等的非匹配设计

设病例数:对照数 = $1:c$, 则需要的病例数为 n。

$$n = (1 + 1/c)\bar{p}\bar{q}(z_\alpha + z_\beta)^2/(p_1 - p_0)^2 \qquad (4-2)$$
其中:$\bar{p} = (p_1 + cp_0)/(1 + c)$
$$\bar{q} = 1 - \bar{p}$$

式中,p_1的计算同公式4-1;对照数 = $c \times n$。

(5) 1:1匹配设计

分析病例与对照暴露状况不一致的对子数对于所研究的问题才有意义。Schlesselman推荐的公式如下:

$$m = \left[z_\alpha/2 + z_\beta \sqrt{p(1-p)} \right]^2/(p - 1/2)^2 \qquad (4-3)$$
$$p = OR/(1 + OR) \approx RR/(1 + RR) \qquad (4-4)$$

其中,m为暴露状况不一致的对子数。因此,总对子数M为:

$$M \approx m/(p_0q_1 + p_1q_0) \qquad (4-5)$$

p_0和p_1分别代表对照组与病例组的估计暴露率:

$$p_1 = p_0 RR/\left[1 + p_0(RR - 1)\right]$$

$$q_1 = 1 - p_1$$

$$q_0 = 1 - p_0$$

（6）1 : r matched design

The number of case:

$$n =$$

$$\frac{\left[z_\alpha \sqrt{(1 + 1/r)\bar{p}(1 - \bar{p})} + z_\beta \sqrt{p_1(1 - p_1)/r + p_0(1 - p_0)}\right]^2}{(p_1 - p_0)^2}$$

$$(4\text{-}6)$$

$$p_1 = (OR \times p_0)/(1 - p_0 + OR \times p_0)$$

$$\bar{p} = (p_1 + rp_0)/(1 + r)$$

The number of controls = $r \times n$.

5. Get the information of factors

The information to be collected in the study include research of factors, suspicious factors and confounding factors. The cases and controls should be using the same questionnaire and asking the same questions.

（1）The selection of variables

Variables related to the purpose are absolutely essential. Variables independent of the purpose needn't to be selected.

（2）The definition of variable

Each variable should have a clear definition and take international or national uniform standards as much as possible.

（3）The measurement of variables

We should use the quantitative or semi-quantitative determination in study as far as possible.

6. Data collection

In case-control studies information collected mainly by asking respondents and filling in the questionnaire, sometimes need to be supplemented by checking back files or getting from the related filed. No matter what method is used, we should implement the quality control for ensuring the quality of investigations.

$$p_1 = p_0 RR/\left[1 + p_0(RR - 1)\right]$$

$$q_1 = 1 - p_1$$

$$q_0 = 1 - p_0$$

（6）　1 : r 匹配设计

病例数：

$$n =$$

$$\frac{\left[z_\alpha \sqrt{(1 + 1/r)\bar{p}(1 - \bar{p})} + z_\beta \sqrt{p_1(1 - p_1)/r + p_0(1 - p_0)}\right]^2}{(p_1 - p_0)^2}$$

$$(4\text{-}6)$$

其中，$p_1 = (OR \times p_0)/(1 - p_0 + OR \times p_0)$

$$\bar{p} = (p_1 + rp_0)/(1 + r)$$

对照数=$r \times n$

5. 获取研究因素的信息

研究中需要收集的信息包括研究因素、可疑因素和混杂因素等。病例组与对照组的资料来源及收集方法应一致，并应使用相同的调查表。

（1）因素的选择

因素的选择与研究目的相关，与研究目的相关的因素必须选择，不相关的因素不选择，应尽可能选择客观、可测量的因素。

（2）因素的定义

每个因素都应有明确的定义，并应尽可能使用国际或国内统一的标准。

（3）因素的测量

在研究中，应尽可能地采用定量或半定量方法进行测定。

6. 资料的收集

病例对照研究中信息的收集主要通过询问调查对象并填写问卷获得，有时还通过查阅档案、采样化验、实地察看或从有关方面咨询获得。无论采用什么方法，都应实行质量控制，以保证调查质量。

4.4 Data Collection and Analysis

4.4.1 Evaluating sources

① Verification of the original data.

② Entry of the original data.

4.4.2 Data analysis

1. Descriptive Statistics

① Describes the general characteristics of research objects.

② Balance test.

2. Statistical inference

The indicator shows the strength of the association between disease and exposure in case - control studies caller odds ratio (OR). The odds in favor of an event or a proposition are the ratio of the probability that the event will happen to the probability that the event will not happen. The OR represents the odds that an outcome will occur given a particular exposure, compared to the odds of the outcome occurring in the absence of that exposure. $OR=1$ exposure does not affect odds of outcome; $OR>1$ exposure associated with higher odds of outcome; $OR<1$ exposure associated with lower odds of outcome.

Table 4-3　Display of data from a case-control study

Risk factor status	Disease status		Total
	Disease (cases)	No disease (controls)	
Exposed	a	b	$a+b=n_1$
Not exposed	c	d	$c+d=n_0$
Total	$a+c=m_1$	$b+d=m_0$	$a+b+c+d=t$

4.4 资料的整理与分析

4.4.1 资料的整理

①原始资料的核查。

②原始资料的录入。

4.4.2 资料的分析

1. 描述性统计

①描述研究对象的一般特征。

②均衡性检验。

2. 统计推断

病例对照研究中，表示疾病与暴露之间关联强度的指标为比值比（OR）。所谓比值（odds），是指某事物发生的可能性与不发生的可能性之比。OR表示特定暴露者的疾病风险为非暴露者的多少倍。$OR=1$，说明疾病的风险不会因暴露而增加或减少；$OR>1$，说明疾病的风险会因暴露而增加；$OR<1$，说明疾病的风险会因暴露而减少。

表4-3　病例对照研究资料整理表

暴露或特征	疾病		合 计
	病例	对照	
有	a	b	$a+b=n_1$
无	c	d	$c+d=n_0$
合计	$a+c=m_1$	$b+d=m_0$	$a+b+c+d=t$

According to Table 4-3, the exposure ratios of cases in case-control study is:

$$\frac{a/(a + c)}{c/(a + c)} = a/c \qquad (4-7)$$

The exposure ratios of controls in case-control study is:

$$\frac{b/(b + d)}{d/(b + d)} = b/d \qquad (4-8)$$

Odds Ratio(OR) =

$$\frac{\text{Exposure ratios of cases}(a/c)}{\text{Exposure ratios of controls}(b/d)} \qquad (4-9)$$

Neither the incidence nor the relative risk could be calculated in case-control studies, and we could only use the OR to reflect the strength of association.

The OR at different prevalence and RR is shown in Table 4-4. The RR at different incidence and OR is shown in Table 4-5.

根据表4-3，病例对照研究中病例组的暴露比为：

$$\frac{a/(a + c)}{c/(a + c)} = a/c \qquad (4-7)$$

对照组的暴露比为：

$$\frac{b/(b + d)}{d/(b + d)} = b/d \qquad (4-8)$$

$$比值比(OR) = \frac{病例组的暴露比(a/c)}{对照组的暴露比(b/d)}$$

$$(4-9)$$

病例对照研究既不能用来计算发病率，也不能用来计算相对危险度，只能使用OR来反映关联强度。

不同患病率和RR时的OR见表4-4，不同发病率和OR时的RR见表4-5。

Table 4-4　The OR at different prevalence and RR

Prevalence in no ex-posed groups/%	RR				
	1.5	2.0	3.0	4.0	5.0
0.1	0.1	0.1	0.2	0.3	0.4
0.5	0.3	0.5	1.0	1.5	2.1
1.0	0.5	1.0	2.1	3.1	4.2
5.0	2.7	5.6	11.8	18.8	26.7
10.0	5.9	12.5	28.6	50.0	80.0

表4-4　不同患病率和RR时的OR

非暴露组患病率/%	RR				
	1.5	2.0	3.0	4.0	5.0
0.1	0.1	0.1	0.2	0.3	0.4
0.5	0.3	0.5	1.0	1.5	2.1
1.0	0.5	1.0	2.1	3.1	4.2
5.0	2.7	5.6	11.8	18.8	26.7
10.0	5.9	12.5	28.6	50.0	80.0

Table 4-5　The RR at different incidence and OR

OR	The incidence in no exposed groups (I_0)			
	0.20	0.10	0.05	0.01
2	1.7	1.8	1.9	2.0
3	2.1	2.5	2.7	2.9
4	2.5	3.1	3.5	3.0
5	2.8	3.6	4.2	4.8
6	3.0	4.0	4.8	5.7
7	3.2	4.4	5.4	6.6
8	3.3	4.7	5.9	7.5
9	3.5	5.0	6.4	8.3
10	3.6	5.3	6.9	9.2

表4-5　不同发病率和OR时的RR

OR	非暴露组发病率(I_0)			
	0.20	0.10	0.05	0.01
2	1.7	1.8	1.9	2.0
3	2.1	2.5	2.7	2.9
4	2.5	3.1	3.5	3.0
5	2.8	3.6	4.2	4.8
6	3.0	4.0	4.8	5.7
7	3.2	4.4	5.4	6.6
8	3.3	4.7	5.9	7.5
9	3.5	5.0	6.4	8.3
10	3.6	5.3	6.9	9.2

3.Non-matched and non-hierarchical data

This is the basic form of data analysis in case-control studies.

（1）Each exposure could be organized a four fold table (Table 4-3)

For example, a case-control study of oral contraceptives （OC） as a risk factors for myocardial infarction （MI）, the result shows in Table 4-6.

Table 4-6　Case-control study of the relationship between OC and MI

The status of OC	Cases	Controls	Total
Yes	39	24	63
No	114	154	268
Total	153	178	331

（2）Chi-square test （χ^2 test）

$$\chi^2 = \frac{(ad - bc)^2 n}{(a + b)(c + d)(a + c)(b + d)} = 7.70$$

$\chi^2_{0.01(1)}$ =6.63, in this study, χ^2=7.70 > 6.63, P< 0.01.

Conclusion: There was a statistical difference in exposure rate between two groups.

（3）Calculate the OR

$OR = ad/bc = 2.20$

（4）Woolf's logit approximation

$$Z = \frac{\ln OR}{\sqrt{1/a + 1/b + 1/c + 1/d}} \quad (4-10)$$

$Z > 1.96$, $P < 0.05$; $Z > 2.58$, $P < 0.01$; $Z > 3.08$, $P < 0.001$. In this study, Z=0.788 5/0.287 4=2.74 > 2.58, so $P < 0.01$. In theory, the conclusion of this test should be same with the Chi-square test.

（5）Calculate the confidence interval （CI） of OR

1）Woolf natural logarithm transformation method

$Var(\ln OR) = 1/a + 1/b + 1/c + 1/d = 0.082\ 6$

$\ln OR\ 95\%CI = \ln OR \pm 1.96 \times \sqrt{Var(\ln OR)} =$

3. 不匹配不分层资料

这是病例对照研究资料分析的基本形式。

（1）整理表格

每个暴露因素都可整理成表4-3所示的形式。

例如，有一项关于口服避孕药与心肌梗死关系的病例对照研究，结果如表4-6所示。

表4-6　口服避孕药(OC)与心肌梗死(MI)关系的病例对照研究结果

是否服药	病例	对照	合计
服药	39	24	63
未服药	114	154	268
合计	153	178	331

（2）卡方 （χ^2） 检验

$$\chi^2 = \frac{(ad - bc)^2 n}{(a + b)(c + d)(a + c)(b + d)} = 7.70$$

已知 $\chi^2_{0.01\ (1)}$ =6.63，本例中 χ^2=7.70 > 6.63，则 P<0.01。

结论：拒绝无效假设，即两组暴露率的差异有统计学意义。

（3）计算暴露与疾病的联系强度 OR

$OR = ad/bc = 2.20$

（4）Woolf对数近似法

$$Z = \frac{\ln OR}{\sqrt{1/a + 1/b + 1/c + 1/d}} \quad (4-10)$$

Z>1.96时，P<0.05；Z>2.58时，$P < 0.01$；Z >3.08时，P<0.001。本例中，Z=0.788 5/0.287 4=2.74 >2.58，则P<0.01。理论上，该检验应当与χ^2检验的结论一致。

（5）计算OR的可信区间 （confidence interval, CI）

1）Woolf自然对数转换法

$Var(\ln OR) = 1/a + 1/b + 1/c + 1/d = 0.082\ 6$

$\ln OR\ 95\%CI = \ln OR \pm 1.96 \times \sqrt{Var(\ln OR)} =$

ln2.2 ± 1.96 × 0.2874 = (0.2252, 1.3218)

Calculate the natural logarithm of above values, exp(0.2252)=1.25, exp(1.3218)=3.75, so the 95% CI of OR is (1.25, 3.75).

2）Miettnen Chi-square method

$OR\,95\%\,\mathrm{CI} = OR^{(1\pm1.96/\sqrt{\chi^2})} = 2.2^{(1\pm1.96/\sqrt{7.7})} =$ (1.26, 3.84)

4. Non-matched and hierarchical data

Stratification analysis is according to certain characteristics or factors of study population, and dividing them into different layers, such as by gender the population can be divided into two layers of men and women, and by age the population can be divided into three layers of 20-39 years old, 40-59 years old, aged 60 and above, then analyzing the association between exposure and disease in each layer. A layered factor is may be a confounding factor, we could use stratification analysis to control the confounding.

（1）Sorting the hierarchical data

Sorting data according to Table 4-7.

Table 4-7　Sorting table of hierarchical data in case-control studies

Exposure or characteristic	Disease situation in the "i" layer		Total
	Cases	Controls	
Yes	a_i	b_i	n_{1i}
No	c_i	d_i	n_{0i}
Total	m_{1i}	m_{0i}	t_i

Table 4-6 as an example, considering that age is associated with the behavior of oral contraceptives, and also relate to MI, it might be a confounding factors. So according to age, the population divided into two layers of less than 40 years old, aged 40 and above （seen in Table 4-8）.

ln2.2 ± 1.96 × 0.2874 = (0.2252, 1.3218)

求上述值的反自然对数，得：exp(0.2252)=1.25，exp(1.3218)=3.75。即 OR 的 95% CI 为（1.25，3.75）。

2）Miettnen 卡方值法

$OR\,95\%\,\mathrm{CI} = OR^{(1\pm1.96/\sqrt{\chi^2})} = 2.2^{(1\pm1.96/\sqrt{7.7})} =$ (1.26, 3.84)

4. 不匹配分层资料

分层分析是根据研究人群的某些特征或因素，将其划分为不同的层次，如按性别将人群分为男性和女性二层，按年龄将人群分为 20~39 岁、40~59 岁、60 岁及以上三层，然后分析各层中暴露与疾病之间的关系。分层因素可能是混杂因素，可以使用分层分析来控制混杂。

（1）分层资料的整理

根据表 4-7 的形式整理资料。

表 4-7　病例对照研究分层资料整理表

暴露或特征	i 层的疾病情况		合计
	病例	对照	
有	a_i	b_i	n_{1i}
无	c_i	d_i	n_{0i}
合计	m_{1i}	m_{0i}	t_i

以表 4-6 的数据为例，考虑到年龄与口服避孕药的行为有关，也与 MI 的发生有关，可能是个混杂因素，故可按年龄将研究对象分为 <40 岁和 ≥40 岁两层，如表 4-8 所示。

Table 4-8　The result of the layered according to age

| | < 40 years old | | | ≥40 years old | | |
| | The status of OC | | Total | The status of OC | | Total |
	Yes	No		Yes	No	
Cases	21 (a_1)	26 (b_1)	47 (m_{11})	18 (a_2)	88 (b_2)	106 (m_{12})
Controls	17 (c_1)	59 (d_1)	76 (m_{01})	7 (c_2)	95 (d_2)	102 (m_{02})
Total	38 (n_{11})	85 (n_{01})	123 (t_1)	25 (n_{12})	183 (n_{02})	208 (t_2)

Note: $OR_1=2.80$, $OR_2=2.78$.

（2）Calculate the value of OR in each layer

$OR_1 = (21 \times 59)/(17 \times 26) = 2.80$

$OR_2 = (18 \times 95)/(7 \times 88) = 2.78$

Further analysis the association between age and incidence of MI in non-exposed group（didn't taking OC）（Table 4-9）.

Table 4-9　The association between age and incidence of MI in people who didn't taking OC

	< 40	≥40
MI	26	88
Controls	59	95

$OR=0.48$, $\chi^2=7.27$, shows that the age are associated with the occurrence of MI（The risk of occurrence of MI was increased with age）.

Analysis the association between age and OC in controls（Table 4-10）.

Table 4-10　The association between age and OC in controls

	< 40	≥40
Taking OC	17	7
Didn't taking OC	59	95

$OR=3.91$, $\chi^2=8.98$, shows that the age are associated with the OC too.

表4-8　按年龄分层的结果

| | < 40 岁 | | | ≥40 岁 | | |
	服OC	未服OC	合计	服OC	未服OC	合计
病例	21 (a_1)	26 (b_1)	47 (m_{11})	18 (a_2)	88 (b_2)	106 (m_{12})
对照	17 (c_1)	59 (d_1)	76 (m_{01})	7 (c_2)	95 (d_2)	102 (m_{02})
合计	38 (n_{11})	85 (n_{01})	123 (t_1)	25 (n_{12})	183 (n_{02})	208 (t_2)

注：$OR_1=2.80$，$OR_2=2.78$。

（2）计算各层的 OR

$OR_1 = (21 \times 59)/(17 \times 26) = 2.80$

$OR_2 = (18 \times 95)/(7 \times 88) = 2.78$

进一步分析非暴露组（未服OC者）中年龄与MI的关系（表4-9）。

表4-9　未服OC者中年龄与MI的关系

	< 40 岁	≥40 岁
MI	26	88
对照	59	95

$OR=0.48$，$\chi^2=7.27$，说明年龄与MI有关（年龄越大，发生MI的风险越高）。

再分析对照组中年龄与服用OC的关系（表4-10）。

表4-10　对照组年龄与服用OC行为的关系

	< 40 岁	≥40 岁
服OC	17	7
未服OC	59	95

$OR=3.91$，$\chi^2=8.98$，说明年龄与服用OC有关。

In addition, age is not the intermediate link between OC and MI, so age is a confounding factor in studying the relationship between OC and MI. In this condition, we could use hierarchical analysis method to control the confounding factor.

When the value of OR in two layers are closed or equal, two layers are homogeneous.

（3）Calculate the total value of OR

Use the formula proposed by Mantel-Haenszel：

$$OR_{MH} = \frac{\sum\left(a_i d_i / t_i\right)}{\sum\left(b_i c_i / t_i\right)} \qquad (4-11)$$

According the data from Table 4-8, the OR_{MH}= 2.79.

（4）Calculate the total Chi-square value

$$\chi^2_{MH} = \frac{\left[\sum a_i - \sum E\left(a_i\right)\right]^2}{\sum Var\left(a_i\right)} \qquad (4-12)$$

$\sum E\left(a_i\right)$ is theoretical value of $\sum a_i$:

$$\sum E\left(a_i\right) = \sum m_{1i} n_{1i} / t_i \qquad (4-13)$$

$\sum Var\left(a_i\right)$ is variance of $\sum a_i$:

$$\sum Var\left(a_i\right) = \sum_{i=1}^{I} \frac{m_{1i} m_{0i} n_{1i} n_{0i}}{t_i^2\left(t_i - 1\right)} \qquad (4-14)$$

According the data of Table 4-8, χ^2_{MH}=11.79. The degree of freedom of Mantel-Haenszel stratification analysis is 1, check the boundary value table of χ^2, P<0.01.

（5）Calculate the total confidence interval（CI）of OR

Use the method of Miettinen：

$$(OR_L, OR_U) = OR_{MH}^{\left(1 \pm 1.96 / \sqrt{\chi^2_{MH}}\right)} = (1.55, 5.01)$$

So the 95% CI of OR_{MH} is（1.55, 5.01）. If we want calculate the 99% CI, we could replace 1.96 with 2.58 in the formula above. The CI wasn't including 1, the OR value was statistically significant in 0.05 or 0.01 level.

另外，年龄也不是OC与MI的中间病理环节，故年龄是研究OC与MI关系时的混杂因素。这种情况下可以用分层分析方法控制年龄的混杂作用。

当两层的OR值接近或相等时，说明两层是同质的（homogeneous），此时可进一步做合并估计。

（3）计算总的OR

用Mantel-Haenszel提出的公式：

$$OR_{MH} = \frac{\sum\left(a_i d_i / t_i\right)}{\sum\left(b_i c_i / t_i\right)} \qquad (4-11)$$

根据表4-8的数据，可得OR_{MH}=2.79。

（4）计算总的卡方值

$$\chi^2_{MH} = \frac{\left[\sum a_i - \sum E\left(a_i\right)\right]^2}{\sum Var\left(a_i\right)} \qquad (4-12)$$

其中，$\sum E\left(a_i\right)$为$\sum a_i$的理论值：

$$\sum E\left(a_i\right) = \sum m_{1i} n_{1i} / t_i \qquad (4-13)$$

$\sum Var\left(a_i\right)$为$\sum a_i$的方差：

$$\sum Var\left(a_i\right) = \sum_{i=1}^{I} \frac{m_{1i} m_{0i} n_{1i} n_{0i}}{t_i^2\left(t_i - 1\right)} \qquad (4-14)$$

根据表4-8的数据，可得χ^2_{MH}=11.79。Mantel-Haenszel分层分析的自由度等于1，查χ^2界值表，P< 0.01。

（5）估计总OR的可信区间

用Miettinen法计算：

$$\left(OR_L, OR_U\right) = OR_{MH}^{\left(1 \pm 1.96 / \sqrt{\chi^2_{MH}}\right)} = (1.55, 5.01)$$

即，OR_{MH}的95% CI是（1.55， 5.01）。如要计算99% CI，将上式中的1.96换成2.58即可。可信区间中不包括1.0，即可认为该OR值在0.05或0.01水平上有统计学意义。

5. Ranked data

If we could get the data from different exposure levels of exposure factor, we could use the data to analyze the dose-response relationship between exposure and disease, and to increase the inferred gist of causality.

（1）Sorting the data to contingency tables

a_0 and in b_0 in contingency table corresponds to the c and d in fourfold table above (Table 4-11).

Table 4-11　Contingency table of ranked data in case-control studies

	Exposure levels						Total
	0	1	2	3	4	...	
Cases	$a_0(=c)$	a_1	a_2	a_3	a_4	...	n_1
Controls	$b_0(=d)$	b_1	b_2	b_3	b_4	...	n_0
Total	m_0	m_1	m_2	m_3	m_4	...	n

（2）Chi-square test

For example, in 1956, Doll and Hill conducted a case-control study about the relationship between smoking and lung cancer in male (Table 4-12).

Table 4-12　The relationship between daily number of smoking and lung cancer in male

	Daily number of smoking				Total
	0	1-	5-	15-	
Cases	2 (c)	33 (a_1)	250 (a_2)	364 (a_3)	649 (n_1)
Controls	27 (d)	55 (b_1)	293 (b_2)	274 (b_3)	649 (n_0)
Total	29 (m_0)	88 (m_1)	543 (m_2)	638 (m_3)	1 298 (n)
OR	1.00	8.10	11.52	17.93	

Results: $\chi^2=43.15$, degree of freedom was 3, $P<0.001$.

5. 有序资料

如能获得某暴露因素不同暴露水平的资料，则可用来分析暴露和疾病的剂量反应关系，以增加因果关系推断的依据。

（1）将资料整理归纳成列联表

表中的a_0与b_0分别对应前面四格表中的c与d（表4-11）。

表4-11　病例对照研究分级资料整理表

	暴露分级						合计
	0	1	2	3	4	...	
病例	$a_0(=c)$	a_1	a_2	a_3	a_4	...	n_1
对照	$b_0(=d)$	b_1	b_2	b_3	b_4	...	n_0
合计	m_0	m_1	m_2	m_3	m_4	...	n

（2）χ^2（卡方）检验

例如，1956年Doll和Hill开展了男性吸烟与肺癌关系的病例对照研究（表4-12）。

表4-12　男性每日吸烟的支数与肺癌的关系

	每日吸烟支数				合计
	0	1～	5～	15～	
病例	2 (c)	33 (a_1)	250 (a_2)	364 (a_3)	649 (n_1)
对照	27 (d)	55 (b_1)	293 (b_2)	274 (b_3)	649 (n_0)
合计	29 (m_0)	88 (m_1)	543 (m_2)	638 (m_3)	1 298 (n)
OR	1.00	8.10	11.52	17.93	

结果显示：$\chi^2=43.15$，自由度为3，$P<0.001$。

（3）Calculate the value of *OR* in each exposure level

Usually use the non-exposure group or the lowest level of exposure group as the control group. In this example, we used the no smoking group as control group, the *OR* in other exposure levels were 8.10, 11.52 and 17.83, the value of *OR* increased with the daily number of smoking, and showing a obviously dose response relationship.

（4）Trend of Chi-square test

When the degree of freedom is 1, the formula of trend test is:

$$\chi^2 = \frac{\left[T_1 - \left(n_1 T_2 / n \right) \right]^2}{Var} \quad (4\text{-}15)$$

$$Var = \frac{n_1 n_2 \left(n T_3 - T_2^2 \right)}{n^2 \left(n - 1 \right)}$$

$$T_1 = \sum_{i=0}^{t} a_i X_i$$

$$T_2 = \sum_{i=0}^{t} m_i X_i$$

$$T_3 = \sum_{i=0}^{t} m_i X_i^2$$

For example, in Table 4-12,

$T_1 = 33 \times 1 + 250 \times 2 + 364 \times 3 = 1\,625$

$T_2 = 88 \times 1 + 543 \times 2 + 638 \times 3 = 3\,088$

$T_3 = 88 \times 1^2 + 543 \times 2^2 + 638 \times 3^2 = 8\,002$

$$Var = \frac{649 \times 649 \times \left(1\,298 \times 8\,002 - 3\,088^2 \right)}{1\,298^2 \times \left(1\,298 - 1 \right)} =$$

164.003 9

$$\chi^2 = \frac{\left[1\,625 - \left(649 \times 3\,088 / 1\,298 \right) \right]^2}{164.003\,9} = 40.01$$

Degree of freedom is 1, *P*<0.01. The trend of dose-response relationship is significant statistical significance.

6. Matching data

In this section we mainly introduced the analysis

（3）计算各暴露分层的*OR*

通常以不暴露或最低水平的暴露组为参照组。本例以不吸烟组为参照组，其余各层*OR*值分别为8.10、11.52和17.83，随着吸烟量的增加而递增，二者呈现出明显的剂量反应关系。

（4）χ^2（卡方）趋势检验

自由度为1的χ^2趋势检验公式为：

$$\chi^2 = \frac{\left[T_1 - \left(n_1 T_2 / n \right) \right]^2}{Var} \quad (4\text{-}15)$$

其中：$Var = \frac{n_1 n_2 \left(n T_3 - T_2^2 \right)}{n^2 \left(n - 1 \right)}$

$$T_1 = \sum_{i=0}^{t} a_i X_i$$

$$T_2 = \sum_{i=0}^{t} m_i X_i$$

$$T_3 = \sum_{i=0}^{t} m_i X_i^2$$

以表4-12的资料为例：

$T_1 = 33 \times 1 + 250 \times 2 + 364 \times 3 = 1\,625$

$T_2 = 88 \times 1 + 543 \times 2 + 638 \times 3 = 3\,088$

$T_3 = 88 \times 1^2 + 543 \times 2^2 + 638 \times 3^2 = 8\,002$

$$Var = \frac{649 \times 649 \times \left(1\,298 \times 8\,002 - 3\,088^2 \right)}{1\,298^2 \times \left(1\,298 - 1 \right)} =$$

164.003 9

$$\chi^2 = \frac{\left[1\,625 - \left(649 \times 3\,088 / 1\,298 \right) \right]^2}{164.003\,9} = 40.01$$

自由度为1，*P*<0.01，结果说明剂量反应趋势有统计学意义。

6. 匹配资料

本节主要介绍匹配资料的分析。

of pair matching data.

（1）Sorting the data to fourfold table (Table 4-13)

Table 4-13　Sorting table of pair matching data in case-control studies

Controls	Cases		Number of pairs
	Had a history of exposure	Had no history of exposure	
Had a history of exposure	a	b	$a+b$
Had no history of exposure	c	d	$c+d$
Number of pairs	$a+c$	$b+d$	t

In 1976, Mack and other reported the relationship between exogenous estrogen and endometrial cancer in case-control study, as this an example (Table 4-14).

Table 4-14　Research data of the relationship between exogenous estrogen and endometrial cancer in a matching case-control study

Controls	Cases		Number of pairs
	Had a history of exposure	Had no history of exposure	
Had a history of exposure	27 (a)	3 (b)	30 ($a+b$)
Had no history of exposure	29 (c)	4 (d)	33 ($c+d$)
Number of pairs	56 ($a+c$)	7 ($b+d$)	63 (t)

（Mack, 1975）

（2）Chi-square test

Use the formula proposed by McNemar:

$$\chi^2 = \frac{(b-c)^2}{(b+c)} \qquad (4-16)$$

This formula is suitable for a larger sample, we could use correction formula proposed by McNemar when the pairs number is less.

$$\chi^2 = \frac{(|b-c|-1)^2}{(b+c)} \qquad (4-17)$$

According to formula 4-17 in this example,

（1）将资料整理成四格表（表4-13）

表4-13　1:1配对病例对照研究资料整理表

对照	病例		对子数
	有暴露史	无暴露史	
有暴露史	a	b	$a+b$
无暴露史	c	d	$c+d$
对子数	$a+c$	$b+d$	t

以1976年Mack等报告的在洛杉矶所做的外源性雌激素与子宫内膜癌关系的病例对照研究为例，整理成的四格表见表4-14。

表4-14　外源性雌激素与子宫内膜癌关系的配比病例对照研究资料

对照	病例		对子数
	有暴露史	无暴露史	
有暴露史	27 (a)	3 (b)	30 ($a+b$)
无暴露史	29 (c)	4 (d)	33 ($c+d$)
对子数	56 ($a+c$)	7 ($b+d$)	63 (t)

（Mack, 1975）

（2）χ^2（卡方）检验

利用McNemar公式计算：

$$\chi^2 = \frac{(b-c)^2}{(b+c)} \qquad (4-16)$$

此公式适用于较大样本。当对子数较少时，可采用McNemar校正公式：

$$\chi^2 = \frac{(|b-c|-1)^2}{(b+c)} \qquad (4-17)$$

本例按式4-17计算可得：

χ^2=19.53, $P < 0.005$.

（3）Calculate the value of OR

$$OR = \frac{c}{b} \ (t \neq 0) \qquad (4\text{-}18)$$

In this example, OR=9.67.

（4）Calculate the 95% CI of OR

Use the formula proposed by Miettinen:

$$\left(OR_L, OR_U\right) = OR^{\left(1 \pm 1.96/\sqrt{\chi^2}\right)} = (3.54, 26.45)$$

7. Attributable fraction（AF）

Attributable fraction of exposure population marked as AF_e.

$$AF_e = \frac{I_e - I_0}{I_e} \approx \frac{OR - 1}{OR} \qquad (4\text{-}19)$$

In the formula, I_e is the incidence of exposure group, I_0 is the incidence of non-exposure group. In a case-control study we couldn't get incidence, and only get OR. AF_e measures the excess event rate or risk fraction in the exposed population that is attributable to the exposure. That is, it is the proportion of event rate or risk in the exposed population that would be reduced if the exposure were not present.

Population attributable fraction marked as AF_p.

$$AF_p = \frac{I_p - I_0}{I_p} \approx \frac{P_e \times (OR - 1)}{1 + P_e \times (OR - 1)} \qquad (4\text{-}20)$$

In the formula, I_p is the incidence of the total population; I_0 is the incidence of non-exposure group; P_e is the exposure rate of the total population (or replaced by exposure rate of control group). AF_p measures the excess event rate or risk fraction in the total population that is attributable to the exposure, AF_p is the proportional reduction in population disease or mortality that would occur if exposure to a risk factor were reduced to an alternative ideal exposure scenario.

χ^2=19.53，$P < 0.005$。

（3）计算 OR

$$OR = \frac{c}{b} \ (t \neq 0) \qquad (4\text{-}18)$$

本例计算得 $OR = 9.67$。

（4）计算 OR 的95%可信区间

仍用Miettinen公式，本例得：

$$\left(OR_L, OR_U\right) = OR^{\left(1 \pm 1.96/\sqrt{\chi^2}\right)} = (3.54, 26.45)$$

7. 归因分值（attributable fraction, AF）

暴露人群的归因分值记为 AF_e，公式如下：

$$AF_e = \frac{I_e - I_0}{I_e} \approx \frac{OR - 1}{OR} \qquad (4\text{-}19)$$

式中，I_e 为暴露组发病率，I_0 为非暴露组发病率。在病例对照研究中不能获得发病率，只能计算 OR。AF_e 指暴露人群中暴露引起的额外发病率或风险值，即暴露引起的发病占总发病的比例。也就是说，它是指消除该暴露后，暴露组发病降低的比例。

人群归因分值记为 AF_p，

$$AF_p = \frac{I_p - I_0}{I_p} \approx \frac{P_e \times (OR - 1)}{1 + P_e \times (OR - 1)} \qquad (4\text{-}20)$$

式中，I_p 为全人群发病率，I_0 为非暴露组发病率，P_e 为全人群暴露率（或以对照组的暴露率代替）。AF_p 反映暴露对全人群发病的影响，表示全人群中由该暴露引起的超额发病率或风险值，即暴露引起的发病占全部发病的比例。也就是说，它是指消除该暴露后，人群中发病率或死亡率降低的比例。

8. Power

Power can be explained by the ability to reject the null hypothesis. When the null hypothesis is not establishment, the probability of the null hypothesis is rejected. For example, to estimate the power of 1:1 matched case-control study.

Assume that the proportion of exposed to the study risk factors in the population is 0.30 ($p_0 = 0.30$); the significance level of statistical test on both sides is 0.05 ($\alpha = 0.05$); the number of cases and controls are 50. Calculate the study power to find the $OR=2$.

First, calculate the value of z:

$$z_\beta = \sqrt{\frac{n(p_1 - p_0)^2}{2\bar{p}\bar{q}}} - z_\alpha \qquad (4\text{-}21)$$

Power= $1-\beta = P(z \leqslant z_\beta)$ (P is probability).

According to the standard normal distribution, we check the probability.

$$p_1 = \frac{p_0 RR}{1 + p_0(RR - 1)}$$
$$= \frac{0.3 \times 2}{1 + 0.3 \times (2 - 1)} = 0.4615$$

In this example, $n=50$, $p_0=0.30$, $\alpha=0.05$ (two-sided test), $z_\alpha = 1.96$, $RR=2$, so

$$\bar{p} = (p_0 + p_1)/2 = (0.3 + 0.4615)/2 = 0.3808$$

$$z_\beta = \sqrt{\frac{50 \times (0.4615 - 0.3)^2}{2 \times 0.3808 \times 0.6192}} - 1.96$$
$$= -0.297 \approx -0.30$$

Check the normal distribution table, when $z_\beta= -0.30$, $\beta =0.62$, power $=P=1-\beta=38\%$.

Conclusion: If the number of cases and controls are 50, under the given conditions, the probability of checking the OR was significantly not equal to 1 is 38% in this study. If $OR \leqslant 2$, this study has little chance of success.

8. 功效

功效（power）也叫作把握度，可以解释为拒绝无效假设的能力，即当无效假设不成立时，该假设被拒绝的概率。此处以1:1匹配病例对照研究资料的功效估计为例进行介绍。

例如，人群中研究因素的暴露率$p_0 = 0.30$，统计学双侧检验的显著性水平$\alpha = 0.05$，病例组与对照组各有50例研究对象，计算该研究有多大的把握度，可得到$OR = 2$。

首先计算z值

$$z_\beta = \sqrt{\frac{n(p_1 - p_0)^2}{2\bar{p}\bar{q}}} - z_\alpha \qquad (4\text{-}21)$$

把握度 $=1-\beta = P(z \leqslant z_\beta)$（$P$为概率）。

根据标准正态分布，可以查到z_β对应的概率P。先利用下面的公示计算p_1，

$$p_1 = \frac{p_0 RR}{1 + p_0(RR - 1)}$$
$$= \frac{0.3 \times 2}{1 + 0.3 \times (2 - 1)} = 0.4615$$

本例中，$n=50$，$p_0=0.30$，$\alpha=0.05$（双侧检验），$z_\alpha = 1.96$，$RR = 2$，则：

$$\bar{p} = (p_0 + p_1)/2 = (0.3 + 0.4615)/2 = 0.3808$$

$$z_\beta = \sqrt{\frac{50 \times (0.4615 - 0.3)^2}{2 \times 0.3808 \times 0.6192}} - 1.96$$
$$= -0.297 \approx -0.30$$

查正态分布表，当$z_\beta=-0.30$时，$\beta=0.62$，功效$=P=1-\beta= 38\%$。

结论：如果病例组和对照组各50例，在给定的条件下，该研究能检出OR不等于1的概率为38%。如果$OR \leqslant 2$，该研究很难得到有统计学意义的结果。

It is generally acknowledged that the power should be higher than 75%.

If the pairs are inconsistent, we could calculate the power by using the following formula:

$$z_\beta = \frac{(n - \frac{1}{2})\sqrt{n} - \frac{z_\alpha}{2}}{\sqrt{\pi(1-\pi)}} \qquad (4-22)$$

In the formula $\pi = OR/(1+OR)$.

4.5　The Common Bias and Its Control

A number of potential biases must be either avoided or taken into account in case control studies. The major biases include the following: selection bias, information bias and confounding bias.

4.5.1　Selection bias

Selection bias is a statistical bias in which there is an error in choosing the individuals or groups to take part in a scientific study.

1. Admission rate bias

Admission rate bias also called Berkson bias. It is a systematic bias in the distribution of disease amongst hospitalized patients. We should randomly select the object of study in design stage, and select the object in multiple hospitals.

2. Prevalence-incidence bias

Prevalence - incidence bias also called Neyman bias. Prevalence - incidence bias — a form of selection bias in case - control studies attributed to selective survival among the prevalent cases (i.e., mild, clinically resolved, or fatal cases being excluded from the case group). It happens when mild or asymptomatic cases as well as fatal short disease episodes are missed when studies are performed late in disease process.

一般认为，一项研究的检验功效应在75%以上。

如果分析的是不一致对子数（n），研究功效可用下式计算：

$$z_\beta = \frac{(n - \frac{1}{2})\sqrt{n} - \frac{z_\alpha}{2}}{\sqrt{\pi(1-\pi)}} \qquad (4-22)$$

式中：$\pi = OR/(1+OR)$。

4.5　常见偏倚及其控制

在病例对照研究中，必须避免或考虑一些潜在的偏倚。主要偏倚包括：选择偏倚、信息偏倚和混杂偏倚。

4.5.1　选择偏倚

选择偏倚是选择个体或群体作为研究对象时存在的系统误差。

1.入院率偏倚

入院率偏倚也称为Berkson偏倚。入院率偏倚是住院患者疾病分布的系统误差，即不同疾病的患者入院率或就诊率不同，导致了病例组和对照组某些特征的系统差异。设计阶段应随机在多家医院选择研究对象。

2.现患-新发病例偏倚

现患-新发病例偏倚也称为Neyman偏倚。现患-新发病例偏倚是一种选择偏倚，归因于现患病例中的选择性生存（即从病例组中排除轻度、临床缓解或致命病例），幸存者可能改变了生活习惯，降低了危险因素水平，从而导致被调查时夸大或缩小了病前生活习惯上的某些特征。在疾病研究过程中，如果遗漏了轻微或无症状病例以及致命的短期发作病例，就会发生这种情况。应尽量选择新发病例。

3. Detection signal bias

Detection signal bias also called unmasking bias. It is a bias in specifying and selecting the study sample. We should select the cases including early, middle and late of the patient.

4. Time effect bias

For chronic disease, such as cancer or coronary heart disease, there is a long time between exposures to risk factors and lesion. So the people who impending lesions after exposure, occurred early lesions but cannot be checked out could be selected to the control group.

4.5.2　Information bias

Information bias occurs in the data collection stage of studies. It happens when estimated effect is distorted either by an error in measurement or by misclassifying the subject for exposure and/or outcome variables.

1. Recall bias

Recall bias is a systematic error caused by differences in the accuracy or completeness of the recollections retrieved ("recalled") by study participants regarding events or experiences from the past. Recall bias happens e. g. when people, having had adverse health outcomes, remember and report past exposure differently from those who did not experience any adverse health outcome.

2. Investigation bias

Investigation bias results when systematic differences occur in the soliciting, recording, or interpreting of information from study subjects. Investigation bias may come from the survey object and researchers.

3．检出征候偏倚

检出征候偏倚也称为暴露偏倚，是在指定和选择研究样本时存在的偏倚。患者常因某些与致病无关的症状就医，从而提高了早期病例检出率，致使过高估计了暴露程度而产生系统误差。应选择早期、中期和晚期各阶段的病例。

4．效应偏倚

肿瘤或冠心病等慢性病患者，从开始暴露于危险因素到出现病变，往往会经历一段较长的时间。因此，暴露后出现早期病变但无法检出的患者可能被错误选入对照组。应采用灵敏的疾病早期检查技术。

4.5.2　信息偏倚

信息偏倚发生在数据收集阶段，是效果评价被错误测量、暴露和/或疾病结局被错误分类时所发生的系统误差。

1．回忆偏倚

回忆偏倚是一种系统误差，由研究对象对过去事件或经历的回忆存在准确性或完整性差异引起。例如，患者与非患者对过去经历或暴露的回忆存在差异。

2．调查偏倚

调查偏倚是从研究对象中获取、记录或解释信息时出现的系统误差。调查偏倚可能来自调查对象和研究者。

4.5.3　Confounding bias

Confounding is essentially a mixing of effects that occurs when a factor (confounder) associated with the exposure of interest is also associated with development of the disease or outcome of interest independently of exposure. Therefore, a distorted estimate of the exposure effect results because the exposure effect is mixed with the effect of extraneous variables.

A confounder must be predictive of disease occurrence independent of its association with the exposure of interest, but cannot be an intermediate in the casual chain of association between exposure and disease development. The confounding variable can effect the association between exposure and disease positively or negatively; the distorted estimate resulting from confounding can overestimate or underestimate the true effect or even change the apparent direction of effect.

4.6　Advantages and Disadvantages

The advantages and disadvantages of case-control studies as follows:

4.6.1　Advantages

①Relatively easy to carry out.

②Rapid and inexpensive (compared with cohort studies).

③Require comparatively few subjects.

④Particularly suitable to investigate rare diseases or diseases about which little is known. But a disease which is rare in the general population (e.g., leukaemia in adolescents) may not be rare in special exposure group (e.g., prenatal X-rays).

⑤No risk to subjects.

4.5.3　混杂偏倚

混杂是一个因素（混杂因子）与暴露因素有关，且独立于暴露因素，与疾病的发展或研究结局也相关时发生的混合效应。因此，暴露效应与外部变量的效应混合导致歪曲了暴露效应。

混杂因素必须独立于暴露因素，能够预测疾病的发生，且与暴露因素有关，但不能是暴露与疾病发展之间关联链的中间环节。混杂变量可以对暴露与疾病之间的关系产生积极或消极的影响，使得研究者高估或低估真实效应，甚至歪曲结果，造成完全相反的效应。

4.6　优点与局限性

病例对照研究的优缺点如下：

4.6.1　优点

①相对容易实施。

②快速而廉价（与队列研究相比）。

③需要相对少的研究对象。

④特别适合罕见病和少见病的研究。但普通人群中的罕见病（如青少年白血病）在特殊暴露（如产前X光）人群中可能并不少见。

⑤研究对象无风险。

⑥Allows the study of several different aetiological factors (e.g., smoking, physical activity and personality characteristics in myocardial infarction).

⑦Risk factors can be identified. Rational prevention and control programmes can be established.

⑧ No attrition problems, because case control studies do not require follow-up of individuals into the future.

⑨Ethical problems minimal.

4.6.2　Disadvantages

① Problems of bias relies on memory or past records, the accuracy of which may be uncertain; validation of information obtained is difficult or sometimes impossible.

②Selection of an appropriate control group may be difficult.

③We cannot measure incidence, and can only estimate the relative risk.

④ Do not distinguish between causes and associated factors.

⑤Not suited to the evaluation of therapy or prophylaxis of disease.

⑥ Another major concern is the representativeness of cases and controls.

4.7　Examples of Case-Control Studies

Case control studies have provided much of the current base of knowledge in epidemiology. Some of the early case control studies centred round cigarette smoking and lung cancer. Recent studies include: maternal smoking and congenital malformations, radiation and leukaemia, oral contraceptive use and hepatocellular adenoma, herpes simplex and Bell palsy, in-

⑥可以开展一果多因的研究（例如，吸烟、体力活动和性格特征与心肌梗死）。

⑦可以识别危险因素。可以制定合理的预防和控制方案。

⑧省钱、省力、省时间。因为病例对照研究不需要随访。

⑨伦理问题较小。

4.6.2　局限性

①回忆偏倚可能造成信息不准确。有时信息的获得会存在困难，甚至不可行。

②合适对照组的选择可能存在困难。

③不能获得发病率，只能利用 OR 估算相对危险度。

④不能确定因果关系。

⑤不适用于疾病防治效果的评价。

⑥另一个主要的问题是病例和对照的代表性。

4.7　病例对照研究实例

病例对照研究是流行病学最基本、最重要的研究方法之一。一些早期的病例对照研究集中在吸烟与肺癌的关系上。近期的研究有：母亲吸烟与胎儿先天性畸形、辐射与白血病、口服避孕药与肝细胞腺瘤、单纯疱疹和贝尔氏麻痹、人工流产与自然流产、体力活动与冠心病、人工甜味剂和膀胱癌等。

duced abortion and spontaneous abortion, physical activity and coronal death, artificial sweeteners and bladder cancer, etc.

A few studies are cited in detail:

【Example 1】Adenocarcinoma of the vagina

An excellent example of a case control study adenocarcinoma of the vagina in young women. It is not only a rare disease, but also the usual victim is over 50 years age. There was an unusual occurrence of this tumor in young women (15 to 22 years) born in one Boston hospital between 1966 and 1969. The apparent time clustering cases—7 occurring within 4 years at a single hospital—led this enquiry. An eighth case occurred in 1969 in a 20 year patient who was treated at another Boston hospital in USA.

The cause of this tumor was investigated by a case control study in 1971 to find out the factors that might be associated with this tumor. As this was a rare disease, for each case, for matched controls were put up. The controls were identified from the birth records of the hospital in which each case was born. Female births occurring closest in time to each patient were selected as controls. Information was collected personal interviews regarding：① maternal age；② maternal smoking；③antenatal radiology；④ diethyl-stilboestrol（DES）exposure in foetal life. The results of the study shown in Table 4-15 which shows that cases differ significantly from the controls in their past history. Seven in the eight cases had been exposed to DES in foetal life. The drug had been given to their mothers during the first trimester of pregnancy to prevent possible miscarriage. But none of mothers in the control group had received DES. Since study, more cases have been reported and the associate with DES has been confirmed. The case control method played a critical role in re-

下面详细举例：

【例1】阴道腺癌

有一个很好的病例对照研究实例——年轻女性的阴道腺癌。阴道腺癌是一种罕见病，通常在50岁以上的女性中发病。1966年至1969年，波士顿一家医院的年轻女性患者（15至22岁）中被发现了一种不寻常的肿瘤。4年内在一家医院聚集发现了7例该肿瘤病例，这一事件引起了相关研究者的重视。1969年，美国波士顿的另一家医院发现了第8例20岁的阴道腺癌患者。

为了探索阴道腺癌的病因，相关研究者于1971年开展了一项病例对照研究。由于这是一种罕见的疾病，因此研究者对每个病例都进行了配对。对照是从每一个病例出生的医院记录中确定的，与每个病例出生日期最接近的女性被选入对照组，且以下相关信息被收集：①孕母年龄；②孕母孕期吸烟情况；③孕母产前放射性检查情况；④胎儿期对二乙基己烯雌酚（DES）的暴露情况。研究结果表明，病例的暴露史与对照组的存在差异（表4-15）。8例病例中有7例在胎儿期暴露于DES（DES主要用于孕前三个月，以防流产），但对照组孕母均未服用DES。自研究以来，更多被证实与DES相关的阴道腺癌病例被报道。病例对照研究对揭示孕母因使用DES造成胎儿暴露，从而引起女婴20年后发生阴道腺癌这一因果关系发挥了关键作用。

vealing exposure to DES in utero the cause of vaginal adenocarcinoma in the exposed child 20 years later.

Table 4-15 Association between maternal DES therapy and adenocarcinoma of vagina amongst female offspring

Information acquired retrospectively	Case (8)	Control (32)	Significant level
Maternal age	26.1	29.3	n.s.
Maternal smoking	7	21	n.s.
Antenatal radiology	1	4	n.s.
Oestrogen exposure	7	—	$P < 0.0001$

【Example 2】 Oral contraceptives and thromboembolic disease

By August 1965, the British Committee on Safety of Di had received 249 reports of adverse reactions and 16 reports of death in women taking oral contraceptives. It because apparent that epidemiological studies were needed determine whether women who took oral contraceptives with at greater risk of developing thromboembolic disease. In 1968 and 1969, Vassey and Doll reported the finding their case control studies in which they interviewed women who had been admitted to hospitals with venous thrombocyte or pulmonary embolism without medical cause and compared the history with that obtained from other women who been admitted to the same hospital with other diseases who were matched for age, marital status and parity.

It was found that out of 84, 42 (50%) of those with venous thrombosis and pulmonary embolism had been using oral contraceptives, compared with 14% of controls (Table 4-16). The studies confirmed that taking the pill and having pulmonary embolism co - existed more frequently than would be expected by chance.

表 4-15　孕妇 DES 治疗与女性后代阴道腺癌之间的关系

追溯性获得的信息	病例组 （8例）	对照组 （32例）	显著水平
孕母年龄	26.1	29.3	n.s.
孕母吸烟人数	7	21	n.s.
产前接受放射学检查人数	1	4	n.s.
雌激素暴露人数	7	—	$P < 0.0001$

【例2】口服避孕药与血栓栓塞性疾病

截至 1965 年 8 月，英国迪村安全委员会收到了 249 份口服避孕药的不良反应报告和 16 份口服避孕药的死亡报告。因此，有必要开展流行病学研究来确定口服避孕药是否会增加女性患血栓栓塞性疾病的风险。1968—1969 年，Vassey 和 Doll 开展了一项病例对照研究。研究以因不明原因的静脉血栓和肺栓塞入院治疗的女性患者为病例组，以年龄、婚姻状况相匹配、因其他疾病入院的女性患者为对照组。

结果发现，84 例静脉血栓和肺栓塞患者中有 42 人（50%）使用口服避孕药，对照组口服避孕药的比例仅为 14%（表 4-16）。研究证实，服用避孕药后发生肺栓塞的频率超过预期。服用者与非服用者发生肺栓塞的相对风险为 6.3∶1，即口服避孕药者发生血栓栓塞的风险约是非服用者的 6 倍。

The relative risk of users to non-users was 6.3 : 1. That is, the investigators found that users of oral contraceptives were about 6 times as likely as non-users to develop thrombo-embolic disease.

Table 4-16   Case control studies on the safety of oral contraceptives

	Total number	Per cent who used oral contraceptives
Cases (venous thrombosis and pulmonary embolism)	84	50
Controls	168	14

表4-16   口服避孕药安全性的病例对照研究

	总人数	使用口服避孕药的占比（%）
病例组（静脉血栓和肺栓塞）	84	50
对照组	168	14

【Example 3】Thalidomide tragedy

Thalidomide was first marketed as a safe, non-barbiturate hypnotic in Britain in 1958. In 1961, at a congress of gynaecologists, attention was drawn to the birth of a large number of babies with congenital abnormalities, which was previously rare. In the same year, it was suggested that thalidomide might be responsible for it.

A retrospective study of 46 mothers delivered of deformed babies showed that 41 were found to have thalidomide during their early pregnancy. This was compared with a control of 300 mothers who had delivered normal babies: None of these had taken thalidomide. Laboratory experiments confirmed that thalidomide was teratogenic in experimental studies.

【例3】反应停事件

1958年，反应停在英国作为一种安全的非巴比妥类催眠药首次出现。1961年，妇产科协会注意到以前罕见的先天畸形在当时频繁发生频发。同年，有人提出反应停的使用可能与此事件有关。

研究人员对46名分娩畸形婴儿的母亲进行回顾性研究，并以300名分娩正常婴儿的母亲作为对照，结果发现娩出畸形儿的孕母中有41人服用了反应停，娩出正常婴儿的孕母均未服用反应停。该研究证实了反应停可致畸。

Chapter 5　Cohort Studies

Cohort study is one of the most important analytical epidemiologic methods, which directly observes the outcomes of population exposed in different status to explore the relationship between risk factor and outcomes. Cohort study is also commonly known as prospective study, incidence rate study, follow‐up study, and longitudinal study.

5.1　Summarize

5.1.1　Conception

Cohort study identifies a subset of human subjects from a defined population, these subjects have been unexposed or exposed, or exposed in varying intensities, to a factor or factors suspected of influencing the probability of occurrence of a disease or other health outcomes such as death. The subjects are then followed up for a sufficiently long time to collect data on the outcomes. The incidence rates can then be estimated and compared in groups that differ in exposure status; the results are used to test the relationship between a risk factor and an outcome. As opposed to case‐control and cross‐sectional studies, cohort study starts from causes and observes the occurrence of outcome prospectively in time. Thus, cohort study provides stronger evidence than other observational studies for the temporal order for a cause‐effect association and is deemed the most rigorous epidemiological method for studying causes of disease.

第5章　队列研究

队列研究是分析流行病学研究中的重要方法之一，它通过直接观察危险因素暴露状况不同人群的结局，来探讨危险因素与所观察结局的关系。队列研究也常被称为前瞻性研究、发病率研究、随访研究及纵向研究。

5.1　概　述

5.1.1　概念

队列研究是将人群按照是否暴露于某个或某些影响疾病或健康结局（如死亡）发生率的可疑因素（或者按照暴露程度）分为不同的亚组，然后随访其结局，估计并比较不同暴露状况亚组之间结局发生率的差异，从而判断暴露因素与结局之间的关系。与病例对照研究和横断面研究不同，队列研究是从病因开始观察结局发生的前瞻性研究，因此，队列研究比其他观察性研究检验病因假设的能力强，被认为是研究病因的最严格的流行病学方法。

Exposure refers to the objects of study had in touched with some substances (such as heavy metals), and possessed some characteristics (such as age, gender, and heredity) or behavior (such as smoking). Exposure has different meaning in different studies; it could be harmful or could be beneficial.

The word cohort was originally used to describe a military unit in ancient Rome. You can see how this retains traces of the word's origins: cohorts are bound together by similar circumstances just like a group of soldiers in a military unit. In epidemiology, cohort is a particular study group of people. According to the specified conditions, cohort usually has two circumstances: one is birth cohort, it refers to a group of people who were born in a specific period of time; another is exposure cohort, it refers to a group of people who have some common exposure or characteristics.

According to the time the people in and out of the cohort, cohort can be divided into two kinds: One is fixed cohort, another is dynamic cohort. Fixed cohort refers to that subjects are recruited and enrolled at a uniform point in the natural history of a disease or by some defining event and that does not permit additional subjects to be added subsequently. Dynamic cohort refers to that after a cohort is established, individuals recruited to or leave the cohort at different times. As shown in Figure 5-1, in the observed cohort, the cohort of A, C, D, E and F called fixed cohort, and the cohort of A, B, C, D, E, F, G, H, I, J and K called dynamic cohort.

暴露（exposure）是指研究对象接触过某种待研究的物质（如重金属），具备某种待研究的特征（如年龄、性别及遗传等）或行为（如吸烟）。暴露在不同的研究中有不同的含意，暴露可以是有害的，也可以是有益的，但都是需要研究的。

队列（cohort）原指古罗马军团中的一个分队，后来流行病学家加以借用，用来表示一个特定的研究人群。根据特定条件的不同，流行病学中的队列一般有两种情况：一种是指特定时期内出生的一组人群，叫出生队列（birth cohort）；另一种是泛指具有某种共同暴露或特征的一组人群，一般称为队列或暴露队列（exposure cohort），如某个时期进入某工厂工作的一组人群。

根据人群进出队列的时间不同，队列又可分为两种：固定队列（fixed cohort），是指人群都在某一固定时间或一个短时期之内进入队列，之后对其进行随访观察，直至观察期终止，成员都没有因为结局事件以外的其他原因退出，队列中也不再加入新的成员，即在观察期内队列保持相对固定；动态队列（dynamic cohort），即在某队列确定之后，原有的队列成员可以不断退出，新的观察对象可以随时加入。如图 5-1 所示，在所观察的队列人群中，由 A、C、D、E、F 组成的队列称为固定队列，而由 A、B、C、D、E、F、G、H、I、J、K 组成的队列则称为动态队列。

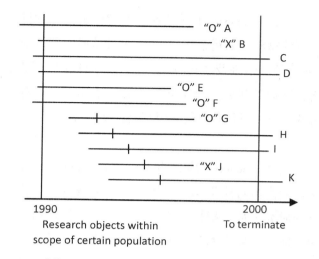

"I" In the cohort; "X" Leave the cohort because of other reason; "O" Outcome.

Figure 5-1 Schematic plot of a cohort

A risk factor is a variable could cause a particular adverse outcome (such as disease) or associated with an increased risk of it, such as individual behavior, life style, environment and heredity.

5.1.2 Basic principle

The basic principle of cohort study is to collect research objects in a specific population, and to divide them into different groups, on the basis of whether research objects exposed into some risk factors in a certain period or on the basis of the different levels of exposure, such as exposure group and non - exposed group, high - dose and low dose exposure groups. The subjects are then followed up for a sufficiently long time to collect data on the outcomes (such as disease, death, or other state of health). The incidence rates can then be estimated and compared in groups that differ in exposure status; the results are used to test the relationship between a risk factor and an outcome. If the incidence of a certain outcome is significantly higher in exposure group than in non-exposed group,

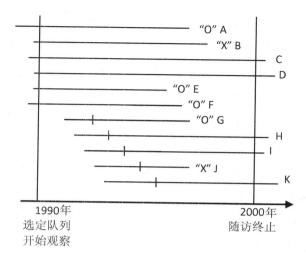

"I" 指进入队列;"X" 指因其他原因退出队列;"O" 指出现终点结局。

图5-1 随访队列示意图

危险因素(risk factor),又称为危险因子,泛指能引起某特定不良结局(outcome)(如疾病)发生,或能使其发生的概率增加的因子。危险因素包括个人行为、生活方式、环境和遗传等多方面的因素。

5.1.2 基本原理

队列研究的基本原理是在一个特定人群中选择所需的研究对象,根据研究对象目前或过去某个时期是否暴露于某个待研究的危险因素或其所处的不同暴露水平,将其分成不同的组(如暴露组和非暴露组、高暴露组和低暴露组等),随访观察一段时间,检查并登记各组人群待研究的预期结局的发生情况(如疾病、死亡或其他健康状况),比较各组结局的发生率,从而评价和检验危险因素与结局的关系。如果暴露组某结局的发生率明显高于非暴露组,则可推测暴露与结局之间可能存在因果关系,其结构模式见图5-2。在队列研究中,所选研究对象必须是在开始时没有出现所要研究的结局,但在随访期内有可能出现该结局(如疾病)的人群。暴露组与非暴露组必须有可比性,非暴露组应该是除了未暴露于某因素之

we could speculated that there may be a causal relationship between exposure and outcomes. The structural model shows in Figure 5-2. In cohort studies, the selected subjects must not appear the outcome at the beginning of the study, however, they may be appear the outcome（such as disease）in the follow-up period. Exposed group and non-exposed group must be comparability, they should be as similar as possible in all aspects except that non-exposed group should not expose to the research factor.

外，其余各方面都尽可能与暴露组相同的一组人群。根据队列研究的基本原理，可以分析出队列研究的一些基本特点。

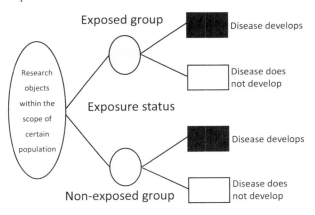

Figure 5-2　The structural model figure of cohort studies

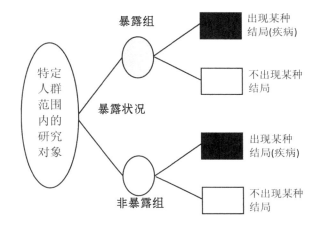

图5-2　队列研究的结构模式图

Basic feature of cohort studies:

① Belongs to observational survey.

② Set up the control group.

③ From causes to effects.

④ Could corroborate the causal relationship between exposure and outcomes.

5.1.3　Research objectives

① Test the hypothesis for the etiology.

② Evaluation of preventive effect.

③ Investigate the natural history of disease.

④ Post-marketing surveillance of new drugs.

队列研究的基本特征：

①属于观察性研究。

②需设立对照组。

③由"因"及"果"。

④可以证实暴露与结局之间的因果关系。

5.1.3　研究目的

①检验病因学假设。

②评价预防效果。

③研究疾病的自然史。

④新药的上市后监测。

5.1.4 Types of cohort studies

According to the different times of individuals recruited to the cohort and termination observation, the cohort studies is divided into prospective cohort studies, historical cohort studies, ambispective cohort studies. As shown in Figure 5-3.

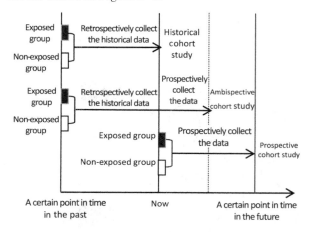

Figure 5-3 Schematic diagram of types of cohort studies

1. Prospective cohort studies

A prospective cohort study is a cohort study that follows over time a group of similar individuals (cohorts) who differ with respect to certain factors under study, to determine how these factors affect rates of a certain outcome. For example, one might follow a cohort of middle-aged truck drivers who vary in terms of smoking habits, to test the hypothesis that the 20-year incidence rate of lung cancer will be highest among heavy smokers, followed by moderate smokers, and then non-smokers. One of the advantages of prospective cohort studies is they can help determine risk factors for being infected with a new disease because they are a longitudinal observation over time, and the collection of results is at regular time intervals, so recall error is minimized. The disadvantage is that prospec-

5.1.4 研究类型

根据研究对象进入队列时间及终止观察的时间不同，队列研究分为前瞻性（prospective）队列研究、历史性（historical）队列研究和双向性（ambispective）队列研究三种。三种队列研究方法的示意图如图5-3所示。

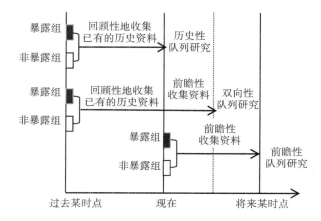

图5-3 队列研究类型示意图

1. 前瞻性队列研究

前瞻性队列研究是队列研究的基本形式。研究对象的分组是根据研究开始时研究对象的暴露状况而定的，此时研究的结局还没有出现，需要前瞻性观察一段时间才能得到。这样的设计模式即称为前瞻性或即时性（concurrent）队列研究。在前瞻性队列研究中，由于研究者可以直接获取关于暴露与结局的第一手资料，因而资料的偏倚较小，结果可信。其缺点是所需观察的人群样本很大，随访观察时间长、花费大，因而影响其可行性。

tive cohort studies requires to observe a large number of population sample, and needs a long time to observe and expensive, all those affecting their viability.

2. Historical cohort studies

A historic cohort study generally means to take a look back at events that already have taken place. For example, the term is used in medicine, describing a look back at a patient's medical history or lifestyle. In the case of a historic cohort study, the investigator collects data from past records and does not follow patients up as is the case with a prospective study. However, the starting point of this study is the same as for all cohort studies. The first objective is still to establish two groups — exposed versus non-exposed; and these groups are followed up in the ensuing time period. In a nutshell, in historic cohort study, all the events-exposure, latent period, and subsequent outcomes (ex. development of disease) have already occurred in the past. We merely collect the data now, and establish the risk of developing a disease if exposed to a particular risk factor. On the other hand, Historic cohort study is conducted by starting with two groups at the current point, and following up in future for occurrence of disease, if any. Historic cohort studies have the following distinct advantages when compared with prospective cohort studies: They are conducted on a smaller scale, they typically require less time to complete, they are better for analyzing multiple outcomes, and in a medical context, they can potentially address rare diseases, which would necessitate extremely large cohorts in prospective studies. The fact that retrospective studies are generally less expensive than prospective studies also can be a key benefit.

2. 历史性队列研究

历史性队列研究中，研究对象的分组是根据研究开始时研究者已掌握的有关研究对象在过去某个时点的暴露状况的历史材料做出的。研究开始时研究的结局已经出现，不需要前瞻性观察，这样的设计模式称为历史性或非即时性（non-concurrent）队列研究。在历史性队列研究中，虽然研究是从现在开始的，但研究对象是在过去某个时点进入队列的；虽然暴露与结局跨时较长，但资料搜集及分析却可以在较短时期内完成；虽然搜集暴露与结局资料的方法是回顾性的，但究其性质而言，其仍属前瞻性观察，仍是从因到果的。因此，该法是一种深受欢迎的快速的队列研究方法，具有省时、省力、出结果快的特点。缺点是因资料积累时未受到研究者的控制，可能存在偏差。

3. Ambispective cohort studies

Ambispective cohort studies are also called mixed cohort study. It means to conduct a study that is a combination of prospective cohort and retrospective cohort designs. With this approach, exposure is ascertained from objective records in the past (as in a historical cohort study), and follow-up and measurement of outcome continue into the future.

5.1.5 The selection principle of different types

1. Prospective cohort studies

When choose the prospective cohort study, we should consider that:

① Should have a definite hypothesis testing.

② The incidence or mortality rate of disease in study should be higher, such as no less than 5‰.

③ Should be clearly stipulated the exposures.

④ Should be clearly stipulated the outcome variable.

⑤ We should be sure to get enough people to observe, and divide them into exposed group and non-exposed group clearly.

⑥ Most of the objects could be followed for a long time.

⑦ Should have enough people, money and material resources to support the work.

2. Historical cohort studies

When choose the historical cohort study, we should consider all notes mentioned above, and also consider if there have enough, complete and reliable historical records or archives about the exposure and outcomes of objects. Such as a hospital's medical re-

3. 双向性队列研究

双向性队列研究也称混合型队列研究，即在历史性队列研究的基础上，继续前瞻性观察一段时间。它是将前瞻性队列研究与历史性队列研究结合起来的一种设计模式，因此兼有上述两类的优点，也在一定程度上弥补了各自的不足。

5.1.5 不同研究类型的选用原则

1. 前瞻性队列研究

选择前瞻性队列研究时，应重点考虑以下条件：

①有明确的病因检验假设。

②所研究疾病的发病率或死亡率应较高，如不低于5‰。

③应明确规定暴露因素，并且应有把握获得观察人群的暴露资料。

④应明确规定结局变量，如发病或死亡，并且要有可确定结局的简便、可靠的手段。

⑤应有把握获得足够的观察人群，并可以明确地将其分成暴露组与非暴露组。

⑥大部分观察人群应能被长期随访，并能取得完整可靠的资料。

⑦应有足够的人力、财力、物力支持该项工作。

2. 历史性队列研究

选择历史性队列研究时，除了应考虑前瞻性队列研究中需要注意的问题外，还应考虑是否有足够数量的、完整可靠的、在过去某段时间内有关研究对象暴露和结局的历史记录或档案材料，如医院的病历、个人的医疗档案及工厂和车间的

cords, personal medical files, and a variety of factories and workshops record.

3. Ambispective cohort studies

When basically have a historical cohort study conditions, and also need to follow-up and measurement of outcome continue for an extended period, in this case, we choose ambispective cohort studies.

5.2   Design and Implementation

5.2.1   The study factors

The study factors (exposure) are usually determined on the basis of descriptive studies and case - control studies. We should consider that how to select, define and measure exposures, and consider the way of exposure, such as intermittent exposure or continuous exposure, exposure directly or indirectly, short - term exposure or long - term exposure. And the way of measure the exposure should be sensitive, accurate, simple and reliable.

5.2.2   The research outcomes

Outcomes means the events of expected result that will appear in follow - up, also means the natural end of cohort study. Outcomes are not only confined to the morbidity, mortality, they also could be the changes in the health and life quality. They could be the ultimate consequence (such as morbidity or mortality), also could be the intermediate outcomes (such as the changes of molecules or serum). The outcomes should have a clear unified standard.

各种记录等。只有具备以上条件, 才适合做历史性队列研究。

3. 双向性队列研究

基本具备历史性队列研究的条件后, 如果从暴露到现在的观察时间还不能满足研究的要求, 还需继续前瞻性观察一段时间才可观察到研究的结局, 则选用双向性队列研究。

5.2   研究设计与实施

5.2.1   确定研究因素

队列研究中的研究因素 (暴露) 通常在描述性研究和病例对照研究的基础上确定。应该考虑如何选择、定义和测量暴露, 并考虑暴露的方式, 如间歇暴露或连续暴露、直接暴露或间接暴露、短期暴露或长期暴露。暴露应尽可能选择客观、可测量的因素, 测量方法应灵敏、准确、简便、可靠。

5.2.2   确定研究结局

结局是指随访中出现的预期结果事件, 也意味着队列研究的自然结束。结局不仅限于发病率、死亡率, 还可能是健康和生活质量的变化。它们可能是最终结局 (如发病率或死亡率), 也可能是中间结局 (如分子或血清的变化)。结局应该有一个明确的统一标准。

5.2.3 The study site and study population

1. The study site

The cohort study site selection requires a sufficient number of qualified objects, also requires local leaders attaches great importance to the study, understanding and support of the masses. It is best that the local educational level is higher, health conditions are better, and the traffic is convenient.Of course, we must consider the representation of site.

2. The study population

（1）The selection of exposure population

① Occupational groups.

② Special exposure population.

③ General population.

④ Organized population.

（2）The selection of control population

① Internal control.

② External control.

③ Total population control.

④ Multiple controls

5.2.4 Size of sample

1. Considerations

① Sampling methods.

② The proportion between exposure group and control group.

③ The rate of lost to follow-up.

2. The influencing factors of sample size

① Incidence of the study disease in control population (p_0).

② Difference between the incidence of exposure group and control group.

③ Significance level (α). α is the probability of

5.2.3 确定研究现场与研究人群

1. 确定研究现场

由于队列研究的随访时间长，因此，队列研究的现场选择除要求有足够数量的、符合条件的研究对象外，还要求当地的领导能够重视，群众能够理解和支持，最好是当地的文化教育水平较高、医疗卫生条件较好、交通较便利的现场。选择符合这些条件的现场，将使随访调查更加顺利，所获资料更加可靠。当然，也要考虑现场的代表性。

2. 确定研究人群

（1）暴露人群的选择

①职业人群。

②特殊暴露人群。

③一般人群。

④有组织的团体。

（2）对照人群的选择

①内对照。

②外对照。

③总人口对照。

④多重对照。

5.2.4 确定样本量

1. 要考虑的因素

①抽样方法。

②暴露组与对照组的比例。

③失访率。

2. 样本量的影响因素

①一般人群（对照人群）中所研究疾病的发病率p_0。

②暴露组与对照组人群发病率之差。

③显著性水平（α）。α是假设检验中出现 I

Error type Ⅰ in hypothesis testing.

④Power ($1-\beta$), β is the probability of Error type Ⅱ in hypothesis testing. Power can be explained by the ability to reject the null hypothesis. When the null hypothesis is not establishment, the probability of the null hypothesis is rejected.

3. Calculation of size of sample

$$n = \frac{\left(z_\alpha \sqrt{2\overline{pq}} + z_\beta \sqrt{p_0 q_0 + p_1 q_1}\right)^2}{\left(p_1 - p_0\right)^2} \qquad (5-1)$$

p_1 and p_0 are expected incidence of exposed group and control group, $\overline{P}$ is mean value of the two incidence, $q=1-p$, z_α and z_β are areas under the standard normal distribution.

Example: Discuss the relation between pregnant women exposed to a particular drug and infants with congenital heart disease in a cohort study. And we had known the incidence of infants with congenital heart disease in non-exposed group was 0.007, and the estimated RR of drug exposure was 2.5, assume that α= 0.05 (two-tailed), β=0.10. Calculate the size of sample.

$z_\alpha = 1.96$, $z_\beta = 1.282$, $p_0 = 0.007$, $q_0 = 0.993$

$p_1 = RR \cdot p_0 = 2.5 \times 0.007 = 0.017\,5$,

$q_1 = 0.982\,5\,\overline{p} = \frac{1}{2}(0.007 + 0.017\,5) = 0.012\,3$,

$\overline{q} = 0.987\,7$

Use the formula 5-1

$n=(1.96\sqrt{2 \times 0.012\,3 \times 0.987\,7} +$

$\quad 1.282\sqrt{0.017\,5 \times 0.982\,5 + 0.007 \times 0.993}\,)^2/$

$(0.017\,5 - 0.007)^2 = 2\,310$

So the number of exposed group and non - exposed are 2 310.

If we consider the possibility of lost to follow - up, the sample sizes are remains to be increased by 10% based on this. So the actual required numbers of two

类错误的概率。

④效力（$1-\beta$），β是假设检验中出现Ⅱ类错误的概率。效力可以用拒绝无效假设的能力来解释，即无效假设未建立时，无效假设被拒绝的概率。

3. 样本量的计算

$$n = \frac{\left(z_\alpha \sqrt{2\overline{pq}} + z_\beta \sqrt{p_0 q_0 + p_1 q_1}\right)^2}{\left(p_1 - p_0\right)^2} \qquad (5-1)$$

式中，p_1与p_0分别代表暴露组与对照组的预期发病率，$\overline{P}$为两组发病率的平均值，$q=1-p$，z_α和z_β为标准正态分布下的面积，可查表获知。

例如，用队列研究探讨孕妇暴露于某药物与婴儿患先天性心脏病之间的联系。非暴露孕妇所生婴儿的先天性心脏病发病率（p_0）为0.007，估计该药物暴露的RR为2.5，设α=0.05（双侧），β= 0.10，求调查所需的样本量。

$z_\alpha = 1.96$，$z_\beta = 1.282$，$p_0 = 0.007$，$q_0 = 0.993$

$p_1 = RR \cdot p_0 = 2.5 \times 0.007 = 0.017\,5$，

$q_1 = 0.982\,5\,\overline{p} = \frac{1}{2}(0.007 + 0.017\,5) = 0.012\,3$，

$\overline{q} = 0.987\,7$

将上述数据代入式5-1：

$n=(1.96\sqrt{2 \times 0.012\,3 \times 0.987\,7} +$

$\quad 1.282\sqrt{0.017\,5 \times 0.982\,5 + 0.007 \times 0.993}\,)^2/$

$(0.017\,5 - 0.007)^2 = 2\,310$

即暴露组与非暴露组各需2 310人。

如果考虑失访的可能性，还需在此基础上增加10%的样本量，即两组实际需要的样本数量各为$n=2\,310\times(1 +0.1) = 2\,541$人。如果抽样方法不

groups are $n = 2\,310 \times (1 + 0.1) = 2\,541$.

是单纯随机抽样，还需适当增加样本量。

5.2.5 Data collection and follow-up

1. Baseline data collection

Baseline data generally include exposure condition, status of disease and health, personal situation such as age, gender, occupation, culture and marriage and so on, family environment, personal lifestyle, family history of disease. The methods of getting baseline data:

① Checking back the records or files of hospital, factory, department or private health insurance.

② Interviewing objects of study.

③ Doing physical examination and laboratory tests to objects.

④ The environmental investigation and detection.

2. Follow-up

① Object and methods of follow-up. We should use the same method to conduct the follow-up in exposed group and non-exposed group, and adhere to trace the end-point. The method of follow-up include face to face interview, telephone interview, self-administered, periodic physical examination, the environment and disease surveillance, etc.

② Content of follow-up. The content of follow-up generally consistent with the baseline data, but follow-up collection focuses on the outcome variables.

③ End-point. End-point means the object of study appeared the expected results. If the object appeared the end-point, it is no longer continuing to follow-up.

④ Terminal time of observation. Terminal time of observation means the cut-off date (or deadline) of the whole research work.

5.2.5 收集资料与随访

1. 基线资料的收集

基线资料一般包括待研究暴露因素的暴露状况，疾病与健康状况，年龄、性别、职业、文化、婚姻等个人状况，家庭环境，个人生活习惯，家族疾病史等。获取基线资料的方式一般有下列4种：

①查阅医院、工厂、单位及个人健康保险的记录或档案。

②访问研究对象或其他能够提供信息的人。

③对研究对象进行体格检查和实验室检查。

④环境调查与检测。

2. 随访

①随访的目的和方法。对暴露组和非暴露组应采用同样的方法进行随访，并坚持追踪至终点。随访方法包括面对面访谈、电话访谈、自填问卷、定期体检、环境与疾病监测等。

②随访内容。随访内容通常与基线数据一致，但随访收集的重点是结局变量。

③观察终点。终点是指研究对象出现了预期的结果。如果研究对象发生了观察终点事件，则不再继续跟踪。

④观察终止时间。观察终止时间是指整个研究工作的截止日期。

⑤ The interval of follow‐up. Generally the interval of follow‐up of chronic disease is 1‐2 year.

⑥Investigators could be general inquiries investigators, or can also be laboratory technicians, clinicians. All investigators must be training seriously.

5.2.6 Quality control

General quality control measures include the following points:

① The choice of the investigator.
② The training of investigators.
③ Making the investigator manual.
④ Supervision.

5.3 Data Collection and Analysis

Before data analysis, we should examine the data firstly, to understand the correctness and integrity of the data. To reinvestigate, correct or eliminate the wrong data; to replenish the incomplete data. And then describe the data to analyze the comparability of two groups and reliability of the data. Finally, analyze the difference between two groups, conclude the effect of exposure.

5.3.1 Mode of data arrangement

The mode of data arrangement shows in Table 5‐1. a/n_1 and c/n_0 are incidence of exposed group and non‐exposed group.

⑤随访时间间隔。一般而言，慢性病的随访时间间隔为1～2年。

⑥调查人员可以是一般调查人员，也可以是实验室技术人员、临床医生。所有调查人员都必须接受统一的严格培训。

5.2.6 质量控制

一般而言，质量控制措施包括以下几点：

①研究者的选择。
②调查人员的培训。
③编制调查人员手册。
④监督。

5.3 资料的整理与分析

分析资料前，首先应对资料进行审查，了解资料的准确性与完整性。对有明显错误的资料应进行重新调查、修正或剔除，对不完整的资料要设法补齐。在此基础上，先对资料做描述性统计，即描述研究对象的组成、人口学特征、随访时间及失访情况等，分析两组的可比性及资料的可靠性，然后再做推断性分析，分析两组率的差异，推断暴露的效应及其大小。

5.3.1 基本整理模式

根据统计分析的要求，队列研究的资料一般整理成表5-1所示的模式。式中，a/n_1和c/n_0分别为暴露组的发病率和非暴露组的发病率，是统计分析的关键指标。

Table 5-1　The mode of data arrangement
in cohort study

	Case	Non-case	Total	Incidence
Exposed group	a	b	$a+b=n_1$	a/n_1
Non-exposed group	c	d	$c+d=n_0$	c/n_0
Total	$a+c=m_1$	$b+d=m_0$	$a+b+c+d=t$	

5.3.2　Calculation of ratio

Indicators commonly used:

（1）Cumulative incidence

Cumulative incidence is defined as the probability that a particular event, such as occurrence of a particular disease, has occurred before a given time. It is equivalent to the incidence, calculated using a period of time during which all of the individuals in the population are considered to be at risk for the outcome. It is sometimes also referred to as the incidence proportion. Cumulative incidence is calculated by the number of new cases during a period divided by the number of subjects at risk in the population at the beginning of the study.

（2）Incidence density

The incidence rate is the number of new cases per population at risk in a given time period. When the denominator is the sum of the person-time of the at risk population, it is also known as the incidence density.

（3）Standardized ratio

Standardized mortality ratio (SMR), this is the ratio of the number of observed deaths in a study group to the number that would be expected if the study group had the same specific rates as in a standard group. This procedure is the same as indirect method of standardization. The ratio is sometimes multiplied by 100 to express it in terms of percentage.

表5-1　队列研究资料的归纳整理表

	病例	非病例	合计	发病率
暴露组	a	b	$a+b=n_1$	a/n_1
非暴露组	c	d	$c+d=n_0$	c/n_0
合计	$a+c=m_1$	$b+d=m_0$	$a+b+c+d=t$	

5.3.2　率的计算

常用以下指标:

（1）累积发病率

累积发病率定义为特定事件（如特定疾病的发生）在特定时间内的发生概率，相当于观察期间的发病率。在此期间，人群中的所有个体都被认为存在发生结局的风险。累积发病率有时也称为发病率比例。累积发病率以观察期内的新发病（死亡）例数为分子，以观察开始时人群中具有发病风险的人数（暴露人口）为分母。累积发病率通常用于固定队列的计算。

（2）发病密度

当研究对象进入队列的时间先后不一致时，即为动态队列。以总人数为单位计算发病率是不合理的，此时需要以观察人时为分母计算发病率，用人时为单位计算出来的率即为发病密度。

（3）标准化比

当研究对象数目较少，结局事件发生率很低时，不易计算率。此时，用研究人群中实际观察到的死亡数与通过标准人口死亡率计算出的预期死亡数相比得到的标准化死亡比作为评价指标。该比率有时乘以100，以百分比表示。

$$SMR = \frac{\text{Observed number of deaths}}{\text{Expected number of deaths}} \quad (5\text{-}2)$$

The denominator is based on the specific rates in the chosen standard population. These are not necessarily age specific but could be gender specific, exposure specific, or specific for any other categorization. An *SMR* greater than 1 is interpreted as indicating that the study group has excess mortality relative to the standard. The study and the standard group can be disease and control groups in a case-control study or general populations of two types or any other groups of interest. In this method, more stable rates of the larger population are applied to the smaller study group to obtain the expected number of deaths. SMR gives a measure of the likely excess or reduction in mortality in the study group.

5.3.3　Significance test

1. *U* test

When the size of sample is bigger, both p and $1-p$ are not too small, for example, both np and $n(1-p)$ are bigger than 5, the frequency distribution of sample rate approximately normal distribution. Now we could use U test to test the difference of rate between exposed group and non-exposed group.

$$U = \frac{p_1 - p_0}{\sqrt{p_c(1 - p_c)(1/n_1 + 1/n_0)}} \quad (5\text{-}3)$$

In this formula, p_1 is the rate of exposed group, p_0 is the rate of control group, n_1 is the number of observation in exposed group, n_0 is the number of observation in control group. $p_c = (X_1 + X_2)/(n_1 + n_0)$, X_1 and X_0 are occurrence number of outcomes in exposed group and control group.

$$SMR = \frac{\text{研究人群中观察到的死亡数}(O)}{\text{以标准人口死亡率计算出的}\atop\text{预期死亡数}(E)} \quad (5\text{-}2)$$

分母基于所选标准总体中的特定比率，可以是年龄别率，也可以是性别、特定暴露或其他专率。*SMR* 大于1表示研究人群的死亡率高于标准人群。研究人群和标准人群可以是病例对照研究中的病例组和对照组，也可以是两种类型的普通人群或任何其他感兴趣的群体。在该方法中，将较大人群中更稳定的比率应用于较小的研究人群，以获得预期的死亡人数。*SMR* 是一种测量死亡率超额或者死亡率减少的指标。

5.3.3　显著性检验

1. *U* 检验

当研究样本量 n 较大，p 和 $1-p$ 都不太小时，如 np 和 $n(1-p)$ 均大于5，样本率的频数分布近似正态分布，此时可应用正态分布的原理来检验率的差异是否有统计学意义，即可用 U 检验法来检验暴露组与对照组之间率的差异。

$$U = \frac{p_1 - p_0}{\sqrt{p_c(1 - p_c)(1/n_1 + 1/n_0)}} \quad (5\text{-}3)$$

式中，p_1 为暴露组的率，p_0 为对照组的率，n_1 为暴露组的观察人数，n_0 为对照组的观察人数，p_c 为合并样本率，$p_c = (X_1 + X_2)/(n_1 + n_0)$，其中 X_1 和 X_0 分别为暴露组和对照组结局事件的发生数。求出 U 值后，查 U 界值表可得 P 值，按所取的检验水准即可作出判断。

2. Other test methods

Exact probability test, binomial test or Poisson distribution test; chi-square test, score test.

5.3.4 Effect estimates

1. Relative risk (RR)

Relative risk (RR) is the ratio of the probability of an event occurring (for example, developing a disease, being injured) in an exposed group to the probability of the event occurring in a comparison, non-exposed group. Rate ratio is the ratio of the incidence density in an exposed group to the incidence density in a comparison, non-exposed group.

$$RR = \frac{I_e}{I_0} = \frac{a/n_1}{c/n_0} \tag{5-4}$$

In this formula, I_e and I_0 are the ratio in exposed group and non-exposed group. The value of RR is bigger, reflects the association between exposure and outcomes is bigger.

Table 5-2　Relative risk (RR) and strength of association

RR		Strength of association
0.9-1.0	1.0-1.1	No
0.7-0.8	1.2-1.4	Weak
0.4-0.6	1.5-2.9	Middle
0.1-0.3	3.0-9.9	Strong
<0.1	10-	Very strong

（Monson, 1980）

The relative risk calculated by formula 5-4 is just a point estimate. We could use the methods of Woolf and Miettinen, and we advocate using the method of Woolf.

$$Var(\ln RR) = \frac{1}{a} + \frac{1}{b} + \frac{1}{c} + \frac{1}{d} \tag{5-5}$$

2. 其他检验方法

其他检验方法包括：精确概率检验，二项检验或泊松分布检验，卡方检验，分数检验。

5.3.4　效应的估计

1. 相对危险度(RR)

相对危险度（RR）是暴露组发生结局事件的概率（如发生疾病、受伤）与非暴露（对照）组发生结局事件的概率之比。率比是暴露组的发病率密度与对照组的发病率密度之比。

$$RR = \frac{I_e}{I_0} = \frac{a/n_1}{c/n_0} \tag{5-4}$$

式中，I_e 和 I_0 分别代表暴露组和对照组的率。RR 表示暴露组发病或死亡的危险是对照组的多少倍。RR 值越大，表明暴露的效应越大，暴露与结局的关联强度越大。

表5-2　相对危险度(RR)与关联的强度

RR		关联的强度
0.9～1.0	1.0～1.1	无
0.7～0.8	1.2～1.4	弱
0.4～0.6	1.5～2.9	中
0.1～0.3	3.0～9.9	强
<0.1	10～	很强

（Monson，1980）

据式5-4算出的相对危险度 RR 只是一个点的估计值，可以使用Woolf法和Miettinen法计算 RR 的可信区间，此处使用Woolf法计算。

$$Var(\ln RR) = \frac{1}{a} + \frac{1}{b} + \frac{1}{c} + \frac{1}{d} \tag{5-5}$$

The 95% confidence interval of lnRR=lnRR ± $1.96\sqrt{Var(\ln RR)}$, and its natural logarithm is the 95% confidence interval of RR.

Odds ratio (OR) is often a good approximation to the relative risk when the disease in question is rare. Referring to Table 5-1, when the disease is rare, it must be that

$a+b \approx b$

$c+d \approx d$

where ≈means "approximately equal to". Hence,

$$OR = ad/bc \approx \frac{a(c+d)}{(a+b)c} = RR$$

2. Attributable risk (AR)

AR is also called risk difference and excess risk. It is the difference in incidence between an exposed population and an unexposed population.

$$AR = I_e - I_0 = \frac{a}{n_1} - \frac{c}{n_0} \qquad (5-6)$$

Because

$$RR = \frac{I_e}{I_0}, \qquad I_e = RR \times I_0$$

So

$$AR = RR \times I_0 - I_0 = I_0(RR-1) \qquad (5-7)$$

3. Relative risk versus a attributable risk

Relative risk is important in etiological enquiries. Its size a better index than is attributable risk for assessing etiological role of a factor in disease. The larger the relative risk, the stronger the association between cause and effect. But relative risk dose not reflect the potential public health importance as does the attributable risk. That is, attributable risk gives a better idea than dose relative risk of the impact of successful preventive or public health programme might have in reducing the problem.

Two examples are cited (Tables 5-3 and 5-4) to

lnRR的95%可信区间=lnRR ± $1.96\sqrt{Var(\ln RR)}$，其反自然对数即为RR的95%可信区间。

当疾病的发病率较低时，OR值与RR值相近，如表5-1所示。当为罕见病时，

$a+b \approx b$

$c+d \approx d$

≈的意思是"近似等同于"。因此

$$OR = ad/bc \approx \frac{a(c+d)}{(a+b)c} = RR$$

2. 归因危险度(attributable risk, AR)

AR是暴露组发病率与对照组发病率之差，它表示危险特异地归因于暴露因素的超额数量。

$$AR = I_e - I_0 = \frac{a}{n_1} - \frac{c}{n_0} \qquad (5-6)$$

由于

$$RR = \frac{I_e}{I_0}, \qquad I_e = RR \times I_0$$

所以

$$AR = RR \times I_0 - I_0 = I_0(RR-1) \qquad (5-7)$$

3. 相对危险度与归因危险度

在病因调查中，相对危险度是很重要的。相对危险度比归因危险度更适合用来评估病因关联的作用。相对风险越大，因果关系越强。归因危险度更适合反映潜在的公共健康重要性。也就是说，归因危险度比相对危险度更具疾病预防和公共卫生学意义。

现引用两个例子（表5-3和5-4）来区分相对

show the practical importance of distinguishing relative and attributable risk. In the first example (Table 5-3), the *RR* of a cardiovascular complication in users of oral contraceptives is independent of age, whereas the *AR* is more than 5 times higher in the older age groups. This epidemiological observation has been the basis for not recommending oral contraceptive in those aged 35 years and over.

Table 5-3　The relative and attributable risks of cardiovascular complications in women taking oral contraceptives

Cardiovascular risk (100 000 patient years)	Ages	
	30-39	40-44
Relative risk	2.8	2.8
Attributable risk	3.5	20

The second example (Table 5-4) shows that smoking is attributable to 92.2 per cent of lung cancer, and 13.3 percent of CHD. In CHD, both *RR* and *AR* are not very high suggesting not much of the disease could be prevented as compared to lung cancer.

Table 5-4　Risk assessment, smokers vs non-smokers

Cause of death	Death rate/‰		RR	AR /%
	Smokers	Non-smokers		
Lung cancer	0.90	0.07	12.86	92.2
CHD	4.87	4.22	1.15	13.3

4. Attributable risk proportion or percent (ARP or AR%)

The attributable risk proportion is also called etiologic fraction (EF) or attributable fraction (AF). It is a calculation that can be derived from attributable risk. It gives the portion of cases attributable (and avoidable) to this exposure in relation to all cases. It can be calculated as (relative risk − 1) / relative risk.

危险度和归因危险度各自的意义。第一个例子（表5-3）显示，服用口服避孕药者心血管并发症的*RR*与年龄无关，而*AR*则在40～44岁组中是30～39岁组的5倍以上。这个研究结果为35岁以上的人不推荐口服避孕药提供了依据。

表5-3　服用口服避孕药的妇女心血管并发症的相对危险度（RR）和归因危险度（AR）

心血管疾病 （1/10万人年）	年龄	
	30～39岁	40～44岁
RR	2.8	2.8
AR	3.5	20

第二个例子（表5-4）显示，肺癌中有92.2%可归因于吸烟，冠心病中有13.3%可归因于吸烟。与肺癌相比，冠心病患者的*RR*和*AR*都不是非常高，并且预防效果不佳。

表5-4　吸烟者与非吸烟者的危险评估

死因	死亡率/‰		RR	AR /%
	吸烟	不吸烟		
肺癌	0.90	0.07	12.86	92.2
冠心病	4.87	4.22	1.15	13.3

4. 归因危险度百分比（attributable risk proportion or percent, ARP, AR%）

归因危险度百分比又称为病因分值（etiologic fraction, EF）或归因分值（attributable fraction, AF），是指暴露人群中的发病或死亡归因于暴露的部分占全部发病或死亡的百分比。

$$AR\% = \frac{I_e - I_0}{I_e} \times 100\% \qquad (5\text{-}8)$$

Or,

$$AR\% = \frac{RR - 1}{RR} \times 100\% \qquad (5\text{-}9)$$

5. Population attributable risk（PAR）and population attributable risk proportion or percent（PAR%）

Population attributable risk proportion or percent is also called population etiologic fraction（PEF）or population attributable fraction. *PAR* has been described as the reduction in incidence that would be observed if the population were entirely unexposed, compared with its current（actual）exposure pattern. Population attributable fraction guides policy makers in planning public health interventions. Population attributable fraction（PAF）, population attributable risk proportion, and population attributable risk percent are all the same as *PAR*.

RR and *AR* are the comparison between exposed group and control group, reflecting biological effect of exposure, which is pathogenic effect of exposure. *PAR* and *PAR%* are the comparison between exposed group and all population, reflecting the harm of exposure to a specific population, and injury extent of exposure to a specific population.

The attributable risk in a population depends on the prevalence of the risk factor and the strength of its association（relative risk）with the disease, and the reduction in incidence or mortality rate that would be observed if the population was entirely unexposed. The formula of *PAR* and *PAR%* as follow：

$$PAR = I_t - I_0 \qquad (5\text{-}10)$$

I_t is the rate of the population, I_0 is the rate of control group.

$$AR\% = \frac{I_e - I_0}{I_e} \times 100\% \qquad (5\text{-}8)$$

或

$$AR\% = \frac{RR - 1}{RR} \times 100\% \qquad (5\text{-}9)$$

5. 人群归因危险度（population attributable risk, PAR）与人群归因危险度百分比（population attributable risk proportion or percent, PAR%）

人群归因危险度百分比也叫人群病因分值（population etiologic fraction, PEF）或人群归因分值。*PAR*是指总人群发病率中归因于暴露的部分，而*PAR%*是指*PAR*占总人群全部发病（或死亡）的百分比。

*RR*和*AR*是暴露组和非暴露组之间的比较，反映了暴露的生物学效应，即暴露的致病效应。*PAR*和*PAR%*是暴露人群和全人群的比较，反映了暴露对特定人群的危害，以及暴露对特定人群的伤害程度。

人群中的归因风险取决于风险因素的流行程度及其与疾病的关联强度（相对风险），以及在人群完全未暴露的情况下观察到的发病率或死亡率的降低。*PAR*和*PAR%*的公式如下：

$$PAR = I_t - I_0 \qquad (5\text{-}10)$$

式中，I_t为全人群的率，I_0为非暴露组的率。

$$PAR\% = \frac{I_t - I_0}{I_t} \times 100\% \qquad (5\text{-}11)$$

Non-exposed group as follow:

$$PAR\% = \frac{P_e(RR - 1)}{P_e(RR - 1) + 1} \times 100\%$$

P_e is the proportion of exposed people in the crowd.

6. Analysis of dose-response relationship

If there is a dose-response relationship between exposure and effect, means the greater the dose of exposure, the greater effect, and the greater likelihood of exposure as the cause.

5.4　The Common Bias and Its Control

A number of potential biases must be either avoided or taken into account in conducting cohort studies. The major biases include the following:

5.4.1　Bias in assessment of the outcome

If the person who decides whether disease has developed in each subject also knows whether that subject was exposed, and if that person is aware of the hypothesis being tested, that person's judgment as to whether the disease developed may be biased by that knowledge. This problem can be addressed by masking the person who is making the disease assessment and also by determining whether this person was, in fact, aware of each subject's exposure status.

5.4.2　Information bias

If the quality and extent of information obtained is different for exposedp ersons than for non-exposed persons, a significant bias can be introduced. This is particularly likely to occur in historical cohort studies,

$$PAR\% = \frac{I_t - I_0}{I_t} \times 100\% \qquad (5\text{-}11)$$

另外，$PAR\%$亦可由下式计算：

$$PAR\% = \frac{P_e(RR - 1)}{P_e(RR - 1) + 1} \times 100\%$$

式中，P_e表示人群中某种暴露者的比例。

6.剂量-反应关系的分析

如果暴露和效应之间存在剂量-反应关系，意味着暴露剂量越大，效应越大，暴露作为病因的可能性也越大。

5.4　常见偏倚及其控制

在进行队列研究时，必须避免或考虑到一些潜在的偏倚。主要偏倚包括：

5.4.1　结果评估的偏倚

如果统计分析者既知道研究对象的事件结局，也知道其暴露情况，那么在进行病因假设检验时，病因推断会因对信息熟知而产生偏倚。利用盲法隐藏有关疾病或暴露的信息可以解决相关问题。

5.4.2　信息偏倚

如果从暴露者中获得的信息的质量和程度与从非暴露者中获得的不同，则可能引入重大偏倚。这种情况尤其可能发生在历史队列研究中，其中的信息是从过去的记录中获得的。正如我们在随

in which information is obtained from past records. As we discussed with regard to randomized trials, in any cohort study, it is essential that the quality of the information obtained be comparable in both exposed and non-exposed individuals.

5.4.3　Biases from nonresponse and losses to follow-up

As was discussed in connection with randomized trials, nonparticipation and nonresponse can introduce major biases that can complicate the interpretation of the study findings. Similarly, loss to follow-up can be a serious problem: If people with the disease are selectively lost to follow-up, the incidence rates calculated in the exposed and non-exposed groups will clearly be difficult to interpret.

5.4.4　Analytic bias

As in any study, if the epidemiologists and statisticians who are analyzing the data have strong preconceptions, they may unintentionally introduce their biases into their data analyses and into their interpretation of the study findings.

5.5　Advantages and Disadvantages

5.5.1　Advantages

①Since comparison groups are formed before disease develops, certain forms of bias can be minimized like misclassification of individuals into exposed and unexposed groups. Generally there is no recall bias in cohort studies.

②We could get the incidence or mortality rate of exposed group and control group directly, and calcu-

机试验中所讨论的，在任何队列研究中，获得的信息质量在暴露和未暴露的个体中都应是可比较的。

5.4.3　无应答和失访偏倚

研究对象无应答或不参加调查可能会引入重大偏倚，使研究结果的解释复杂化。类似的，失访也可能是一个严重的问题。如果研究对象因为疾病而失访，暴露组和非暴露组发病率的差异显然很难解释。

5.4.4　分析偏倚

与任何研究一样，如果分析数据时有强烈的先入之见，数据分析和结果解释过程中可能会引入偏见。

5.5　优点与局限性

5.5.1　优点

①暴露资料是在疾病结局发生之前收集的，并且是按照设计由研究者亲自观察得到的，所以资料完整可靠，可以将个体被错误地分为暴露组和非暴露组的错分偏倚最小化，使信息偏倚相对较小。队列研究为前瞻性研究，因此不存在回忆偏倚。

②可以直接得到暴露组和对照组的发病率或死亡率，并可由此计算出反映疾病强度、风险的

late the index reflected strength of disease, risk such as RR and AR.

③ Dose-response ratios can also be calculated.

④ Cohort studies give direct information on the sequence of happenings. This is ideal for demonstrating causality and natural history of disease.

⑤ Several possible outcomes related to exposure can be studied simultaneously — that is, we can study the association of the suspected factor with many other diseases in addition to the one under study. For example, cohort studies designed to study the association between smoking and lung cancer also showed association of smoking with coronary heart disease, peptic ulcer, cancer esophagus and several others.

5.5.2 Disadvantages

① Cohort studies are not suitable for rare disease. If the disease is rare, then we would either need to take an enormous baseline sample or to monitor for a very long time.

② Loss to follow-up bias may occur. It is not unusual to loss a substantial proportion of the original cohort — they may migrate, lose interest in the study or simply refuse to provide any required information.

③ Cohort studies are often very expensive and time-consuming. Certain administrative problems such as loss of experienced staff, loss of funding and extensive record keeping are inevitable.

④ In the process of follow-up, the unknown variables or the change of the known variables all affected the outcomes, and complicated the analysis. Selection of comparison groups which are representative of the exposed and unexposed segments of the population is a limiting factor. Those who volunteer for the study may not be representative of all individuals with the

指标，如 RR 和 AR。

③可以分析剂量-反应关系。

④队列研究符合时间先后顺序，检验病因假设的能力较强，有助于研究者了解疾病自然史。

⑤可以同时观察一种暴露与多种结局的关系，也就是说，可以进行一因多果的研究。例如，用于研究吸烟和肺癌之间关联的队列研究，也可以用于分析吸烟与冠心病、消化性溃疡、食管癌和其他疾病之间的关系。

5.5.2 局限性

①队列研究不适用于罕见病的病因研究。研究罕见病时所需的样本量较大，随访观察的时间也较长。

②可能产生失访偏倚。由于需要随访，因此容易产生失访偏倚，如研究对象可能会迁移，也可能会失去对研究的兴趣，或者干脆拒绝提供任何必要的信息。

③队列研究通常耗费的人力、物力、财力和时间较多，其组织管理比较困难，如会缺乏经验丰富的工作人员和资金，而且还有大量的记录需要保存。

④在随访过程中，未知变量或已知变量的变化都会影响结果，使分析复杂化。队列研究是依据人们是否暴露于某因素而分组的，自愿参加研究的研究对象可能代表性不足。在长期随访中，疾病的诊断标准和暴露因素都可能发生变化，但研究必须按照制定的研究计划实施。

characteristic of interest. There may be changes in the standard methods on diagnostic criteria of the disease over prolonged follow-up. In long-term follow-up, the diagnostic standards and exposure factors of the disease may change, but the research must be implemented in accordance with the formulated research plan.

⑤ The study itself may alter people's behavior. If we are examining the role of smoking in lung cancer, an increased concern in the study cohort may be created. This may induce the study subjects to stop on decrease smoking.

⑥ With any cohort study we are faced with ethical problems of varying importance. As evidence accumulates about the implicating factor in the etiology of disease, we are obliged to intervene and if possible reduce or eliminate this factor.

5.6　Examples of Cohort Studies

【Example1】Smoking and lung cancer

At least eight prospective studies on the relation of smoking to lung cancer had been done. Doll and Hill, Hammond and Horn and Dorn were the first to report their findings.

In October 1951, Doll and Hill sent aquestionnaires to 59 600 British doctors listed in the Medical Register of the UK enquiring about their smoking habits. This enabled them to form two cohorts (smokers and non-smokers) who were similar in all other respects like age, education and social class. They received usable replies from 40 701physicians — 34 494 men and 6 207 women.

These were followed for 4 years and 5 months by obtaining notifications of physicians' deaths from the Registrar General, the General Medical Council and

⑤研究可能会改变人们的行为。如果研究吸烟在肺癌中的作用，对研究队列的关注可能会导致原本吸烟的人戒烟。

⑥在任何一项队列研究中，都要面临伦理学问题。对已有证据证明的致病因素，必须采取干预措施，减少或消除这一暴露因素。

5.6　队列研究实例

【例1】吸烟与肺癌

目前，关于吸烟与肺癌关系的前瞻性研究有多项。其中，Doll 和 Hill、Hammond 和 Horn 还有 Dorn 的研究结果在较早的时间就已报道。

1951 年 10 月，Doll 和 Hill 给英国医学登记册上的 59 600 名英国医生发放问卷来调查他们的吸烟习惯，据此将这些医生分成了两个队列（吸烟和不吸烟），这些医生在年龄、受教育程度和社会地位等其他方面都是相似的。最终，40 701 名医生给予了有效回复，包括 34 494 名男性和 6 207 名女性。随访 4 年零 5 个月后，他们从注册主任、总医务委员会和英国医学会获得部分医生死亡的通知。对于每一个因肺癌而死的病例，他们都向医生书面确认了其死因，并在必要时向医院或（顾问）医生询问了其基本情况。

the British Medical Association. For every death certified as due to lung cancer, confirmation was obtained by writing to the physician certifying the death and also, when necessary to the hospital or consultant to whom the patient had been referred.

【Example 2 】The Framingham Heart Study

The Framingham heart study was initiated in 1948 by the United States Public Health Service to study the relationship of a number of (risk) factors (e.g., serum cholesterol, blood pressure, weight, smoking) to the subsequent development of cardiovascular disease. The town of Framingham (Massachusetts) had a population of 28 000 in 1948. The study was planned for 20 years in view of the slow development of heart disease.

The lower and upper limits of the study population were set at 30 and 59 years. Out of 10 000 people in this age group a sample of 6 507 persons of both sexes were invited to participate in the study, out of which 5 209 participated. The initial examination revealed that 82 subjects had clinically evident CHD. These were excluded from the sample leaving a total of 5 127.

4 469 (69 percent) of the 6 507 in the initial sample actually underwent the first examination. After the first examination, the study population was examined every 2 years for a 20 years period. Information was obtained with regard to serum cholesterol, blood pressure, weight and cigarette smoking. Although biennial examinations were the main source of follow up-information, other means were also adopted to detect CHD (e.g., death certificate records).

Among other things, the study showed increasing risk of CHD with increasing serum cholesterol levels in the 45-54 age group. The study also showed that the

【例2】弗明汉心血管病研究

弗明汉心血管病研究于1948年由美国公共卫生局发起，目的是研究一些（危险）因素（如血清胆固醇、血压、体重、吸烟）与心血管疾病的关系。1948年，马萨诸塞州的弗明汉镇有28 000人。由于心脏病发展缓慢，这项研究计划了20年。

研究对象的年龄被限定在30岁到59岁之间，当时弗明汉镇共有10 000人处于这一年龄段，其中6 507人（男女都有）被邀请参加这项研究，最终5 209人参加了这项研究。基线调查发现82人有冠心病，故最终保留了其余5 127名没有冠心病的人作为队列研究的研究对象。

实际上，6 507人中有4 469人（69%）有第一次血检的信息。基线调查后，每隔2年对研究人群进行一次调查，为期20年，主要记录血清胆固醇、血压、体重与吸烟等信息。2年一度的调查是随访信息的主要来源，通过其他手段获得的信息也可以作为补充，如通过死亡证明确定的冠心病。

研究表明，45～54岁年龄组中，随血清胆固醇水平的升高，发生冠心病的风险也在增加。这项研究还表明，吸烟与冠心病的关系因疾病的表

association between smoking and CHD varied with manifestations of the disease. Thus, smoking was more strongly associated with sudden death from CHD than with less fatal forms of the disease. Risk factors have been found to include male sex, advancing age, high serum lipid concentration, high blood pressure, cigarette smoking, diabetes mellitus, obesity, low vital capacity and certain ECG abnormalities. The predictive value of serum lipids, blood pressure and cigarette smoking have been repeatedly demonstrated. The Framingham heart study become a prototype of similar studies in US and other countries.

【Example 3】 Oral contraceptives and health

Another example is the cohort study of oral contraceptives and health conducted by the Royal College of General Practitioners in England (1974). It was initiated in 1968, after 2 years of planning. 23 000 users of the pill aged 15-49 years together with a similar number of controls using other methods or no method of contraception were brought under observation of 1 400 general practitioners. During follow‐up doctors recorded the diagnoses of episodes of illness, and information about pregnancies and deaths.

The study brought out the risks and benefits of oral contraceptive use. For example, the study showed that the risk of hypertension increases, and the risk of benign breath disease decreases with the dose of norethisterone acetate (progestogen) in the combined pill which is an important finding. The study found an increased mortality from disease of cardiovascular system in pill users confirming the results of retrospective case control studies.

现而不同，吸烟与因冠心病猝死的关系比吸烟与非致命性疾病的关系更为密切。心血管病的危险因素有男性、高龄、高血脂、高血压、吸烟、糖尿病、肥胖、低肺活量和心电图异常等，其中血脂、血压和吸烟已多次被证实为冠心病的高危因素。后来，弗明汉心血管病研究成了美国和其他国家类似研究的典范。

【例3】口服避孕药与健康

另一个例子是皇家全科医师学院在英国进行的口服避孕药与健康之间关系的队列研究（1974）。经过2年的规划，该学院于1968年开始实施该研究。在15～49岁年龄组中，选取23 000名避孕药使用者为暴露组，选取相同数量的使用其他方法避孕或没有避孕的人为对照组，1 400名全科医生作为调查员实施调查。在随访过程中，医生记录了疾病的诊断，以及怀孕和死亡的信息。

这项研究揭示了口服避孕药的危险和益处。结果发现，随着醋酸炔诺酮（孕激素）剂量的增加，高血压的风险增加，而良性呼吸疾病的风险则降低。同时，还发现服用避孕药增加了心血管疾病的致死率，这也证实了回顾性病例对照研究的结果。

Chapter 6　Experimental Epidemiology

6.1　Summarize

6.1.1　Definition

Intervention or experimentation involves attempting to change a variable in one or more groups of people. This could mean the elimination of a dietary factor thought to cause allergy, or testing a new treatment on a selected group of patients. The effects of an intervention are measured by comparing the outcome in the experimental group with that in a control group. Since the interventions are strictly determined by the protocol, ethical considerations are of paramount importance in the design of these studies. For example, no patient should be denied appropriate treatment as a result of participation in an experiment, and the treatment being tested must be acceptable in the light of current knowledge.

6.1.2　Basic characteristic

① It belongs to prospective study.

② Random allocation.

③ Set up the control group.

④ It has the intervene measures.

The principle schematic diagram of experimental epidemiology is given in Figure 6-1.

第6章　实验流行病学

6.1　概述

6.1.1　定义

干预或实验是人为施加或去除某种因素，进而观察研究对象发生的改变，由此评价人为措施的效果。这可能意味着消除一种导致过敏的饮食因素，或者在选定的患者群体中评价一种新疗法的效果。通过比较和分析试验组和对照组的结局，从而判断干预措施的效果。但在设计研究方案中，出于伦理学的考虑，不能迫使人群暴露于某种危险因素。例如，对任何患者都不能因为其参与实验而不给予适当的治疗，并且被评价的干预措施必须是有益、无害且可接受的。

6.1.2　基本特点

①属于前瞻性研究。

②随机分组。

③设立对照组。

④有干预措施。

实验流行病学研究原理示意图见图6-1。

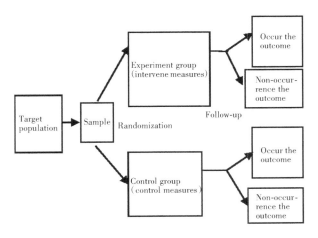

Figure 6-1　The principle schematic diagram of experimental epidemiology

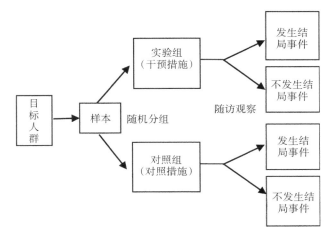

图 6-1　实验流行病学研究原理示意图

6.1.3　Types of experimental epidemiology

1. Clinical trial

There are two types:

① Randomized controlled trials (i. e., those involving a process of random allocation).

② Non-randomized or "non-experimental" trials (i. e., those departing from strict randomization for practical purposes, but in such a manner that non-randomization does not seriously affect the theoretical basis of conclusions).

2. Field trial

3. Community trial

6.2　Clinical Trial

6.2.1　Main application

① Treatment study.

② Diagnosis study.

③ Screening study.

④ Prognosis study.

⑤ Pathogenesis study.

6.1.3　实验流行病学的类型

1. 临床试验

有两种类型：

①随机对照试验（即涉及随机化分组）。

②非随机或"准实验"研究（即因为可行性，无法进行随机化分组的实验研究，需要注意非随机化不能影响研究的结论）。

2. 现场试验

3. 社区试验

6.2　临床试验

6.2.1　主要用途

①治疗研究。

②诊断研究。

③筛检研究。

④预后研究。

⑤发病机制研究。

6.2.2　Basic principle of clinical trial

① Randomly.

② Control.

③ Repeat.

④ Objective.

⑤ Multi-center.

⑥ Behave ethically.

6.2.3　Basic design types of clinical trial

① Parallel design.

② Cross-over design.

③ Factorial design.

④ Sequential design.

6.2.4　Issues that requires attention

① Patient compliance.

② Clinical disagreement.

③ Placebo effect.

④ Regression to the mean.

⑤ Contamination and interference.

⑥ Adverse event.

6.2.5　Design of Randomized controlled trials

Too often physicians are guided in their daily work by clinical impressions of their own or their teachers. These impressions, particularly when they are incorporated in textbooks and repeatedly quoted by reputed teachers and their students were acquired authority, just as if they were proved facts. Similarly many public health measures are introduced on the basis of assumed benefits without subjecting them to rigorous testing. The history of medicine amply illustrates

6.2.2　临床试验的基本原则

①随机。

②对照。

③重复。

④客观。

⑤多中心。

⑥符合伦理道德要求。

6.2.3　临床试验的基本设计类型

①平行设计。

②交叉设计。

③析因设计。

④序贯设计。

6.2.4　需要注意的问题

①患者依从性。

②临床分歧。

③安慰剂效应。

④向平均值回归。

⑤污染和干扰。

⑥不良事件。

6.2.5　随机对照试验的设计步骤

医生往往根据自己的经验或上级医生的临床指导开展临床医疗的日常工作。尤其教科书上的知识，被很多专家和医生视作权威而在临床实践中广泛应用，就好像这些知识被证明是事实一样。同样，许多公共卫生措施也是在假定有益的基础上实施的，并没有通过严格的测试去证明。医学史上的很多实例也充分阐明了这一点。例如，目前被医学界证明并摒弃的治疗性放血和剧烈催泻。

this. For instance, it took centuries before therapeutic blood letting and drastic purging were abandoned by the medical profession.

It is mainly in the last many years, determined effort have been made to use scientific techniques to evaluate methods of treatment and prevention. An important advance in this field has been the development of an assessment method, known as Randomized Controlled Trial (RCT). It is really an epidemiologic experiment. Since its introduction, the RCT has questioned the validity of such widely used treatments as oral hypoglycemic agents, varicose vein stripping, and tonsillectomy, hospitalization of all patients with myocardial infarction, multiphasic screening, and toxicity and applicability of many preventive and therapeutic procedures.

The design of a randomized controlled trial is given in Figure 6-2. For new programmes or new therapies, the RCT is the No.1 method of evaluation. The basic steps in conducting a RCT include the following :

在过去的许多年中，研究人员在利用科学方法评价治疗和预防措施效果方面做了大量研究工作。其中，随机对照试验（RCT）的开发是评价治疗和预防措施效果的科学方法的重要进展。RCT出现以后，已经对曾广泛使用的一些治疗方法进行了评价，如口服降糖药、静脉曲张剥脱术、扁桃体摘除术、所有心肌梗死患者的住院治疗及多项筛查，以及许多预防和治疗方法的毒性和适用性。

随机对照试验的设计如图6-2所示。对新方案或新疗法的效果进行评价时，RCT是首选的评估方法。RCT的基本使用步骤包括以下内容：

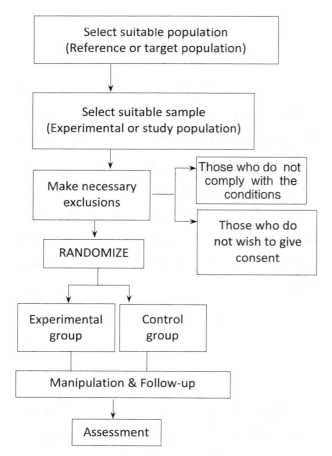

Figure 6-2　Design of a randomized controlled trial

1. The protocol

One of the essential features of a randomized controlled trial is that the study is conducted under a strict protocol. The protocol specifies the aims and objectives of the study, questions to be answered, criteria for the selection of study and control groups, size of the sample, the procedures for allocation of subjects into study and control groups, treatments to be applied — when and where and how to what kind of patients, standardization of working procedures and schedules as well as responsibilities of the parties involved in the trial, up to the stage of evaluation of outcome of the study. A protocol is essential especially when a number of centres are participating in the trial. Once a protocol has been evolved, it should be strictly adhered to through out the study. The protocol aims at preventing

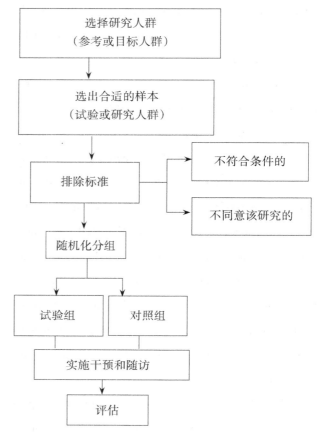

图 6-2　随机对照试验的设计

1. 制定研究方案

根据严格的计划方案开展研究是随机对照试验的一个基本要求。严格的计划方案应包括研究目的、试验组和对照组研究对象的选择标准、样本含量、将受试者分成试验组和对照组的过程、具体治疗方案（什么样的病人在何时何地接受何种治疗）、工作程序的标准化、时间进度安排、参与到该项试验的各方责任及研究结果的分析和评价等内容。计划书是必不可少的，特别是在多中心临床试验中。为了避免偏倚和减少研究中的误差来源，一旦确定了统一的计划方案，整个研究过程就必须严格遵守计划书中的要求和操作步骤。

bias and to reduce the sources of error in the study.

Preliminary test runs: Sometimes, before a protocol is completed, preliminary (pilot) studies have to be made to find out the feasibility or operational efficiency of certain procedures, or unknown effects, or on the acceptability of certain policies. Sometimes it is useful to have a short test run of the protocol to see whether it contains any flaws. It is important that the final version of the protocol should be agreed upon by all concerned before the trial begins.

2. Selecting reference and experimental populations

（1）Reference or target population

It is the population to which the findings of the trial, if found successful, are expected to be applicable (e.g., a drug, vaccine or other procedure). A reference population may be as broad as mankind or it may be geographically limited or limited to persons in specific age, sex, occupational or social groups. Thus the reference population may comprise the population of a whole city, or a population of school children, industrial workers, and obstetric population and so on according to the nature of the study.

（2）Experimental or study population

The study population is derived from the reference population. It is the actual population that participates in the experimental study. Ideally, it should be randomly chosen from the reference population, so that it has the same characteristics as the reference population. If the study population differs from the reference population, it may not be possible to generalise the findings of the study to the reference population. When an experimental population has been defined, the members are invited to participate in the study. It

预实验的进行：有时，在计划书完成之前，必须进行初步（试点）研究，以查明某些过程的可行性或运行效率，或未知效果，或某些政策的可接受性。有时一个简短的预实验对于检查该计划是否包含其他缺陷是非常有用的。在试验正式开始前，计划书的最终版本应由所有相关单位和机构一起商定。

2.选择研究人群

（1）参考或目标人群

如果试验成功，预期的结果（如药物、疫苗或其他研究过程）适用或结果可外推使用的人群称为目标人群。目标人群可能是一般人群，也可能是局限于某地区的人群，或局限于特定年龄、性别、职业或社会群体的人群。因此，根据研究目的不同，目标人群可能是整个城市的人口，也可能是学生、工人、孕妇等。

（2）试验或研究人群

参与试验的研究人群来自目标人群（总体）。参与试验研究的人群应该从目标人群中随机抽取，使其具有与目标人群相同的特征。如果试验人群是目标人群以外的人群，那么就不能把研究结果推广到目标人群。试验人群确定后，试验人群中的每个人都应该被邀请参加研究。为了减少失访，应选择一个稳定的、配合的、依从性较高的研究人群。参加者或志愿者必须符合以下三项标准：

is important to choose a stable population whose cooperation is assured to avoid losses to follow-up. The participants or volunteers must fulfil the following three criteria:

① They must give "informed consent", that is they make agree to participate in the trial after having been fully informed about the purpose, procedures and possible dangers of the trial.

② They should be representative of the population to which they belong (i.e., reference population).

③They should be qualified or eligible for the trial. That is, let us suppose that, we are testing the effectiveness of a new drug for the treatment of anaemia. If the volunteers are not anaemic, we will then say, they are not eligible or qualified for the trial. Similarly, let us suppose, we are going to test the effectiveness of a new vaccine against whooping cough. If the volunteers are already immune to the disease in question, we will then say, they are not qualified for the trial. In other words, the participants must be fully susceptible to the disease under study.

It must be recognized that persons who agree to participate in a study are likely to differ from those who do not, in many ways that may affect the outcome under investigation.

3. Randomization allocation

Randomization is a statistical procedure by which the participants are allocated into groups usually called "study" and "control" groups, to receive or not to receive the experimental preventive or therapeutic procedure, manoeuvre or intervention. Randomization is an attempt to eliminate "bias" and allow for comparability. Theoretically it is possible to assure comparability by matching. But when one matching can only be matched those factors which are known to very im-

①必须签署"知情同意书"，意味着这是研究对象在被告知试验的目的、过程以及可能存在的危险后，做出的同意参加试验的决定。

②研究对象应能代表其来源和所属的人群，即目标人群（总体）。

③研究对象必须是有资格参加试验研究的群体。也就是说，假设要测试一种治疗贫血的新药有效性，志愿者如果不是贫血患者，就不适合参加该研究。同样，假设要测试一种新的百日咳疫苗的效果，如果志愿者已经对该病免疫了，那么就没有资格参加该研究。总而言之，参与者必须是所要研究疾病的易感者或受益者。

需要注意的是，如果同意参加研究的志愿者与没有参加研究的人存在某些特征的差异，那么这些差异会带来偏倚，从而影响研究结果的评价。

3. 随机化分组

随机化分组是一个统计过程。研究对象有相同的机会或概率被分到试验组或对照组，接受或不接受实验性预防或治疗过程。随机化分组的目的是使试验组与对照组具有可比性，减少混杂偏倚。理论上可以通过匹配来保证两组的可比性，但匹配的因素往往是已知的影响因素，对于其他未知的影响因素无法进行匹配，而且匹配的因素也不宜过多，否则可能引起过度匹配的问题。随机化分组不仅可以使已知因素在两组中均衡分布，

portant, there may be other factors which are important but whose effect is not recognized or cannot be determined. By a process of randomization, hopefully, these factors will be distributed equally between the two groups.

Randomization is the "heart" of a control trial. It will give the greatest confidence that the groups are comparable, so that it can be compared with like. It ensures that the investigator is no control over allocation of participants to either study or control group, thus eliminating what is known as "selection bias". In other words, by random allocation, every individual gets an equal chance of being allocated into either group or on of the trial groups.

It is crucial that both the groups should be alike with retain to certain variables or characteristics that might affect the outcome of the experiment（e.g., age, sex）, the entire study population can be stratified into subgroups according to the variable, and individuals within each subgroup can therefore randomly allocated into study and control groups. It is almost desirable to check that the groups formed initially are based on similar in composition. Randomization is done only after the participant has entered the study, that is after having been qualified for the trial and has given his informed consequence to participate in the study. Randomization is best done by taking a table of random numbers.

The essential difference between a randomized controlled trial and an analytical study is that in the latter, there is no randomization because a differentiation into diseased and non-diseased（exposed or non-exposed）groups has already taken place. The only option left to ensure comparability in analytical studies is by matching.

也可以使未知因素在两组中均衡分布。

随机化分组是对照试验的核心环节，可最大限度地保证组间具有可比性。另外，随机化分组后进行的分组隐藏，可以确保调查者不能控制参与者的分组，从而消除选择偏倚。随机化分组可以使每个参与者都有平等的机会被分配到试验组或对照组。

应该保留那些可能会影响试验结果的变量或特征（如年龄、性别）的信息，可以根据这些变量将研究对象分为不同层，这样每层中的研究对象就可以被随机分到试验组或对照组。分层因素就是那些在组间存在差异且对结果可能有影响的因素，即混杂因素。随机化分组是在参与者进入研究之后进行的，也就是说，在确定了研究对象具有参加该试验的资格并且签署了知情同意书之后，就要开始随机化分组。随机化分组的基础是随机数字表。

随机对照试验和分析性研究的本质区别在于后者没有随机化分组，而是在研究前根据客观状况将研究对象分为病例组和无病组（或暴露组和非暴露组）。在分析性研究中，设计阶段确保两组具有可比性的唯一途径是匹配。

4. Manipulation

Having formed the study and control groups, the next step is to intervene or manipulate the study (experimental) group by the deliberate application or withdrawal or reduction of the suspected causal factor (e.g., this may be a drug, vaccine, dietary component, a habit, etc.) as laid down in the protocol.

This manipulation creates an independent variable (e.g., drug, vaccine, a new procedure) whose effect is then determined by measurement of the final outcome, which constitutes the dependent variable (e.g., incidence of disease, survival time, recovery period).

5. Follow-up

This implies examination of the experimental and control group subjects at defined intervals of time, in a standard manner, with equal intensity, under the same given circumstances, in the same time frame till final assessment of outcome. The duration of the trial is usually based on the expectation that a significant difference (e.g., mortality) will be demonstrable at a given point in time after the start of the trial. Thus the follow - up may be short or may require many years depending upon the study undertaken.

It may be mentioned that some losses to follow - up are inevitable due to factors, such as death, migration and loss of interest. This is known as attrition. If the attrition is substantial, it may be difficult to generalize the results of the study to the reference population. Every effort, therefore, should be made to minimize the losses to follow - up.

6. Assessment

The final step is assessment of the outcome of the trial in terms of：

4.干预

通过随机化分组确定好试验组和对照组后，下一步需要按照计划书中的规定人为地施加或减少某些可疑的致病因素（如药物、疫苗、饮食成分、习惯等）进行试验干预。

干预（如药物、疫苗、一个新的程序）也是影响最终疗效的独立变量，应尽量选择可以客观测量和量化的评价指标。效果评价还受到其他变量（如疾病发生率、生存时间、恢复期）的影响。

5.随访

随访就是在规定的时间内，以标准的方法，在相同的时间内，用相同的关注度，在相同的试验环境下，对试验组和对照组的受试者进行追踪观察，直到观察终止期。随访时间通常以试验开始后，预期可能出现组间统计学差异（如死亡率）的某一特定时间点来确定。因此，随访的时间可能很短，也可能很长，甚至长达几年，这取决于所进行的研究。

死亡、迁移和对研究失去兴趣等因素可能导致失访，这是前瞻性随访研究中不可避免的。如果失访率过大，会对研究结果的外推带来影响。因此，应尽一切努力减少失访。

6.评估

试验结束后，需要从以下方面对结果进行评价分析：

（1）Positive results

Positive results, that is, benefits of the experimental measure such as reduced incidence or severity of the disease, cost to the health service or other appropriate outcome in the study and control groups.

（2）Negative results

Negative results, that is, severity and frequency of side - effects and complications, if any, including death. Adverse effects may be missed if they are not sought.

The incidence of positive/negative results is rigorously compared in both the groups, and the differences, if any, are tested for statistical significance. Techniques are available for the analysis of data as they are collected（sequential analysis）, but it is more useful to analyze the results at the end of the trial.

Bias may arise from errors of assessment of the outcome due to human element. These may be from three sources: Firstly, there may be bias on the part of the participants, who may subjectively feel better or report improvement if they knew they were receiving a new form of treatment. This is known as "subject variation". Secondly, there may be observer bias that is the investigator measuring the outcome of a therapeutic trial may be influenced if he knows beforehand the particular procedure or therapy to which the patient has been subjected. This is known as "observer bias". Thirdly, there may be bias in evaluation — that is, the investigator may subconsciously give a favorable report of the outcome of the trial. Randomization cannot guard against these sorts of bias, nor the size of the sample. In order to reduce these problems, a technique known as "blinding" is adopted, which will ensure that the outcome is assessed objectively.

（1）有利的结果

有利的结果即试验措施产生的益处，如降低发病率或疾病严重程度、减少卫生服务费用等。

（2）不利的结果

不利的结果即副作用和并发症的严重程度及发生频率，也可能包括死亡。对试验措施的安全性评价是试验研究中必不可少的部分，只有进行了安全性评价，才能全面评价干预措施的效果。

对两组之间的有利/不利结果的发生率进行比较，如果两组之间的结果有差异，应进行统计学显著性检验。数据收集过程中可以使用序贯分析技术，也就是说，只要出现统计学差异即可终止试验，但在试验结束时对结果进行分析更好。

由人为因素导致的评估结果的错误可能产生偏倚。偏倚通常有三种：第一，来自研究对象的偏倚。研究对象知道自己接受了新的治疗方法，可能会主观感觉好一些，此时出现的正向效应与干预措施的特异作用无关，即"研究对象变异"。第二，观察者偏倚，即如果研究者事先知道试验的过程或治疗方法，可能会影响干预措施效果的测量。第三，结果评估中存在的偏倚。统计分析者知道分组后，在统计分析中可能会有意识地做出对试验结果有利的报告。以上这些偏倚无法通过随机化分组消除，也无法通过增大样本量减少，但可以通过盲法减少，从而确保能够客观地评估结果。

（3）Blinding

Blinding can be done in three ways：

① Single blind trial：The trial is so planned that the participant is not aware whether he belongs to the study group or control group.

②Double blind trial: The trial is so planned that neither the doctor nor the participant is aware of the group allocation and the treatment received.

③Triple blind trial: This goes one step further. The participant, the investigator and the person analyzing the data are all "blind". Ideally, of course, triple blinding should be used, but the double blinding is the most frequently used method when a blind trial is conducted.

When an outcome such as death is being measured, blinding is not so essential.

6.2.6　Some study designs

It is useful to consider here some of the study designs of clinical trials.

1. controlled trials

（1）Concurrent parallel study design

In this situation, comparisons are made between two randomly assigned groups, one group exposed to specific treatment, and the other group not exposed. Patients remain in the study group or the control group for the duration of the investigation.

（2）Cross-over type of study designs

This is illustrated in Figure 6-3. With this type of study design, each patient serves as his own control. As before, the patients are randomly assigned to a study group and control group. The study group receives the treatment under consideration. The control

（3）盲法

有三种盲法：

①单盲：研究对象不知道自己的分组情况。

②双盲：医生和研究对象都不知道分组情况。

③三盲：研究对象、调查人员和数据分析者均不知道分组情况。当然，理想的做法是使用三盲，但双盲是最常用的盲法。

当研究的结果是死亡时，没有必要选择盲法，可采用开放性试验。当研究对象出现一些严重不良反应或突发严重问题急需救治时，需要开盲。

6.2.6　研究类型

临床试验的分类有多种方法，有一种就是根据对照的方式分类。

1. 对照试验

（1）平行设计的临床试验

在随机分配的两组之间进行比较，一组采用要研究的特定治疗方法，另一组采用其他治疗方法。在干预后的观察期间，按照研究方案，所有患者仍待在原分组中。

（2）交叉设计的临床试验

图6-3展示了平行对照试验和交叉对照试验的设计模式。交叉对照试验中的每个研究对象都以自身为对照。与平行对照试验一样，研究对象先被随机分配到试验组或对照组，在第一阶段分别接受对应的干预措施，经过一段时间后，两组

group receives some alternate form of active treatment or placebo. The two groups are observed over time. Then the patients in each group are taken off their medication or placebo to allow for the elimination of the medication from the body and for the possibility of any "carry over" effects, as shown in Figure 6-3. By the diagonal lines, after this period of medication (the length of this interval is determined by the pharmaco-logic properties of the drug being tested), the two groups are switched. Those who received the treatment under study are changed to the control group therapy or placebo, and vice versa.

Cross-over studies offer a number of advantages. With such a design, all patients can be assured that sometime during the course of investigation, they will receive the new therapy. Such studies generally econo-mize on the total number of patients required at the ex-pense of the time necessary to complete the study. This method of study is not suitable if the drug of inter-est cures the disease, if the drug is effective only dur-ing a certain stage of the disease or if the disease changes radically during the period of time required for the study.

的患者都停止使用各自的干预措施（服药或安慰剂），以消除治疗药物的滞留影响，如图6-3中对角线所显示的时期，这一过程称为洗脱期，其长短取决于被测试药物的药理特性。然后将两组的干预措施进行交换，进入第二阶段的干预，即原来试验组研究对象的治疗药物改为对照组研究对象的治疗药物或安慰剂，反之亦然。

交叉试验的优点如下：因为所有患者都将接受两种干预措施（试验组措施和对照措施），所以最终都会接受新的治疗方法。因为个体内变异小于个体间变异，所以交叉设计的自身对照所需的样本量小于平行对照。当所研究的干预措施确实可以有效治疗疾病或对疾病某个阶段有效时，如果干预后疾病因发生变化而无法恢复到交叉试验的第一阶段，就无法开展第二阶段的试验，也不适合进行交叉试验。由此，交叉试验适用于反复发作疾病的研究。

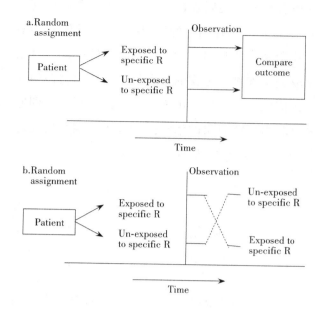

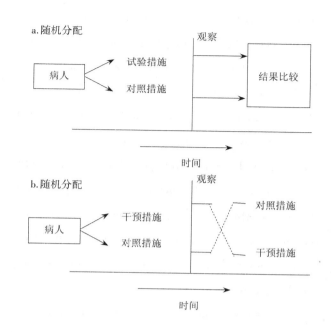

Figure 6-3　Schematic diagram of the design of concurrent parallel and cross-over controlled therapeutic trials

图6-3　平行对照试验和交叉对照试验设计示意图

2. Types of randomized controlled trials

Clinical trials are classified by objective and subjects of study.

（1）Clinical trials

For the most part, "clinical trials" have been concerned with evaluating therapeutic agents, mainly drugs. The last decades have been clearly the utility of clinical trials. Some of the recent examples include — evaluation of beta-blockers in reducing cardiovascular mortality in patient surviving the acute phase of myocardial infarction; trials of folate treatment / supplementation before conception to prevent recurrence of neural tube defects; trials of aspirin on cardiovascular mortality and beta carotene on cancer incidence; efficacy of tonsillectomy for recurrent throat infection; randomized controlled trial of coronary bypass surgery for the prevention of myocardial infarction, etc. The list is endless.

Unfortunately, not all clinical trials are susceptible to being blinded. For example, there is no suscepti-

2. 随机对照试验的类型

临床试验还可以根据研究目的和研究对象分类。

（1）临床试验

通常，"临床试验"用于评价治疗措施（尤其是药物）对患者的效果。过去几十年的研究，充分显示了临床随机对照试验的优势。例如，评估β受体阻滞剂在降低急性心肌梗死患者死亡率方面的价值；评估孕前叶酸补充对预防胎儿神经管畸形的影响；评估阿司匹林对心血管致死率的影响；评估β-胡萝卜素对癌症发病率的影响；评估扁桃体切除对咽喉感染复发的疗效；评估冠状动脉搭桥对预防心肌梗死再发的影响；等等。

不幸的是，并非所有的临床试验都可以使用盲法。例如，进行扁桃体和腺样体切除术效果评

ble to being blinded. For example, there is no way to perform a clinical trial of tonsillectomy and adenoidectomy without its being obvious who received surgery and who did not, a reason why the value of these procedures continues to be uncertain. Many ethical, administrative and technical problems are involved in the conduct of clinical trials. Nevertheless, they are a powerful tool and should be carried out before any new therapy, procedure or service is introduced.

（2）Preventive trials

In general usage, prevention is synonymous with primary prevention, and the term "preventive trials" implies trials of primary preventive measures. These rials are purported to prevent or eliminate disease on an experimental basis. The most frequently occurring type of preventive trials are the trials of vaccines and chemo — prophylactic drugs. The basic principles of experimental design are also applicable to these trials. It may be necessary to apply the trial to groups of subjects instead of to individual subjects. For example, in 1946, the Medical Research Council of UK conducted an extensive trial to test whooping cough vaccine from three manufacturers in ten separate field trials. Those children between 6-18 months who were entered into the trial were randomly allocated in study and control groups. The vaccine was given in three, monthly injections, and the children were followed up at monthly intervals to detect the occurrence of whooping cough. The study group comprised of 3 801 children, and 687 of them developed the infection which wre control group consisted of 3 757 unvaccinated children, and 687 of them developed the infection. This gave an attack rate of 3.9 percent in the vaccinated group and 18.3 percent in the control group. The difference was significant.

价时，无法使用盲法开展试验，导致这些方法的价值仍不明确。临床试验过程还涉及伦理、组织管理和技术等问题。然而，临床随机对照试验作为强有力的科研方法，在任何新的治疗、方法或服务被广泛推广使用前都有必要开展。

（2）预防试验

一般来说，预防是初级预防的同义词，"预防试验"就是采用一级预防措施的试验。这些试验的本意是通过干预，预防或消除疾病。最常见的预防试验是疫苗和药物化疗试验。临床试验设计的基本原则也适用于预防试验。当预防试验是对群体而不是个体进行干预时，为社区试验；当预防试验是对疾病的高危个体进行干预时，为现场试验。例如，在1946年，英国医学会在10个现场对3家工厂生产的百日咳疫苗进行了预防性的现场试验。参加试验的研究对象为6～18月龄、未患过百日咳但可能患百日咳的儿童，这些研究对象被随机分为试验组和对照组。试验组共注射疫苗三次，1次/月，并且每月都随访百日咳发生情况。最终，试验组的3 801名儿童都接种了疫苗，其中149人发生了百日咳；对照组的3 757名儿童都未接种疫苗，其中687人发生了百日咳。试验组的发病率为3.9%，对照组的发病率为18.3%，两组的发病率具有统计学差异。

Analysis of a preventive trial must result in a clear statement about:

① The benefit the community will derive from the measure.

② The risks involved.

③ The costs to the health service in terms of money, men and material resources. Since preventive trials involve larger number of subjects and sometimes a longer time span to obtain results, there may be greater number of practical problems in this organization and execution.

（3）Risk factor trials

A type of preventive trial is the trial of risk factors in which the investigator intervenes to interrupt the usual sequence to the development of disease for those individuals who have "risk factor" for developing the disease; often this involves risk factor modification. The concept of "risk factor" gave a new dimension to epidemiological research.For example, the major risk factors of coronary heart disease are elevated blood cholesterol, smoking, hypertension and sedentary habits. Accordingly, the four main possibilities of intervention in coronary heart disease are: reduction the blood cholesterol, the cessation of smoking, control the hypertension and promotion of regular physical activity. Risk factor trials can be "single - factor" or "multi-factor" trial. Both the approaches are complementary, and both are needed.

The WHO promoted a trial on primary prevention of coronary heart disease using clofibrate to lower serum cholesterol, which was accepted as a significant risk factor of CHD. This study is the largest preventive trial yet conducted comprising more than 15 000 men of whom one - third received clofibrate and two - third received olive oil as a control treatment. The study was

对预防试验进行分析时，还应阐明以下几点：

①预防措施的实施所获得的社会效益。

②可能带来的风险。

③由此产生的卫生服务费用，包括财力、人力和物力。预防试验往往需要通过较大样本、花费较长时间才能观察到预防措施的效果，在组织和实施过程中可能存在较多可行性方面的问题。

（3）危险因素试验

危险因素试验是预防试验的一种，是指通过控制或减少疾病的某些危险因素，防止疾病的进展，从而预防疾病的发生。"危险因素"是流行病学研究中重要的概念。例如，冠心病的主要危险因素是血胆固醇升高、吸烟、高血压和久坐习惯。因此，对冠心病进行干预的方法是降低血胆固醇、戒烟、控制高血压和坚持定期体育活动。危险因素试验可以是"单因素"试验或"多因素"试验，这两种方法是互补的，也都是必要的。

WHO曾开展过一项冠心病一级预防试验。高胆固醇是公认的冠心病重要危险因素，这项研究使用氯贝丁酯降低胆固醇水平，从而预防冠心病的发生。该研究是当时最大的预防性试验，在欧洲有三个研究中心（爱丁堡、布拉格和布达佩斯），超过15 000名男性参与了该研究，其中1/3使用氯贝丁酯（作为试验组），2/3使用橄榄油

conducted in 3 centres in Europe (Edinburgh, Prague, and Budapest). The design was double blind and randomization was successfully achieved. The mean observation was 9.6 years. The trial showed a significant reduction in non‐fatal cardiac infarction, but unfortunately there were 25 percent more deaths in the clofibrate‐treatment group than in the control group possibly due to long‐term toxic effect of the drug. The trial illustrates the kind of contribution that an epidemiological approach can make to protect the public health against possible adverse effects on long‐term medication with potent drugs.

The other widely reported risk factor intervention trials of coronary heart disease are: the Stanford Third Community study; the North Karelia project in Finland; the Oslo study ; the multiple risk factor intervention trial (MRFIT) in USA.

（4）Cessation experiments

Another type of preventive trial is the cessation experiment. In this type of study, an attempt is made to evaluate the termination of a habit (or removal of suspected agent), which is considered to be causally related to a disease. If such action is followed by a significant reduction in the disease, the hypothesis of cause is greatly strengthened. The familiar example is cigarette smoking and lung cancer. If in a randomized controlled trial, one group of cigarette smokers continues to smoke and the other group has given up, the demonstration of a decrease in the incidence of lung cancer in the study group greatly strengthens the hypothesis of a causal relationship. A large randomized controlled trial has been mounted to study the role of smoking cessation in the primary prevention of coronary heart disease.

（作为对照组）。作为一项双盲随机对照试验，该研究的平均随访时间为9.6年。结果显示，试验组非致命性心肌梗死率显著低于对照组，但试验组由于长期使用氯贝丁酯（氯贝丁酯会导致毒性反应），死亡率比对照组高25%以上。该试验说明了流行病学方法在保护公众健康方面可以做出的贡献，即提醒人们防止长期使用药物产生的不利影响。

关于冠心病危险因素的干预试验还有很多报道：斯坦福第三社区的研究；芬兰的North Karelia项目；Oslo研究；在美国进行的多危险因素干预试验（MRFIT）。

（4）终止试验

终止试验是预防试验的另一种类型。这种类型的研究试图评价终止一种习惯（或去除可疑病原体）后疾病的变化。如果疾病伴随着行为（或病原体）的消失而显著减少，那么病因假设的验证就会加强。例如，研究人员曾开展过一项随机对照试验检验吸烟和肺癌关系的病因假设，对照组的吸烟者继续吸烟，试验组戒烟。结果发现，戒烟组的肺癌发病率比对照组的低，这一证据大大加强了吸烟与肺癌存在因果关系的假设。此外，还有一项大型随机对照试验研究证实了戒烟在冠心病一级预防中的作用。

（5）Trial of etiological agents

One of the aims of experimental epidemiology is to confirm or refute an etiological hypothesis. The best known example of trial of an aetiological agent relates to retrolental fibroplasia（RLF）. Retrolental fibroplasia, as a cause of blindness, was non-existent prior to 1938. It was originally observed and reported by T.L. Terry, a Boston ophthalmologist in 1942, and later in many other countries outside the USA.

（6）Evaluation of health services

Randomized controlled trials have been extended to assess the effectiveness and efficiency of health services. Often choices have to be made between alternative policies or health care delivery. The necessity of choice arises from the fact that resources are limited, and priorities must be set for the implementation of a large number of activities which could contribute to the welfare of the society. An excellent example of such an evaluation is the controlled trials in the chemotherapy of tuberculosis in India, which demonstrated that "domiciliary treatment" of pulmonary tuberculosis was an effective as the more costly "hospital or sanatorium" treatment. The results of the study have gained international acceptance and ushered in a new era — the era of domiciliary treatment, in the treatment of tuberculosis.

Another example is that related to studies which have shown that many of the health care delivery tasks traditionally performed by physicians can be performed by nurses and other paramedical workers, thus saving physician time. These studies are also labelled as "health services research" studies.

3.Non-randomized trials

Although the experimental method is almost always to be preferred, it is not always possible for ethi-

（5）病因学试验

实验流行病学研究的一个目的是证实或驳斥某个病因假设。最著名的一个例子是研究晶状体后纤维增生症（RLF）的病因试验。1938年之前，人们并不知道晶状体后纤维组织增生是致盲的原因之一。直到1942年，波士顿的眼科医生T.L. Terry才做了最早的观察和报道，随后美国以外的其他国家也有了相关的报道。

（6）卫生服务评价

随机对照试验已扩展到评估卫生服务的效果和效益。在卫生服务中，经常需要对卫生政策和提供的卫生服务做出抉择。选择应该是在有限的卫生资源基础上，优先资助有益于社会福利的项目。例如，印度的结核病化疗对照试验。该试验表明，肺结核的"家庭式治疗"与"医院或疗养院治疗"相比，同样有效，但更廉价。这一结果已获得国际认可，也为肺结核的治疗迎来了一个新的时代——家庭治疗的时代。

另一项研究表明，许多以往由医生执行的传统医疗保健工作也可以由护士和其他医务工作者完成，从而节省医生的时间。这些研究也被称为"卫生服务研究"。

3.非随机试验

研究中往往会优先选择随机对照试验，但由于伦理、组织管理和其他原因，无法在人体上直

cal, administrative and other reasons to resort to a randomized controlled trial in human beings. For example, smoking and lung cancer and induction of cancer by viruses have not lent themselves to direct experimentation in human beings. Secondly, some preventive measures can be applied only to groups or on a community — wide basis (e.g., community trials of water fluoridation). Thirdly, when disease frequency is low and the natural history long (e.g., cervix cancer), randomized controlled trials require follow - up of thousands of people for a decade or more. The cost and logistics are often prohibitive. These trials are rare. In such situations, we must depend upon other study designs — these are referred to as non - randomized (or quasi) trials.

Where the approach is sophisticated in randomized controlled trials, it is rather crude in non - randomized trials. As there is no randomization in non - experimental trials, the degree of comparability will be low and the chances of a spurious result higher than where randomization had taken place. In other words, the validity of causal inference remains largely a matter of extra - statistical judgement. Nevertheless, vital decisions affecting public health and preventive medicine have been made by non - experimental studies. A few examples of non - randomized trials are discussed below:

(1) Uncontrolled trials

There is room for uncontrolled trials (i.e., trials with no comparison group). For example, there were no randomized controlled studies of the benefits of the Pap test (cervical cancer) when it was introduced in 1920s. Today, there is indirect epidemiological evidence from well over a dozen uncontrolled studies of cervical cancer screening that the Pap test is effective

接进行随机对照试验，这时就需要采用其他的研究设计——非随机试验（准试验）。例如，吸烟和肺癌以及由病毒引起的癌症都不能直接进行人体试验。另外，一些预防措施只适用于群体或社区整体干预（如水氟化的社区试验）。还有一些疾病发病率较低，病史较长（如宫颈癌），开展随机对照试验需要的样本量大，可能需随访10年或更长时间。由于研究成本巨大和组织管理工作难度大，从可行性角度考虑，在这种情况下，可以采用非随机试验（准试验）。

随机对照试验比非随机试验要复杂，但非随机试验由于缺乏随机化分组，组间可比性低，出现虚假结果的可能性高于随机对照试验，会造成非随机试验因果推断的真实性受到很大影响，最终会影响公共卫生和预防医学决策。下面举几个非随机试验的例子：

（1）无对照试验

无对照试验指没有平行对照的试验（即没有对照组的试验）。例如，20世纪20年代还没有随机对照试验证实巴氏检测（宫颈癌）的益处。如今，已有10多个没有对照组的宫颈癌筛查研究间接证明了巴氏试验能有效降低宫颈癌患者的死亡率。研究初期，没有对照的试验可能有助于评估某一疗法治疗某一特定疾病的有效性、确定适当

in reducing mortality from this disease. Initially uncontrolled trials may be useful in evaluating whether a specific therapy appears to have any value in a particular disease, to determine an appropriate dose, to investigate adverse reactions, etc. However, even in these uncontrolled trials, one is using implied "historical controls", i.e., the experience of earlier untreated patients affected by the same disease.

（2）Natural experiments

Where experimental studies are not possible in human populations, the epidemiologist seeks to identify "natural circumstances" that mimic an experiment. For example, in respect of cigarette smoking, people have separated themselves "naturally" into two groups, smokers and non-smoker. Epidemiologists have taken advantage of this separation and tested hypothesis regarding lung cancer and cigarette smoking. Other populations involved in natural experiments comprise the following groups: migrants, religious or social groups, atomic bombing of Japan, famines and earthquakes, etc. A major earthquake in Athens in 1981 provided a "natural experiment" to epidemiologists who studied the effects of acute stress on cardiovascular mortality. They showed an excess of deaths from cardiac and external causes on the days after the major earthquake, but no excess deaths from other causes.

John Snow's discovery that cholera is a water-borne disease was the outcome of a natural experiment. Snow in his "grand experiment" identified two randomly mixed populations, alike in other important respects, except the source of water supply in their households. The results of the experiment are given in Table 6-1.

剂量和评价不良反应等。需要注意的是，即使在这些没有对照组的试验中，人们也使用了"历史对照"，即早期未经治疗的同种疾病患者。

（2）自然试验

在人群中进行试验研究具有一定的难度，所以流行病学家试图模拟"自然环境"开展实验。例如，根据吸烟情况，将人群分成吸烟组和非吸烟组。流行病学家利用这种自然的分组，验证了吸烟与肺癌关系的假设。也可以利用其他人群开展自然试验，例如，移民、宗教或社会团体、日本受原子弹爆炸影响的人群以及受饥荒和地震等影响的人群等。1981年，雅典大地震为研究急性应激对心血管死亡率的影响提供了"自然试验"，结果显示：地震之后，因心脏和外伤原因死亡的人数过多，但因其他原因死亡的人数并不多。

约翰·斯诺发现霍乱是一种通过疫水传播的疾病，这也是通过自然试验得到的结论。这一庞大的试验中包含了两个随机人群，这两个人群除了家庭水源不同外，其他方面都是相似的。研究结果见表6-1。

Table 6-1　Deaths from cholera per 10 000 houses and sources of water supply of these houses, London 1853

Sources of water supply	Number of houses	Deaths from cholera	Deaths in each 10 000 houses
Southwark & Vauxhall Co.	40 046	1 263	315
Lambeth Co.	26 107	98	37

It will be seen from Table 6-1 that deaths were fewer in houses supplied by Lambeth company compared to houses supplied by Southwark and Vauxhall company. The inference was obvious — the Lambeth company water came from an intake on the River Thames well above London, whereas the Southwark and Vauxhall company water was derived from the sewage polluted water basin. The great difference in the occurrence of cholera among these two populations gave clear demonstration that cholera is a water-borne disease. This was demonstrated long before the advent of the bacteriological era; it also led to the institution of public health measures to control cholera.

（3）Before and after comparison studies

These are community trials which fall into two distinct groups:

1）Before and after comparison studies without control

These studies centre round comparing the incidence of disease before and after introduction of a preventive measure. The events which took place prior to the use of the new treatment or preventive procedure are used as a standardize comparison. In other words, the experiment serves as its own control; this eliminates virtually all group differences. The classic examples of "before and after comparison studies" were the prevention of scurvy among sailors by James Lind in 1750 by providing fresh fruit; studies on the transmis-

表6-1　1853年伦敦每10 000个家庭的霍乱致死情况和水源供应情况

供水来源	家庭数量	霍乱导致的死亡人数	每10 000个家庭中的死亡人数
萨瑟克-沃克斯霍尔水公司	40 046	1 263	315
兰贝斯水公司	26 107	98	37

从表6-1中可以看出，由兰贝斯水公司供水的家庭，其死亡数比由萨瑟克-沃克斯霍尔水公司供水的家庭少。兰贝斯公司的水来自泰晤士河畔的上游，而萨瑟克-沃克斯霍尔水公司的水来自泰晤士河畔被污染的下游。这两组人群霍乱发生率的巨大差异清楚表明了霍乱是一种水传播疾病。这一研究的结果，早在用显微镜发现细菌之前，就为通过净化水源的公共卫生措施来控制霍乱提供了依据。

（3）前后对比研究

社区试验可以分为两种类型：

1）无对照组的自身前后对比研究

这些研究是通过比较预防措施实施前后发病率的变化开展的，将新治疗或预防措施干预前事件的发生作为参照进行比较，即只有一组人进行干预前后自身比较，这样的设计没有组间差异。典型范例包括：1750年James Lind通过提供新鲜的水果来预防海员的坏血病；1854年约翰·斯诺对于霍乱传播的研究；Salk和Sabin通过疫苗来预防小儿麻痹症。

sion of cholera by John Snow in 1854; and more recently, prevention of polio by Salk and Sabin vaccines.

In order to establish evidence in before and after comparison studies, the following are needed:

① Regarding the incidence of disease, before and after introduction of a preventive measure must be available.

② There should be introduction or manipulation of only one factor or change relevant to the situation, other fact remaining the same, as for example, addition of fluorine in drinking water to prevent dental caries.

③ Diagnostic criterion of the disease should remain the same.

④ Adoption of preventive measures should be over a wide area.

⑤ Reductive in the incidence must be large following the introduction of the preventive measure, because there is no control and a several trials may be needed before the evaluation be considered conclusive.

Table 6-2 gives an example of a "before and after comparison study" in Victoria following introduction of seat-belt legislation for prevention of deaths and injuries caused by motor vehicle accidents.

Table 6-2 Effect of adoption of compulsory seat-belt legislation in Victoria, Australia-1971

	1970	1971	change/%
Deaths	564	464	−14.8
Injuries	14 620	12 454	− 17.7

Table 6-2 shows a definite fall in the numbers of deaths and injuries in occupants of cars, following the introduction of compulsory seat-belts in one state of Australia.

进行自身前后对比试验时需要注意以下几点：

①必须收集实施预防措施前后疾病的发病率。

②除了实施干预措施以外，其他方面应尽可能保持不变，例如，在饮用水中添加氟以预防龋齿。

③疾病的诊断标准应保持不变。

④所有研究对象应尽可能都使用该预防措施，尽量扩大措施的实施范围。

⑤由于缺乏对照组，要想得到措施有效的结论，应该多开展几次试验，且施加预防措施后，发病率应有大幅度的下降。

表6-2是"自身前后对比研究"的一个示例，是关于维多利亚州实行安全带立法以控制机动车事故造成的伤亡的研究。

表6-2 1971年澳大利亚的维多利亚州在实施安全带立法后的变化

	1970年	1971年	变化幅度/%
死亡人数	564	464	−17.7
受伤人数	14 620	12 454	−14.8

表6-2显示,澳大利亚的维多利亚州在强制实行驾车系安全带的措施后,汽车乘员死亡和受伤人数明显减少。

2）Before and after comparison studies with control

In the absence of a control group, comparison between observations before and after the use of a new treatment procedure may be misleading. In such situations, the epidemiologist tries to utilize a "natural" control group i.e., one provided by nature or natural circumstances. If the preventive programme is to be applied to an enjoy community, he would select another community as similarity possible, particularly with respect to frequency and characteristics of the disease to be prevented. One of them be arbitrarily chosen to provide the study group and the others control group. In the example cited (e.g., seat-belt legislate in Victoria, Australia), a natural "control" was sought out comparing the results in Victoria with other states in Australian where similar legislation was not introduced. The findings be given in Table 6-3.

Table 6-3 Effect of adoption of compulsory seat-belt legislation in Victoria. 1971 compared with other states where similar legislation was not introduced

	1970	1971	change/%
Deaths			
Victoria	564	464	−17.7
Other States	1 426	1 429	0.2
Injuries			
Victoria	14 620	12 454	−14.8
Other States	39 980	40 396	1.0

In the example cited above, the existence of a control with which the results in Victoria could be compared strengthens the conclusion that there was definite fall in the number of deaths and injuries in Occupants of cars after the introduction of compulsory seat-belt legislation.

In the evaluation of preventive measures, three questions are generally considered:

2）有对照组的前后对比研究

由于自身前后对比研究缺乏对照组，用干预前后的差值确定措施效果会导致错误，因此流行病学家尝试使用"自然"对照组，即以自然状态或自然环境下的人群作为对照。如果将应用预防措施的社区作为试验组，另选与试验组社区疾病频率和特征相似的其他社区作为对照组，那么对照社区就是一个自然社区，且没有施加任何干预措施。试验组和对照组社区均是随机抽样选择的。比如在澳大利亚的维多利亚州采取安全带立法控制意外伤害和死亡的研究，就是一个自然对照试验的实例。该研究比较了维多利亚州与其他特征类似但没有实行安全带立法州的车祸引起的意外伤害和死亡，具体结果见表6-3。

表6-3 1971年维多利亚州实行强制性安全带立法后与未实行类似立法的其他州的比较

	1970年	1971年	变化幅度/%
死亡人数			
维多利亚	564	464	−17.7
其他州	1 426	1 429	0.2
受伤人数			
维多利亚	14 620	12 454	−14.8
其他州	39 980	40 396	1.0

上例中，通过设立对照组与维多利亚州进行比较，进一步增强了前面自身前后比较结论的强度，即在实行强制性安全带立法后，由车祸引起的死亡和意外伤害都减少了。

在开展预防措施效果评估的试验研究前，首先要考虑以下三个方面的问题：

① How much will it benefit the community? This will depend upon the effectiveness of the preventive measure and the acceptance of the measure by the community. The combined outcome of effectiveness and acceptability is measured by the difference in the incidence rate among the experimental and control groups.

② What are the risks to the recipients? These include the immediate and long term risks.

③ Cost are in money and man power? This is done to find out whether the preventive measure is economical and practical in terms of money spent.

It is now conceded that no health measure should be introduced on a large scale without proper evaluation. Recent problems that have engaged the attention of epidemiologists are studies of medical care and health services, planning and evaluation of health measures, services and research.

6.3　Field Trial and Community Trial

6.3.1　Definition

Field trials, in contrast to clinical trials, involve people who are disease - free but presumed to be at risk; data collection takes place "in the field", usually among non - institutionalized people in the general population. Since the subjects are disease - free and the purpose is to prevent the occurrence of diseases that may occur with relatively low frequency, field trials are often huge undertakings involving major logistic and financial considerations.

In community trial the treatment groups are communities rather than individuals. This is particularly appropriate for diseases that have their origins in so-

①该措施是否会给社会带来益处？带来的社会效益有多大？这取决于预防措施的有效性和可接受性。可以通过试验组和对照组发病率的差异来衡量措施效果和可行性的联合效应。

②干预措施对研究对象是否有风险？风险应该包括当前的和长期的风险。

③开展试验需要多少人力和财力？预防措施应该经济实惠，具有可行性。

只有对以上三个方面的问题进行充分评估后，才可以开展大规模人群健康措施的干预试验。目前，流行病学领域关注的问题还包括：医疗保健、卫生服务研究，卫生措施、服务和研究的规划和评价。

6.3　现场试验和社区试验

6.3.1　定义

与临床试验不同，现场试验涉及无病但有发病风险的高危人群。现场试验是指在"现场"对个体施加干预并收集数据，通常在社区自然人群中进行。由于受试者没有疾病，试验的目的是预防疾病发生或者降低疾病发病率，因此现场试验需要充足的财力和物力的支持。

社区试验与现场试验类似，目的都是预防疾病的发生，研究对象也是无病但可能发病的人。与现场试验不同的是，社区试验中干预措施的施

cial conditions, which in turn can most easily be influenced by intervention directed at group behavior as well as at individuals.

6.3.2   Objectives

① Evaluate the effect of vaccine, drug or other measures to prevent the disease.

② Evaluate the pathogenesis and risk factors.

③ Evaluate the quality of health services.

④ Evaluate the public health strategy.

6.3.3   Types of design

1. Randomized controlled trial（RCT）

A randomized controlled trial is an epidemiological experiment to study a new preventive or therapeutic regimen. Subjects in a population are randomly allocated to groups, usually called treatment and control groups, and the results are assessed by comparing the outcome in the two or more groups. The outcome of interest will vary but may be the development of new disease or recovery from established disease.

2. Cluster randomized trial

3. Quasi-experiment

6.3.4   Issues that requires attention in design and implement

① To determine the variable of outcome.

② Data collection.

③ Decrease the loss to follow-up.

④ To avoid the contamination.

⑤ To avoid the confounding factors.

加对象是整个社区群体，而不是个体。社区试验尤其适用于研究由社会状况引起的疾病，以及容易受群体和个人行为干预影响的情况。例如，水中加氟预防龋齿，盐中加碘预防地方性甲状腺肿。

6.3.2   目的

①评估疫苗、药物或其他疾病预防措施的效果。

②评估发病机制和疾病危险因素。

③评估卫生服务的质量。

④评估公共卫生策略。

6.3.3   设计类型

1. 随机对照试验（RCT）

随机对照试验是研究新的预防措施或治疗方案的流行病学试验。随机对照试验将人群中的受试者随机分为治疗组和对照组，通过比较两组或更多组的结果来评估干预的效果。研究结果指标根据研究目的的不同而不同，可能是疾病的进展或其过程中的指标，也可能是已有疾病的康复。

2. 整群随机试验

3. 准实验

6.3.4   设计和实施中需要注意的问题

①确定结果变量。

②数据收集。

③减少失访。

④避免沾染。

⑤避免混杂因素。

6.4 Study Design and Implement

① Ascertain the study purpose.

② Ascertain the types of study and design.

③ Choose the field.

④ Choose the study subjects (inclusion criteria, exclusion criteria).

⑤ Ascertain the intervene measures.

⑥ Size of sample.

⑦ Randomization (simple randomization, stratified randomization, cluster randomization).

⑧ The types of control (standard method control, placebo control, self-control, cross-over control).

⑨ Blinding (single blind, double blind, triple blind).

⑩ Deadline of observation.

⑪ The outcome variable and measuring method.

⑫ Baseline data and monitoring systems.

⑬ Follow-up and data collection.

⑭ Ascertain the method of statistical analysis.

6.5 Data Arrangement and Analysis

Common indexes: effective rate, cure rate, case fatality rate, adverse event rate, survival rate, protective rate, index of effectiveness (IE), relative risk reduction(RRR), absolute risk reduction(ARR), number needed to treat (NNT).

6.6 Advantages and Disadvantages

6.6.1 Main advantages

①Randomized group is a good way to control con-

6.4 研究的设计与实施

①确定研究目的。

②确定研究和设计的类型。

③选择现场。

④选择研究对象（纳入标准、排除标准）。

⑤确定干预措施。

⑥确定样本大小。

⑦随机化分组（简单随机、分层随机、整群随机）。

⑧确定对照类型（标准疗法对照、安慰剂对照、自身对照、交叉对照）。

⑨确定盲法（单盲、双盲、三盲）。

⑩确定观察期限。

⑪确定结果变量和测量方法。

⑫确定基线数据和随访监测。

⑬随访和收集数据。

⑭确定统计分析的方法。

6.5 数据的整理与分析

常用指标包括：有效率、治愈率、病死率、不良事件率、生存率、保护率、效果指数（IE）、降低的相对风险（RRR）、降低的绝对风险（ARR）、需要治疗的人数（NNT）。

6.6 优点与局限性

6.6.1 主要优点

①随机化分组可以很好地控制混杂偏倚。

founding bias.

② Field trial and community trial are belong to prospective study, the strength of causal argument are high.

③ They help to understand the natural history of disease.

6.6.2 Main disadvantages

① The problem of compliance.

② The problem of the representativeness of subjects.

③ Easy to lost to follow-up.

④ Expensive.

⑤ The problems of ethics.

②现场试验和社区试验属于前瞻性研究，因果论证强度高。

③有助于了解疾病的自然史。

6.6.2 主要局限性

①存在依从性问题。

②存在研究对象的代表性问题。

③很容易失访。

④花费大。

⑤存在伦理道德问题。

Chapter 7　Cause of Disease and Causal Inference

7.1　Concept of Disease

There have been many attempts to define disease. Webster defines disease as "a condition in which body health is impaired, a departure from a state of health, an alteration of the human body interrupting the performance of vital functions". *The Oxford English Dictionary* defines disease as "a condition of the body or some part or organ of the body in which its functions are disrupted or deranged". From an ecological point of view, disease is defined maladjustment of the human organism to the environment. From a sociological point of view, disease considered a social phenomenon, occurring in all society and defined and fought in terms of the particular forces prevalent in the society. The simplest definition course, that disease is just the opposite of health — i.e., deviation from normal functioning or state of common physical or mental well - being — since health and disease mutually exclusive. These definitions are considered inadequate because they do not give a criterion by who decide when a disease state begins, nor do they themselves to measurement of disease.

The WHO has defined health but not disease. That because disease has many shades, "spectrum" of disease ranging from inapparent (subclinical) cases to severe manifest illness. Some diseases commence acutely (e.g., food poisoning), and some insidiously

第7章　病因和病因推断

7.1　疾病的概念

很多人曾试图定义疾病。韦伯斯特将疾病定义为"与健康的状态相反，疾病指身体健康受到损害及人体重要功能受到干扰的状态"；《牛津英语词典》将疾病定义为"身体或身体某部分、器官受到破坏而发生变化"。从生态学的角度来看，疾病的定义是"人类机体对环境的不适应现象"。从社会学的角度来看，疾病被认为是一种社会现象，发生在社会内部，并与社会中普遍存在的特定力量在斗争。疾病最简单的定义为"与健康相对立的状态"，即偏离正常功能或身体、心理健康的状态。以上有关疾病的定义都不充分，因为没有给出一个标准，即没有给出由谁决定疾病状态何时开始，也没有对疾病进行最精确的测量。

WHO 也只是对"健康"进行了定义，并未定义"疾病"，主要是因为疾病具有复杂性，"疾病谱"的范围可以从隐性（亚临床）疾病状态到严重疾病状态。有些疾病是急性开始的（如食物中毒），有些则是隐性开始的（如精神病、类风湿

(e.g., mental illness, rheumatoid arthritis). In some diseases, a "carrier" state occurs in which the individual remains outwardly healthy, and is able to infect others (e. g., typhoid fever). In some instances, the same organism may cause more than one clinical manifestation (e. g., streptococcus). In some cases, the same disease may be caused by more than one organism (e. g., diarrhea). Some diseases have a short course, and some a prolonged course. It is easy to determine illness when the signs and symptoms are manifest, but in many diseases the border-line between normal and abnormal is indistinct as in the case of diabetes, hypertension and mental illness. The end-point or final outcome of disease is variable — recovery, disability or death of the host.

Distinction is also made between the words disease, illness and sickness which are not wholly synonymous. The term "disease" literally means "without ease" (uneasiness) — disease, the opposite of ease — when something is wrong with bodily function. "Illness" refers not only to the presence of a specific disease, but also to the individual's perceptions and behavior in response to the disease, as well as the impact of that disease on the psychosocial environment. "Sickness" refers to a state of social dysfunction. Susser has suggested the following usage:

Disease is a physiological / psychological dysfunction;

Illness is a subjective state of the person who feels aware of not being well;

Sickness is a state of social dysfunction, i.e., a role that the individual assumes when ill ("sickness role").

The clinician sees people who are ill rather than the diseases which he must diagnose and treat. Howev-

性关节炎）。某些疾病会出现"携带者"，即表面健康，没有明显的症状和体征，但具有传染性（如伤寒）。在某些情况下，同一病原体（如链球菌）可能引起多种临床表现，同一疾病也可能由多种病原体引起（如腹泻）。有些疾病病程较短，有些则病程较长。当患者出现明显的症状和体征时，疾病的诊断相对简单，但很多疾病正常和异常的界限并不明显，如糖尿病、高血压和精神疾病。疾病的终点或最终结果是可变的——有康复、残疾或死亡。

在英语中，disease、illness和sickness尽管都有"疾病"的意思，但这是完全不同的三个单词，其含义也不同。disease一词的字面意思是"不适"（不舒服），即身体机能出现问题。illness不仅指某一特定疾病的临床表现，还包括个体对疾病的主观感受和行为，以及疾病对社会心理环境的影响。sickness指的是一种社会功能障碍状态。Susser对这三个单词的区别有以下观点：

disease是一种存在生理/心理功能障碍的状态；

illness是人感觉到身体不舒服的主观状态；

sickness是一种存在社会功能障碍的状态，即个人生病时所扮演的角色（"疾病角色"）。

医生看到的是生病的人，而不是必须诊断和治疗的疾病（disease）。然而，有些患者可能没有

er, it is possible to be victim of disease without feeling ill, and to be ill without signs of physical impairment. In short, an adequate definition of disease is yet to be found a definition that is satisfactory or acceptable to the epidemiologist, clinician, sociologist and the statistician.

明显的症状和体征，或者在自身还没有感受到疾病时就已经生病了。简而言之，亟需确定一个在流行病学、临床医学、社会学和统计学中都适合应用并可以被接受的"疾病"的定义。

7.2　Concept of Cause

Cause: A cause is something that brings about an effect or a result. In medicine, cause is usually discussed under such headings as etiology, pathogenesis, mechanisms or risk factors. Cause is an important concept for understanding disease prevention, diagnosis and treatment in clinical practices. "Causality" refers to the process relating causes to the effects they produce, and much of the work of research epidemiologists' concerns attempts to establish causality. Epidemiological studies can provide powerful evidence on causality, but epidemiologic evidence alone is rarely sufficient to establish causality.

A "risk factor" is an attribute or exposure that is associated with an increase in the probability of occurrence of disease or other specified outcomes. It can be a genetic characteristic, an environmental exposure, an aspect of personal life-style, and/or a social characteristic. A risk factor may be a cause of a disease, but it also may be a characteristic whose association with a disease is non-causal.

K. Rothman, in his textbook, *Modem Epidemiology*, defined a cause of a disease as: an event, condition, or characteristic that precedes the disease event and without which the disease event either would not have occurred at all or would not have occurred until some later several types of causes can be distin-

7.2　病因的概念

病因是指产生结局或结果的因素。在医学中，病因通常出现在病因学、发病机制、其他机制或危险因素等内容中。病因是临床实践中有助于理解疾病预防、诊断和治疗的重要概念。"因果关系"指的是将病因与其产生的影响联系起来的过程，流行病学的许多研究工作都涉及建立因果关系。流行病学研究可以为因果关系提供强有力的证据，但仅凭流行病学证据不足以确定因果关系。

"危险因素"是指使疾病或其他特定结果发生概率增加的特征或暴露。危险因素可以是遗传特征、环境暴露、个人生活方式和/或社会特征。危险因素可能是疾病的病因，也可能是与疾病相关的非因果特征。

K.Rothman 在他的《现代流行病学》一书中，将疾病的病因定义为：在疾病发生之前存在的某种不利事件、条件或特征。如果没有病因，疾病也不会发生。Last 在《流行病学词典》（Last，2001）中将病因定义为：使疾病发生概率增加的因素。当有相应疾病发生时，之前一定有该病因

guished. According to Last's *Dictionary of Epidemiology* (Last, 2001): A cause is termed "necessary" when it must always precede an effect, although the effect need not be the sole result of the one cause. A cause is termed "sufficient" when it inevitably initiates or produces an effect. Any given cause may be necessary, sufficient, neither, or both. These possibilities are explained below.

In reality, many factors that contribute to disease occurrence are neither necessary nor sufficient. According to the English philosopher, John Stuart Mill, the cause of any effect must consist of a constellation of components that act in concert. A "sufficient cause", which means a complete causal mechanism or a sufficient cause model, can be defined as a set of minimal conditions and events that inevitably produce disease; "minimal" implies that all of the conditions or events are necessary. In the sufficient-cause model, sets of one or more factors act as sufficient causes (illustrated as "pies" by Rothman).

For example, tuberculosis is defined as a disease caused by Mycobacterium tuberculosis (the necessary cause); yet this bacillus is not sufficient for the clinical illness to occur. Whether or not an infected individual will develop clinical tuberculosis is determined by the characteristics of tuberculosis strains, the number of infecting bacilli, and a number of characteristics of the patient including genetic susceptibility, immune status, living conditions and socioeconomic status, access to preventive treatment for latent infection, etc. Each of above factors can be a component of a sufficient causal model, and there may be several sufficient causal models of clinical tuberculosis.

In a sufficient-cause model, any factor that appears in at least one sufficient causal model is called a

存在，称为"必要病因"，此时该疾病不一定是该病因的唯一结果。当该病因存在时，必定导致疾病的发生，称为"充分病因"。病因可分为：充分且必要病因，必要但不充分病因，充分但不必要病因，不充分又不必要病因。

事实上，导致疾病发生的许多因素既不必要也不充分。根据英国哲学家 John Stuart Mill 的说法，任何结果的起因都由一系列联合作用的因素组成。"充分病因"是指一个完整的病因机制或充分病因模型，可以定义为必然导致疾病发生的最少条件和事件的组合。其中，"最少"意味着所有条件或事件都是必要的。在充分病因模型中，一个或多个因素集合作为充分病因（Rothman 以"pies"表示）。

例如，结核病被定义为由结核分枝杆菌（必要病因）引起的疾病。然而，这种芽孢杆菌并不足以导致临床疾病的发生。受感染个体是否会发展为临床结核病，取决于结核分枝杆菌菌株的特征、感染杆菌的数量以及患者的一些特征，包括遗传易感性、免疫状态、生活条件、社会经济状况及预防潜在感染的防治措施等。上述每一个因素都可能是结核病充分病因的组成部分。

在充分病因模型中，任何因素只要在一个充分病因模型中至少出现一次，就是组分病因；在

component cause, and any component cause that appears in all sufficient models is a necessary cause. Each sufficient cause has an independent effect on occurrence of the disease in population. Rothman's sufficient-cause model helps us to understand the multifactorial nature of disease etiology and represents fundamental theory about the causes of a specific disease and the biological interrelations among these causes.

所有充分病因模型中都存在的事件、特征或条件，就是必要病因。每一个充分病因对人群中疾病的发生都有独立影响。Rothman 的充分病因模型有助于理解疾病的多病因，并可作为研究特定疾病的病因及病因间生物学关系的理论基础。

7.3 Etiology Theory and Etiology Model

Up to the time of Louis Pasteur（1822—1895），various concepts of disease causation were in vogue, e.g., the supernatural theory of disease, the theory of humors, the concept of contagion, miasmatic theory of disease, the theory of spontaneous generation, etc. Discoveries in microbiology marked a turning point in our aetiological concept.

7.3 病因理论与病因模型

直到路易·巴斯德（1822—1895）时代，各种病因理论仍在盛行。例如，超自然病因理论、体液理论、传染理论、疾病的瘴气理论、自发产生理论等。微生物学的发现是病因学概念的转折点。

7.3.1 Germ theory of disease

This concept gained momentum during the 19th and the early part of 20th century. The emphasis had shifted from empirical causes（e.g., bad air）to microbes as the sole cause of disease. The concept of cause embodied in the germ theory of disease is generally referred to as a one-to-one relationship between causal agent and disease. The disease model accordingly is：

Causative agent → Man → Disease

The germ theory of disease, though it was a revolutionary concept, led many epidemiologists to take one-sided view of disease causation. That is, they could not think beyond the germ theory of disease. It is now recognized that a disease is rarely caused by a single agent alone, but rather depends upon a number

7.3.1 微生物学说

这一概念在 19 世纪和 20 世纪初得到了发展，重点已从传统的经验病因（如瘴气）转向了微生物作为疾病的唯一病因。在疾病的微生物学说中，病因通常被定义为病原体和疾病之间的一对一关系。相应的疾病模型为：

病原体→ 人 → 疾病

疾病的微生物学说虽然是一个革命性的概念，但它对疾病的病因解释得比较片面，微生物学说认为疾病由单一的病原体引起。现在人们已经认识到，一种疾病很少由一种因素单独引起，而是取决于促成其发生的许多因素。因此，现代医学已经不再严格遵循疾病的微生物学说。

of factors which contribute to its occurrence. Therefore modern medicine has moved away from the strict adherence to the germ theory of disease.

7.3.2 Epidemiological triad

The germ theory of disease has many limitations. For example, it is well - known, that not everyone exposed to tuberculosis develops tuberculosis. The same exposure however, in an undernourished or otherwise susceptible person may result in clinical disease. Similarly, not everyone exposed to beta - hemolytic streptococci develops acute rheumatic fever. There are other factors relating to the host and environment which are equally important to determine whether or not disease will occur in the exposed host. This demanded a broader concept of disease causation that synthesized the basic factors of agent, host and environment（Figure 7-1）.

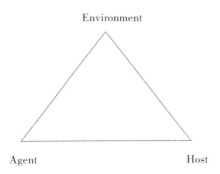

Figure 7-1 Epidemiological triad

The above model — agent, host and environment — has been in use for many years. It helped epidemiologists to focus on different classes of factors, especially with regard to infectious diseases.

7.3.3 Multifactorial causation

The concept that disease is due to multiple factors is not a new one. Pettenkofer of Munich（1819—1901）was an early proponent of this concept. But the

7.3.2 流行病学的三角模型

疾病的微生物学说有许多局限性。比如，众所周知，并非所有接触结核分枝杆菌的人都会患上结核病。然而，在同样的暴露下，营养不良的人群或其他易感人群就可能患上结核病。同样，并非所有接触β-溶血性链球菌的人都会患上急性风湿热，其他与宿主和环境相关的因素也同样会影响疾病的发生。因此，需要一个涉及病原体、宿主和环境因素的更全面的疾病模型（图7-1）。

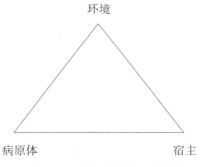

图7-1 流行病学的三角模型

上述三角模型明确显示影响传染病在人群中发生、发展的因素是多种的，即宿主、病原体和环境。该三角模型优于朴素的单病因学说，揭示了在病原体以外存在可用来预防和控制的病因。

7.3.3 多病因论

疾病的多病因论并不是新的概念，慕尼黑的Pettenkofer（1819—1901）很早就提出了这一观点。但到了19世纪末，多病因论受到微生物学说

"germ theory of disease" or "single cause idea" in the late 19th century overshadowed the multiple cause theory.

As a result of advances in public health, chemotherapy, antibiotics and vector control communicable diseases began to decline — only to be replaced by new types of diseases, the so-called "modern" diseases of civilization, e g., lung cancer, coronary heart disease, chronic bronchitis, mental illness, etc. These diseases could not be explained on the basis of the germ theory of disease nor could they be prevented by the traditional methods of isolation, immunization or improvements in sanitation. The realization began to dawn that the "single cause idea" was an oversimplification and that there are other factors in the etiology of diseases, social, economic, cultural, genetic and psychological which are equally important. As already mentioned, tuberculosis is not merely due to tubercle bacilli; factors such as poverty, overcrowding and malnutrition contribute to its occurrence. The doctrine of one-to-one relationship between cause and disease has been shown to be untenable, even for microbial diseases, e.g., tuberculosis, leprosy.

It is now known that diseases such as coronary heart disease and cancer are due to multiple factors. For example, excess of fat intake, smoking, lack of physical exercise and obesity are all involved in the pathogenesis of coronary heart disease. Most of these factors are linked to lifestyle and human behavior. Epidemiology has contributed significantly to our present day understanding of multifactorial causation of disease. Medical men are looking beyond the "germ theory" of disease into the total life situation of the patient and the community in search of multiple (or risk) factors of disease.

等单病因论的影响而沉寂。

随着公共卫生、化疗、抗生素和病媒控制的进步，传染病逐渐减少，慢性非传染病（即所谓的"现代"文明病，如肺癌、冠心病、慢性支气管炎、精神病等）成为人类健康的主要威胁。慢性非传染病不像传染病那样存在明确的病原体，也无法通过传统的隔离、增强免疫或改善卫生条件等措施来预防。"单一病因"过于简单，无法解释慢性病致病因素的多样性；"三角模型"把每个因素独立且等量齐观，也不适合解释慢性病各因素间存在的交叉复杂的关联，以及展示慢性病直接病因和间接病因间主次的区别。比如，社会、经济、文化、遗传和心理因素等致病因素在疾病中共同起作用，且相互之间存在关系，作用大小也存在差别。例如，结核病不仅由结核分枝杆菌引起，贫困、过度拥挤和营养不良等因素也对结核病的发生起到一定作用。因此，单病因论无法解释疾病，即使是对微生物疾病（如结核病、麻风病）。

目前，众所周知，冠心病和癌症均是多病因疾病。例如，脂肪摄入过多、吸烟、缺乏体育锻炼和肥胖等都与冠心病的发病有关，且这些因素大多与人们的生活方式和行为有关。了解这些可改变因素有助于采取对应措施，从而预防冠心病的发生。流行病学重要的应用之一就是探索疾病的病因，为疾病防治措施的确定提供依据。目前，很多医务工作者都利用流行病学方法观察患者和社会的各方面特征，以寻找疾病病因。

Therefore new models of disease causation have been developed（e.g., multifactorial causation, web of causation）which de-emphasize the concept of disease "agent" and stress multiplicity of interactions between host and environment. Many epidemiologists prefer to regard the agent as an integral part of the total environment. The purpose of knowing the multiple factors of disease is to quantify and arrange them in priority sequence（prioritization）for modification or amelioration to prevent or control disease. The multifactorial concept offers multiple approaches for the prevention/control of disease.

7.3.4　Web of causation

This model of disease causation was suggested by MacMahon and Pugh in their book: *Epidemiologic Principles and Methods*. This model is ideally suited in the study of chronic disease, where the disease agent is often not known, but is the outcome of interaction of multiple factors.

The "web of causation" considers all the predisposing factors of any type and their complex interrelationship with each other. Figure 7-2 illustrates the complexities of a causal web of myocardial infarction（which is by no means complete）. The basic tenet of epidemiology is to study the clusters of causes and combinations of effects and how they relate to each other. It can be visualized that the causal web（Figure 7-2）provides a model which shows a variety of possible interventions that could be taken which might reduce the occurrence of myocardial infarction.

The web of causation does not imply that the disease cannot be controlled unless all the multiple causes or chains of causation or at least a number of them are appropriately controlled or removed. This is

因此，新的病因模型（如病因链、病因网）应运而生。这些模型不再强调病原体的作用，而是更关注宿主和环境之间相互作用的多样性，并将病原体视为生物环境中的一个部分。了解多病因论有助于量化病因，并按照其作用的重要性排列，为疾病的预防和控制措施的改进和调整提供依据。

7.3.4　病因网络模型

病因网络模型由 MacMahon 和 Pugh 在《流行病学原理和方法》一书中提出，病因网是指联系病因与发病的整体网状结构，因为慢性病没有明确的病原体，而是多种因素相互作用的结果，因此该模型非常适合慢性病的研究。

病因网络模型考虑了所有类型疾病的致病因素以及因素间复杂的相互关系。图7-2显示了心肌梗死的病因网络模型的复杂性（仅展示了部分病因和效应）。流行病学的基本用途是研究病因和其组合效应以及相互之间的关系。病因网络模型（图7-2）显示的内容，为制定心肌梗死的防制措施提供了依据。

病因网络模型的复杂性，似乎使疾病的防制非常难以实施。而事实上，切断或控制任何一个或几个病因链中相对危险度较大的病因，就能切断所有与其相关的病因链和病因网，从而有效防

not the case. Sometimes removal of elimination of just only one link or chain may be sufficient to control disease, provided that link is sufficiently important in the pathogenic process. In a multifactorial event, therefore, individual factors are by no means equal weight. The relative importance of these factors expressed in terms of "relative risk".

制疾病。因此，多病因疾病中，不同病因链对疾病发生的作用可能不同，病因链中不同因素的作用也可能不同，这些因素的相对重要性用"相对危险度"表示。

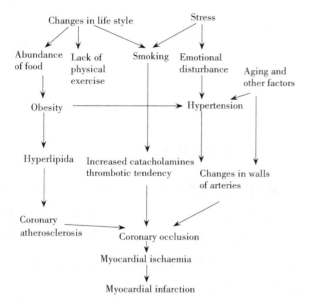

Figure 7-2　Web of causation for myocardial infarction

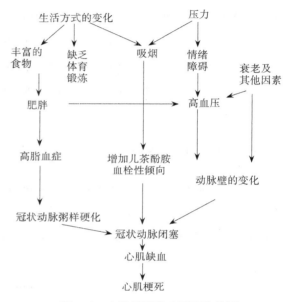

图 7-2　心肌梗死的病因网络模型

7.4　Association and Causation

Descriptive studies help in the identification of the disease problem in the community; and by relating disease to host, agent and environmental factors, it endeavours to suggest an aetiological hypothesis. Analytical and experimental studies test the hypotheses derived from descriptive studies and confirm or refute the observed association between suspected causes and disease. When the disease is multifactorial (e.g., coronary heart disease) numerous factors or variables become implicated in the web of causation, and the notion of "cause" becomes confused. The more associations are, the more investigations are to disentangle

7.4　关联与因果关系

描述性研究有助于社区诊断，将疾病与宿主、病原体和环境因素联系起来，提出病因假设。分析性研究和试验研究检验描述性研究建立的假设，证实或驳斥观察到的可疑病因和疾病之间的联系。对于多病因疾病（如冠心病），病因网中有许多因素或变量，"病因"的确定相对复杂。关联越多，越需要更多的研究去厘清病因网。流行病学主要的目的是建立"因果关系"，以有效预防疾病，也就是从谷物中筛选出谷壳。流行病学研究是从统计关联到因果关系的论证过程。

the web of causes. The epidemiologist whose primary interest is to establish a "cause and effect" relationship has to sift the husk from the grain. He proceeds from demonstration of statistical association to demonstration that the association is causal.

The terms "association" and "relationship" are often used interchangeably. Association may be defined as the concurrence of two variables more often than would be expected by chance. In other words, events are said to be associated when they occur more frequently together than one would expect by chance. Association does not necessarily imply a causal relationship.

It will be useful to consider here the concept of correlation. Correlation indicates the degree of association between two characteristics. The correlation coefficient ranges from − 1.0 to + 1.0. A correlation coefficient of 1.0 means that the two variables exhibit a perfect linear relationship. However, correlation cannot be used to invoke causation, because the sequence of exposure preceding disease (temporal association) cannot be assumed to have occurred. Secondly, correlation does not measure risk. It may be said that causation implies correlation, but correlation does not imply causation.

Association can be broadly grouped under three headings:

7.4.1　Spurious association

Sometimes an observed association between a disease and suspected factor may not be real. For example, a study in UK of 5 174 births at home and 11 156 births in hospitals showed perinatal mortality rates of 5.4 per 1 000 in the home births and 27.8 per 1 000 in the hospital births. Apparently, the perinatal mortality

术语"关联"和"关系"经常互换使用。关联可以定义为两个变量同时出现的频率超过了偶然性。换言之，当事件的发生比预期要频繁时，就被认为是有关联的。但关联并不一定意味着存在因果关系。

在确定因果关系的过程中，有必要确定疾病与因素的相关性。相关性表示两个特征之间的关联程度。相关系数的取值范围是[-1,+1]，相关系数为 1 意味着变量间呈线性关系。然而，相关性只是统计学上的关联。首先，相关性并不能用来确定因果关系，因为无法确定疾病和暴露的先后顺序（关联的时序性）。其次，相关性不能用来度量风险。存在因果关系表明一定存在相关性，但存在相关性并不表明一定存在因果关系。

关联可以分为以下三种：

7.4.1　虚假关联

有时，观察到的疾病和可疑因素之间的关联可能并不是真的。例如，英国进行的一项研究（包括 5 174 个家庭分娩和 11 156 个医院分娩）结果显示，在家分娩的围产期死亡率为 5.4‰，医院分娩的围产期死亡率为 27.8‰。显然，医院分娩的围产期死亡率比家庭分娩的高，因此得出结论，

was higher in hospital births than in the home births. It might be concluded that homes are a safer place for delivery of births than hospitals. Such a conclusion is spurious or artificial, because in general, hospitals attract women at high risk for delivery because of their special equipment and expertise, whereas this is not the case with home deliveries. The high perinatal mortality rate in hospitals might be due to this fact alone, and not because the quality on care was inferior. There might be other factors also such as differences in age, parity, prenatal care, home circumstances, general health and disease state between the study and control groups. This type of bias where "like" is not compared with "like" (confounding bias) is very important in epidemiological studies. It may lead to a spurious association or an association when none actually existed.

7.4.2 Indirect association

Many associations which at first appeared to be causal have been found on further study to be due to indirect association. The indirect association is a statistical association between a characteristic (or variable) of interest and a disease due to the presence of another factor, knowns or unknowns that is common to both the characteristic and the disease. This third factor (i. e., the common factor) is also known as the "confounding" variable. Since it is related both to the disease and to the variable, it might explain the statistical association between disease and a characteristic wholly or in part. Such confounding variables (e. g., age, sex) are potentially and probably present in all data and represent a formidable obstacle to overcome in trying to assess the causal nature of the relationship. Two examples of an indirect association are given below.

家庭比医院更适合分娩。产生这样虚假结论的原因是，医院因其专业的设备和技术而吸引更多的高危产妇前去分娩，而在家中分娩的孕妇高危情况很少见，这就造成了医院分娩的高围产期死亡率。可能还有其他因素，如两组对象的年龄、胎次、产前护理、家庭环境、一般健康和疾病状态等也存在差异，这些差异会带来混杂偏倚，从而导致虚假关联。偏倚在流行病学研究中非常重要，需要控制，否则可能带来虚假关联。

7.4.2 间接关联

研究发现，许多因果关系是间接关联引起的。间接关联指研究因素与疾病之间本来不存在统计学关联，但是它们都与其他因素（第三因素）有关，从而导致两者在统计学上存在关联。这里的第三因素（即共同因素）也被称为混杂因素，指既与疾病有关，又与研究因素有关，但不是研究因素与疾病因果链的中间变量，可以用来解释疾病的全部或部分的统计联系。混杂因素（如年龄、性别等）可能潜在存在于所有数据中，是评估因素与疾病的因果关系时需要克服的困难。下面是两个间接关联的例子。

1.Altitude and endemic goitre

Endemic goitre is generally found in high altitudes showing thereby an association between altitude and endemic goitre（Figure 7-3）. According to current knowledge, we know that endemic goitre is not due to altitude but due to environmental deficiency of iodine. Figure 7-3 illustrates how common factor（i.e., iodine deficiency）can result in an apparent association between two variables, when no association exists. This amplifies the earlier statement that statistical association does not necessarily mean causation.

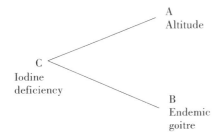

Figure 7-3　Model of an indirect association

2.Sucrose and CHD

Yudkin and Roddy found a higher intake of sugar by patients with myocardial infarction. Their study was based on an enquiry by questionnaire method into dietary habits of cases and controls. They put forward an attractive hypothesis that people who consume lot of sugar are far more likely to have a heart attack — than those who take little.

Further studies were undertaken to test whether sugar intake was associated with other variables such as cigarette smoking, which might be causally related to CHD. Bennet and others found that heavy cigarette smoking was positively associated with an increase in the number of cups of hot drinks consumed daily and the amount of sugar consumed. They concluded that it was cigarette smoking and not sugar consumption which was implicated in the aetiology of CHD. In their

1.海拔高度与地方性甲状腺肿

地方性甲状腺肿一般都发生在高海拔地区，因此海拔高度与地方性甲状腺肿存在关联（图7-3）。目前，根据相关知识，地方性甲状腺肿不是由海拔高度而是由环境中碘缺乏引起的。图7-3说明了共同因素（即碘缺乏）是如何导致这两个本身没有关系的变量存在明显关联的。这种间接关联是一种放大的统计关联，并不等同于因果关系。

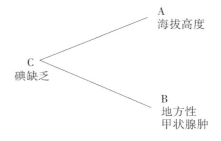

图7-3　间接关联模型

2.蔗糖与冠心病

Yudkin和Roddy发现心肌梗死患者都有高糖饮食的习惯。他们通过问卷调查了病例组心梗患者和对照组无心梗者的饮食习惯，目的是检验高糖摄入者比低糖摄入者更易患心脏病这一假设。

为了检验糖摄入是否与冠心病的其他病因（如吸烟）有关，研究人员做了进一步的研究。Bennet等人发现，吸烟量及每天的热饮杯数和糖摄入量呈正相关，但没有发现随着糖摄入量增加而冠心病风险增加的现象。因此得出的结论是，吸烟（而不是摄入糖分）与冠心病有关。最后，实验研究证明，高蔗糖喂养不会诱发动物的动脉硬化性疾病。

study, they did not find any evidence of increasing trend of CHD with increasing consumption of sugar. Finally, proof came from experimental studies that high sucrose feeding did not induce arteriosclerotic disease in animals.

Sometimes knowledge of indirect associations can be applied towards reducing disease risk. Before the discovery of the cholera vibrio, elimination of certain water supplies achieved a marked decrease in new cases of the disease. Such indirect associations must be pursued, for it is likely that they may provide aetiological clues.

7.4.3 Direct (causal) association

1. One-to-one causal relationship

Two variables are stated to be causally related (AB) if a change in A is followed by a change in B. If it does not, then their relationship cannot be causal. This is known as "one-to-one" causal relationship. This model suggests that when the factor A is present, the disease B must result. Conversely, when the disease is present, the factor must also be present. Measles may be one disease in which such a relation exists.

Epidemiologists are interested in identifying the "cause". The most satisfactory procedure to demonstrate this would be by direct experiment. But this procedure is scarcely available to the epidemiologist. And, in some cases, the "cause" is not amenable to manipulation.

The above concept of one-to-one causal relationship was the essence of Koch's postulates. The proponents of the germ theory of disease insisted that the cause must be:

① Necessary.

② Sufficient for the occurrence of disease, before

关于间接关联的知识也可以用于减少疾病风险。在发现霍乱弧菌之前，停止疫水供应可以使霍乱的新发病例明显减少。在因果关联推断的过程中，对间接关联的研究也是必要的，因为它可以提供病因线索。

7.4.3 直接（因果）关联

1."一对一"因果关联

如果A随着B的改变而改变，那么这两个变量（AB）间就存在着因果关系；如果没有发生改变，那么它们之间可能不存在因果关系，这就是所谓的"一对一"因果关系。该模型表明，当A因素存在时，就会引起疾病B；相反，当疾病B出现时，这个因素A也存在。麻疹就是存在"一对一"关系的疾病。

流行病学的研究目的是确定"病因"，要想确定病因，最有力的方法是直接开展实验。但在某些情况下，病因是不可控制的，因此开展流行病学试验不可行。

上述"一对一"因果关系的概念是Koch法则的核心。微生物学说的支持者认为病因必须是：

①必要的。

②足以导致疾病的发生。病因应发生在疾病

it can qualify as cause of disease. In other words, whenever the disease occurs, the factor or cause must be present.

Although Koch's postulates are theoretically sound, the "necessary and sufficient" concept does not fit well for many diseases. Taking for example tuberculosis, tubercle bacilli cannot be found in all cases of the disease but this does not rule out the statement that tubercle bacilli are the cause of tuberculosis. That the cause must be "sufficient" is also not always supported by evidence. In tuberculosis, it is well-known that besides tubercle bacilli, there are additional factors such as host susceptibility which are required to produce the disease.

The concept of one‐to‐one causal relationship is further complicated by the fact that sometimes, a single cause of factor may lead to more than one outcome, as shown on Figure 7–4. In short, one‐to‐one causal relationship, although ideal in disease aetiology, does not explain every situation.

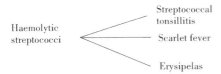

Figure 7-4　Model in which one factor is shown to lead to more than one disease

2.Multifactorial causation

The causal thinking is different when we consider a near communicable disease or condition (e. g., CHD) where the aetiology is multifactorial. Two models are presented to Figures 7–5 and 7–6 to explain the complex situation. In one model (Figure 7–5), there are alternative causal factors (Factor 1, 2 and 3) each acting independently. This situation is exemplified in lung cancer where more than one aetiological factor (e.g., smoking, air pollution, exposure to asbes-

之前。也就是说，每当疾病发生时，因素或病因必须存在。

虽然 Koch 法则在理论上是正确的，但"必要且充分"病因并不适合大部分疾病。以肺结核为例，并不是所有肺结核病例中都能检测出结核分枝杆菌，但也不能认为"结核分枝杆菌是肺结核病因"的说法是错误的。病因必须是充分的，这也不一定有证据的支持。众所周知，在结核病中，除了结核分枝杆菌外，还有其他因素是结核病发生的必要条件，如宿主易感性。

有时，一个病因可能导致多种结果，即一因多果（图7-4）；也会存在多种病因导致一个结果的情况，即一果多因，这比"一对一"因果关系要复杂。简而言之，"一对一"因果关系在疾病病因学中是理想状况，但并不常见。

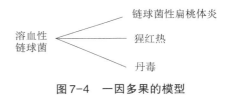

图7-4　一因多果的模型

2. 多因素因果关联

多病因的非传染病（如冠心病）的病因推断与"一对一"因果关系的传染病有所不同。图7-5和图7-6提供了两个实例来解释复杂的情况。在第一个实例中（图7-5），每个因素（因子1、2和3）对疾病都有各自独立的作用。以肺癌为例，许多病因（如吸烟、空气污染、接触石棉）都可以单独导致肺癌发生。目前，随着对癌症了解的不断增加，大量研究发现，在细胞水平上，各种不同的病因能够引起相同的生化反应。参与肺癌发

tos）can produce the disease independently. It is possible as the knowledge of cancer is increasing, we may discover a common biochemical event at the cellular level that can be produced by each of the factors. The cellular or molecular factor then be considered necessary as a causal factor.

病机制的细胞因子或分子因素是导致肺癌的必要病因。

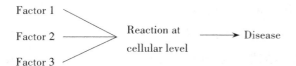

Figure 7-5　A model of multifactorial causation

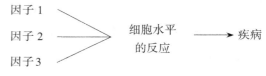

图7-5　多因素因果关联的模型

In the second model（Figure 7-6）the causal factors can cumulatively to produce disease. This is probably the correct model for many diseases. It is possible that each of the several factors act independently, but when an individual is exposed to 2 or more factors, there may be a synergistic effect.

第二个实例（图7-6）显示因素的累积作用可导致疾病的发生。可能许多疾病的发生都符合该模型，也有可能每个因素的致病作用是独立的，当同时暴露于两个或更多的因素时，这些因素可能产生协同效应。

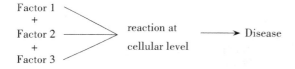

Figure 7-6　A model of multifactorial causation showing synergism

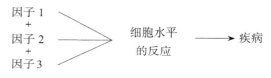

图7-6　多因素协同作用的模型

From the above discussion, it is reasonable to conclude that "one-to-one" relationship in causation is very oversimplification. In biological phenomena, the requirement that "cause" is both "necessary" and "sufficient" condition is not easily reached, because of the existence of multiple factor in disease aetiology. This has created a serious problem to the epidemiologist, who is in search of causes of disease.

综上，"一对一"的因果关系过于简单，无法解释复杂的生物现象。实际上，疾病的多病因很难使病因同时满足"必要"和"充分"两个条件，这也给流行病学寻找疾病的病因带来了困难。

7.5   Criteria for judging causality

In the absence of controlled experimental evidence can incriminate the "cause", certain additional criteria have been evolved for deciding when an association may be considered a causal association. Scientists and philosophers have developed strategies and criteria for determining when a causal relationship exists. Three of these are discussed briefly below.

7.5.1   Mill's Canons

Mill's Canons represent logical strategies ("canons") developed by John Stuart Mill for inferring a causal relationship between a circumstance (e. g., a risk factor) and a phenomenon (e. g., an health outcome). In a Dictionary of Epidemiology (Last, 4th ed. 2001), four of Mill's five strategies are described as especially pertinent to epidemiology.

1.Agreement canon

If two or more instances of the phenomenon under investigation have only one circumstance incommon, the circumstance, in which alone all the instances agree, is the cause (or effect) of the given phenomenon.If an instance in which the phenomenon under investigation occurs, and an instance in which it does.

2.Difference canon

Occur and not occur, have every circumstance in common save one, that one occurring only in the former, the circumstance in which alone the two instances differ is the effect, or cause or a necessary part of the cause, and of the phenomenon.

7.5   病因推断的标准

在缺乏对照实验证据的前提下，需要制定其他病因推断的标准以确定因果关系。因此，在科学和哲学领域已经发展了一些用来确定因果关系的策略和标准。下面简要阐述其中三个标准：

7.5.1   Mill 准则

Mill 准则是英国哲学家John Stuart Mill 为推断环境（如风险因素）和现象（如健康结果）之间的因果关系而制定的逻辑策略（或称准则）。在《流行病学词典》（第4版，2001年）中，Mill 准则中有以下4条准则与流行病学的病因推断相关：

1.求同法

比较某现象出现的不同场合，如果不同场合除了一个条件相同外，其他条件都不同，那么这个相同的条件可能就是某研究现象的原因。在病因研究中，如果患有相同疾病的患者都有某一共同因素，而其他因素并非每个患者都具备，那么该因素可能就是该病的病因。

2.求异法

比较某现象出现的场合和不出现的场合，如果两个场合除一点不同外，其他都相同，那么这个不同点就是该现象的原因。在病因研究中，如果未患病的个体与患病个体相比，除了某一因素外，其他因素均相同，那么这个因素可能就是该病的病因。

3.Residues canon

Subducing from any phenomenon such part as is known by previous inductions to be the effect of certain antecedents, and the residue of the phenomenon is the effect of the remaining antecedents.

4.Concomitant variation canon

Whatever phenomenon varies in any manner whether another phenomenon varies in some particular manner, is either a cause or an effect of that phenomenon, or is connected with it through some fact of causation.

7.5.2　Koch's Postulates

Koch's Postulates refer to a set of criteria promulgated by Robert Koch (with contributions of F. G. Jacob Henle) in the 19th century. Koch devised the postulates for determining whether an infectious agent is the cause of disease, with the assumption that a particular disease has one cause and a particular cause results in one disease. He stated that these four postulates should be met before a causative relationship can be accepted between a particular bacterial parasite or disease agent and the disease in question.

① The agent must be shown to be present in every case of the disease by isolation in pure culture.

② The agent must not be found in cases of other disease.

③ Once isolated, the agent must be capable of reproducing the disease in experimental animals.

④ The agent must be recovered from the experimental disease produced.

Koch's postulates had a great impact on the development of etiological theory, especially during the

3. 剩余法

从现象中去除已经确认有因果联系的部分，剩余的现象应由剩余部分的因素解释。在病因研究中，剩余法很少用于直接发现病因的逻辑推断中，但对于判断是否发现了疾病主要病因是有帮助的。

4. 共变法

当某一现象发生变化时，另一现象也相应发生变化，那么二者可能存在因果关系，也可能通过因果关系的某方面而相关。

7.5.2　Koch 法则

Koch 法则是由德国科学家 Robert Koch 在 19 世纪提出的用来确定病原体是传染病病因的一套标准。假设特定疾病必定存在某个病因，那么该特定病因也必将引发该疾病。在确定某细菌或病原体与相关疾病存在因果关系之前，应该存在以下 4 个前提条件：

① 在该病的每个患者中都能检出该病原体，而在健康者体内则不能。

② 在其他疾病的患者中不能检出该病原体。

③ 从患者体内分离的病原体，经过培养能引起实验动物发生相应疾病。

④ 从患该病的动物体内能分离得到相同病原体。

Koch 法则对病因学理论的发展产生了重大影响，尤其在流行病学发展的早期，Koch 法则被用

early years of epidemiology when interest focused on acute infectious diseases. For most chronic or non‑infectious diseases, however, a single cause cannot be simply established by Koch's postulates, and often many factors appear to act together to cause disease.

7.5.3 Hill's Criteria

Hill's Criteria were proposed by the British medical statistician, Austin Bradford Hill in a paper dealing with the question of whether cigarette smoking was a cause of lung disease. These criteria for causation were adapted by the United States Surgeon General in his 1964 report that determined that smoking causes lung and laryngeal cancer. Hill's criteria are now commonly cited when attempting to distinguish causal from non‑causal associations. Hill suggested consideration of the following aspects of an association:

① Temporal association.

② Strength of association.

③ Specificity of the association.

④ Consistency of the association.

⑤ Biological plausibility.

⑥ Coherence of the association.

The Surgeon‑General's Report (1964) stated that the causal significance of an association is a matter of judgement which goes beyond any statement of statistical probability. To judge or evaluate the causal significance of an association, all the above criteria must be utilized, no one of which by itself is self‑sufficient or a sine qua‑non for drawing causal inferences from statistical associations, but each adds to the quantum of evidence, and all put together contribute to a probability of the association being causal.

来确定急性传染病的病因。然而，对于大多数慢性病或非传染病，Koch法则无法确定其中的因果关系，因为这些疾病往往是多因素共同作用所导致的。

7.5.3 Hill准则

Hill准则是由英国医学统计学家Austin Bradford Hill在一篇讨论吸烟是否为肺部疾病病因的论文中提出的。1964年，当时的美国卫生部部长在某篇报告中采用了这些因果关系标准，该报告明确指出吸烟会导致肺癌和喉癌。现在，Hill准则在人群研究中仍被广泛使用，用来判断因果关系。Hill准则包括以下几个方面：

①关联的时序性。

②关联的强度。

③关联的特异性。

④关联的可重复性。

⑤生物学合理性。

⑥关联的一致性。

1964年的这份报告指出，因果关联是一个超出了任何统计概率的判断问题。为了判断或评估因果关系，必须使用Hill准则。其中，关联的时序性、关联的强度和生物学合理性必须具备，其他每一条都增加了因果关联的可能性，所有的条件集合在一起有助于增加因果关系的可能性。

7.6 Examples: Association Between Cigarette Smoking and Lung Cancer

Cigarette smoking and lung cancer hypothesis provides an excellent example to illustrate the epidemiological criteria for establishing whether or not an observed association plays a causal role in the aetiology of a disease. The data fulfilling the criteria were covered adequately in smoking and health, the initial report of the Advisory Committee to the Surgeon General of the Public Health Service in 1964. The later reports of US Public' Health Service from 1964—1973, and similar other reports (e.g., report of the Royal College of Physicians, London: Smoking or Health, 1977) summarised newer data supporting the validity of the hypothesis. Let us examine the cigarette smoking and lung cancer hypothesis in the light of the above criteria.

7.6.1 Temporal association

This criterion centers round the question: Does the suspected cause precede the observed effect? A causal association requires that exposure to a putative cause must precede temporarily the onset of a disease which it is purported to produce to allow for any necessary period of induction and latency. This requirement is basic to the causal concept.

In certain acute diseases such as water and food-borne outbreaks, discovery of temporal sequence of two variables (e.g., drinking contaminated water and diarrhoea) is not often a serious problem. However, in many chronic diseases, because of insidious onset and ignorance of precise induction periods, it becomes hard to establish a temporal sequence as to which came first—the suspected agent or the disease, be-

7.6 举例：吸烟与肺癌的关系

吸烟和肺癌的关系假说是确定观察到的关联是否为因果关联的流行病学经典案例。1964年，美国咨询委员会向卫生部部长提交的关于吸烟和健康的初步报告就充分体现了Hill准则的应用。1964—1973年，美国公共健康服务后期的报告和其他类似的报告（如1977年英国皇家学院关于吸烟或健康的报告）所总结的新数据都支持了该假说。下面利用Hill准则来检验吸烟和肺癌存在因果关系的假说。

7.6.1 关联的时序性

这条标准围绕着一个问题：可疑因素先于观察结果出现吗？因果关系要求暴露因素必须发生在疾病之前，即先有因，后有果。因素的效应需要一定的诱导期或潜伏期。时间的先后顺序是因果关系的基本条件。

在某些急性病中（如水和食源性疾病），判断两个变量（如饮用受污染的水和腹泻）的时间顺序相对而言不是很困难。然而，在许多起病隐匿且无法预知准确的诱导期或潜伏期的疾病中，很难判断时间上的先后顺序。也就是说，因为疾病在不断地演变、发展，所以无法确定可疑因素和疾病发生时间的先后顺序。

cause one is dealing with a continuous evolving process.

Lung cancer occurs in smokers of long-standing; this satisfies the temporal requirement. Further, the increase in consumption of cigarettes preceded by many years the increase in death rates from lung cancer. These observations are compatible with the long latent period characteristic of carcinogenesis.

7.6.2　Strength of association

The strength of association is based on answers to two questions:

①Relative risk — is it large?

②Is there a dose-response, duration-response relationship?

In general, the larger the relative risk is, the greater the likelihood of a causal association is. Furthermore, the likelihood of a causal relationship is strengthened if there is a biological gradient or dose-response relationship i.e., with increasing levels of exposure to the risk factor, an increasing rise in incidence of the disease is found. If there is no dose-response or dose-response ralationship, that whould be an argument against the relationship being causal.

In the absence of experimental data on humans, the causal relationship of cigarette smoking and lung cancer has been based on three points:①relative risk; ②dose-response relationship, and;③the decrease in risk on cessation of smoking. Table 7-1 presents data showing relative risk and dose-response relationship. Such high relative risks are rarely seen in epidemiological studies. It has been stated that the relationship between lung cancer and smoking is one of the most impressive demonstrations of a dose-response relationship that can be found in epidemiology. The dose re-

肺癌往往发生在长期吸烟者中，这符合时间要求。另外，早期研究也发现，随着香烟消费量的增加，肺癌的死亡率也有所上升。这些观察结果与吸烟暴露引起癌变的长潜伏期特征相一致。

7.6.2　关联的强度

下面这两个问题是关联强度的基础：

①相对危险度的大小？
②是否存在剂量–反应、时间–反应关系？

一般来说，相对危险度越大，存在因果关系的可能性就越大。此外，如果存在生物梯度或剂量–反应关系，那么因果关系的可能性就得到加强，即随着可疑因素暴露水平的增加，疾病的发病率提高。如果关联强度不存在统计学意义，那么就可以否定因果关系的存在。

在缺乏人类实验证据的情况下，吸烟和肺癌因果关系的推断主要基于以下三点：①相对危险度；②剂量–反应关系；③戒烟后肺癌风险的降低。表7-1显示了相对危险度和剂量–反应关系的数据。可以看到不同吸烟水平的相对危险度都比较高，这在流行病学研究中很少见。有学者提出，吸烟水平与肺癌死亡率之间的剂量–反应关系是流行病学研究中的典型实例。实际上，剂量–反应关系在因果推断中具有重要作用，是支持因果关系的重要论据。该研究结果还证实了中度吸烟者肺癌死亡率居于轻度吸烟者和重度吸烟者之间。

sponse relationship has, in fact, played a major role in acceptance of relationship as causal. If there has been no dose-response relationship, that would have been a strong argument against the causal hypothesis. Another factor that has added to the weight of evidence is the fact that lung cancer death rates among moderate smokers were intermediate between those among light smokers and heavy smokers.

Table 7-1　Death rate and relative risk for smokers and non-smokers

Daily average cigarettes smoked	Death rate per 1 000 Smokers Non-smokers		Relative Risk
1-14	0.47	0.07	6.7
15-24	0.86	0.07	12.3
25+	1.66	0.07	23.7

表 7-1　吸烟者和非吸烟者的肺癌死亡率和相对危险度（RR）

日均吸烟量 /支	死亡率/‰		RR
	吸烟者	非吸烟者	
1～14	0.4	0.07	6.7
15～24	0.8	0.07	12.3
25+	1.6	0.07	23.7

Cessation experiment:

Another piece of evidence is provided by the cessation experiment. Table 7-2 shows the Mortality ratio in ex-cigarette smokers by number of years stopped smoking among British doctors. The results confirmed that the mortality ratio was reduced in a way that would be expected if smoking were the cause of the disease. This is a strong point in the evidence favouring the hypothesis.

终止实验进一步为因果推断提供了证据。表 7-2显示了英国医生中不同戒烟年限者的肺癌死亡率。结果证实，如果吸烟是肺癌的病因，那么肺癌死亡率的下降是可以预期的。这是支持病因假设的强有力证据。

Table 7-2　Lung cancer mortality ratios in ex-cigarette-smokers, by number of years stopped smoking, British physicians

Years stopped smoking	Mortality ratio/‰
Still smoking	15.8
1-4	16.0
5-9	5.9
10-14	5.3
15 +	2.0
Non-smokers	1.0

表7-2　英国医生中不同戒烟年限者的肺癌死亡率

戒烟年限	死亡率/‰
一直吸烟	15.8
1～4年	16.0
5～9年	5.9
10～14年	5.3
15年以上	2.0
不吸烟	1.0

7.6.3　Specificity of association

The concept of specificity implies a "one-to-one" relationship between the cause and effect. In the recent past much of the controversy over cigarette smoking and lung cancer centred round lack of specificity of the association. That is, cigarette smoking is linked with not only lung cancer but several others such as coronary heart disease, bronchitis, emphysema, cancer cervix, etc. This was used, for several years, as an argument against the acceptance of the association as causal. It is true that cigarette smoking is associated with so many diseases reflecting an apparent lack of specificity, but that cannot be a strong argument, so as to dismiss the causal hypothesis. This is because the requirement of specificity is a most difficult criterion to establish not only in chronic disease but also in acute diseases and conditions. The reasons are : First, a single cause or factor can give rise to more than one disease. Secondly, most diseases are due to multiple factors with no possibility of demonstrating one-to-one relationship.

The lack of specificity can be further explained by the fact that tobacco smoke is a complex of substances containing several harmful ingredients or factors such as nicotine, carbon monoxide, benzpyrene, particulate matter and many other ingredients with possible additive and synergistic action. The different components of tobacco smoke could as well be responsible for different states. In spite of this, it can be seen from Table 7-3 that the association of lung cancer with cigarette smoking is far more striking than any other association, reflecting a definite causal association. In short, specificity supports causal interpretation but lack of specificity does not negate it.

7.6.3　关联的特异性

特异性往往意味着"一对一"的因果关系。吸烟和肺癌关系的争议曾经集中在关联的特异性上。众所周知，吸烟不仅与肺癌有关，还与其他疾病有关，如冠心病、支气管炎、肺气肿、宫颈癌等，也就是说，吸烟与肺癌的关系不满足关联的特异性，这也因此成为驳斥吸烟与肺癌因果关系的理由。但值得一提的是，关联的特异性并不是因果推断的必要论据，因此，也不能据此推翻吸烟与肺癌的因果假设。特异性不仅在慢性疾病的因果推断中是最难满足的条件，在急性疾病的因果推断中也是。原因是：首先，单一因素可以引起多种疾病；其次，大多数疾病都是由多种因素造成的，"一对一"的病因关系几乎很少见。

吸烟与肺癌的关系缺乏特异性，但并不意味着二者没有因果关系。烟草中含有多种有害成分，如尼古丁、一氧化碳、苯并芘、有害颗粒物和添加剂，而且这些物质存在协同作用。烟草的不同成分可能引起不同的健康问题，从表7-3可以看出，吸烟与肺癌的关联比吸烟与其他死因的关联都要显著，这在一定程度上也反映了其因果联系的存在。简而言之，有特异性能支持因果关系，但缺乏特异性不能否定因果关系。

Table 7-3 Expected and observed deaths for smokers of cigarettes compared to non-smokers; eight prospective studies combined, for selected causes of death

Underlying cause of death	Expected deaths (E)	Observed deaths (O)	Mortality ratio (O/E)
Cancer of lung	170.3	1 833	10.8
Bronchitis and emphysema	89.5	546	6.1
Cancer of larynx	14.0	75	5.4
Cancer oesophagus	37.0	152	4.1
Peptic ulcer	105.1	294	2.8
Cancer bladder	111.6	216	1.9
CHD	6 430.7	11 177	1.7
Cancer rectum	207.8	213	1.0
All causes of death	15 653.9	23 223	1.7

表 7-3 吸烟者与非吸烟者的预期和实际死亡人数：八项死因的前瞻性研究

死因	预期死亡数 (E)	实际死亡数 (O)	标准化死亡比 (O/E)
肺癌	170.3	1 833	10.8
支气管炎和肺气肿	89.5	546	6.1
喉癌	14.0	75	5.4
食管癌	37.0	152	4.1
消化性溃疡	105.1	294	2.8
膀胱癌	111.6	216	1.9
冠心病	6 430.7	11 177	1.7
直肠癌	207.8	213	1.0
所有死因	15 653.9	23 223	1.7

The concept of specificity cannot be entirely dissociated from the concept of association. It has been estimated that about 80-90 percent of lung cancer can be attributed to cigarette smoking. To say this, it is assumed that the association between smoking and lung cancer is causal. Under the heading of specificity, two more observations require comment: ① Not everyone who smokes develops cancer; ②Not everyone who develops lung cancer has smoked. The first apparent paradox is related to the multifactorial nature of lung cancer. It may well be that there are other factors as yet unidentified which must be present in conjunction with smoking for lung cancer to develop. As for lung cancer in non-smokers, it is known that there are factors other than smoking which increase the risk of lung cancer such as occupational exposure to chromates, asbestos, nickel, uranium and exposure to air pollution. Deviations from one-to-one relationship between cigarette smoking and lung cancer therefore cannot be said to rule out a causal relationship.

特异性的概念不能与关联的概念完全脱离。据估计，80%～90%的肺癌患者都吸烟。这么说来，可以假设吸烟和肺癌有因果关系。在特异性的指导下，下面两个观点需要说明：①不是每个吸烟者都会患肺癌；②不是每个肺癌患者都吸烟。第一个矛盾点就是肺癌是由多病因引起的，意味着可能还有其他因素与吸烟共同导致肺癌的发生。至于不吸烟也会患肺癌，众所周知，除了吸烟外，还有一些因素可以导致肺癌的发生，如职业接触铬酸盐、石棉、镍、铀等，以及暴露于污染的空气。因此，吸烟和肺癌间的关系不存在特异性，并不能就此排除它们之间的因果关系。

7.6.4　Experimental evidence of association

If a factor is a cause of a disease, the risk of the disease could be expected to decline when exposure to the factor is reduced or eliminated. Evidence from cessation of exposure strongly supports the existence of causation. However, adequate evidence from experiments in human subjects is seldom available, and evidence from animals may not be relevant to human beings.

7.6.5　Coherence of association

A causal association should not conflict with what is known of the natural history and biology of the disease.

7.6.6　Consistency of association

If a relationship is causal, consistent findings should be obtained from different studies in different populations and under differing circumstances.

7.6.7　Dose-response relationship

As the dose of exposure increases, the risk of disease occurrence also increases. The existence of a clear dose - response relationship strongly indicates a causal relationship, although the absence of a dose - response relationship does not necessarily rule out a causal relationship.

7.6.8　Biologic plausibility

A causal association should have a biologically plausible explanation. When there is a lack of biologic plausibility, interpreting the association is difficult.

7.6.4　关联的实验证据

如果某因素是疾病的病因，那么当减少或消除该因素的暴露时，疾病的风险也会降低。停止接触的证据强烈支持因果关系的存在。然而，很少有来自人体实验的充分证据，来自动物实验的证据不能直接应用于人。

7.6.5　关联的一致性

因果关系不应与已知的疾病自然史和生物学情况相冲突。

7.6.6　关联的可重复性

如果关联是因果关联，那么在不同人群、不同环境中开展的研究应该得到一致的结果。

7.6.7　剂量-反应关系

随着接触剂量的增加，疾病发生的风险也增加。存在明确的剂量-反应关系强烈表明存在因果关系，然而没有剂量-反应关系不能否定因果关系的存在。

7.6.8　生物学合理性

因果关系应该在生物学上可以合理解释。当缺乏生物学上的合理性时，很难解释这种关联。

Chapter 8 Screening and Diagnostic Tests

"Health should mean a lot more than escape from death or, for that matter, escape from disease."

8.1 Iceberg Phenomenon of Disease

Epidemiologist and others who study disease find that the pattern of disease in hospitals is quite different from that in a community. That is, a far larger proportion of disease (e.g, diabetes, hypertension) is hidden from view in the community than is evident to physicians or to the general public. The analogy of an iceberg, only the tip of which is seen, is widely used to describe disease in the community.

The concept of the "iceberg phenomenon of disease" gives a better idea of the progress of a disease from its subclinical stages to overt or apparent disease than the familiar spectrum of disease. The submerged portion of the iceberg represents the hidden mass of disease (e.g, subclinical cases, carriers, undiagnosed cases). The floating tip represents what the physician sees in his practice. The hidden part of the iceberg thus constitutes the mass of unrecognized disease in the community, and its detection and control is a challenge to modern techniques in preventive medicine.

8.2 Concept of Screening

The active search for disease among apparently healthy people is a fundamental aspect of prevention. This is embodied in screening. Which has been de-

第8章 筛检与诊断试验

"健康应该包含更多含义，而不仅仅是免于死亡或疾病。"

8.1 疾病的冰山现象

许多医务工作者发现，医院和社区的疾病模式存在很大差异。很大一部分比例的疾病（如糖尿病、高血压）隐藏于社区中，而不被医生或大众所发现，就像只能看到冰山一角的冰山现象，这种现象可用于社区疾病的描述。

与疾病谱相比，疾病的冰山现象有助于人们更好地理解疾病从亚临床阶段到显性疾病的发展过程。冰山的沉没部分代表了隐藏的疾病（如亚临床疾病、携带的病毒、未诊断的疾病），漂浮的顶端代表在临床实践中所看到的疾病，冰山的隐藏部分组成了社区中大部分没有被发现的疾病，而它的检测和控制对于现代预防医学来说是一个挑战。

8.2 筛检的概念

在表面健康的人群中主动地找出患者是疾病三级预防中的二级预防，即筛检，指"运用快速、简便的试验、检查或其他方法在表面健康的个体

fined as "the search for unrecognized disease or defect by means of rapidly applied tests, examination or other procedures in apparently healthy individuals".

Historically the annual health examinations were meant for the early detection of "hidden" disease. To bring such examinations within the reach of large masses of people with minimal expenditures of time and money, a number of alternative approaches have come into use. They are based primarily conserving the physician‐time for diagnosis and treatment and having technicians to administer simple, inexpensive laboratory tests and operate other measuring devices. This is the genesis of screening programmes were for individual diseases such as tuberculosis, syphilis or selected groups such as antenatal mothers, school children and occupational groups. Over the years, the screening tests have steadily grown in number. Today screening is considered a preventive care function, and some consider it a logical extension of health care.

Screening differs from periodic health examination in the following respects:

① Capable of wide application.

② Relatively inexpensive.

③ Requires little physician‐time. In fact the physician is not required to administer the test, but only to interpret it.

8.3 Screening and Diagnostic Tests

A screening test is not intended to be a diagnostic test but only an initial examination. Those who are found to be positive test results are referred to a physician for full diagnostic work‐up and treatment. Screening and diagnostic tests may be contrasted as in Table 8‐1.

中找出那些未被识别的、可能有病或缺陷的人"。

每年的健康体检就是为了及时发现"隐性"疾病。为了在大样本人群中花费最少的时间和经费进行检查，有必要使用一些可替代的、廉价且操作简单的方法，这是筛检计划的起因。当时主要针对结核病、梅毒等个别疾病患者或产前孕妇、学校儿童和职业团体等特定群体，现在筛检范围逐渐扩大，已经作为一种医疗保健的方法，被认为是医疗卫生服务的一种合理延伸。

筛检与定期体检的区别在于：

①筛检应用的范围更广泛。

②筛检的方法相对更便宜。

③筛检需要医生花费的时间相对较少。事实上，医生不需要进行检查，只需要对检查结果进行解释说明。

8.3 筛检与诊断试验

筛检试验不是诊断试验，筛检只是一个初步的检查，无法对疾病进行诊断。如果筛检试验显示阳性，需要对患者进行进一步的诊断和治疗。筛检试验和诊断试验的区别如表8-1所示。

Table 8-1　Screening and Diagnostic tests contrasted

Screening test	Diagnostic test
1. Done on apparently healthy	Done on those with indications or sick
2. Applied to groups	Applied to single patient and all diseases are considered
3. Test results are arbitrary and final	Diagnosis is not final but modified in light of new evidence, diagnosis is the sum of all evidences
4. Based on one criterion or cut-off point (e.g,diabetes)	Based on evaluation of a number of symptoms, sign and laboratory findings
5. Less accurate	More accurate
6. Less expensive	More expensive
7. Not a basis for treatment	Used as a basis for treatment
8. The initiative comes from the investigator or agency providing care	The innitiative comes from a patient with a complaint

表 8-1　筛检试验和诊断试验的区别

筛检试验	诊断试验
1.在表面健康的人中进行	1.在有临床症状的人或病人中进行
2.适用于群体	2.适用于病人个体或所有疾病
3.结果呈阳性或阴性	3.病例或非病例
4.基于标准或诊断点(如糖尿病),区分可能患病者与可能未患病者	4.基于对一些症状、体征和实验室检查的综合评估,区分病人与可能患病者
5.准确性低	5.准确性高
6.经济、廉价	6.花费高
7.不作为治疗的基础	7.作为治疗的基础
8.由研究者或提供护理的机构启动	8.起始于病人的主诉

However, the criteria in Table 8-1 are not hard and absolute. There are some tests which are used both for screening and diagnosis, e.g, test for anaemia and glucose tolerance test. Screening and diagnosis are not competing, and different criteria apply to each.

8.4　Concept of " Lead Time"

Figure 8-1 shows the possible outcomes for a given disease process. There is nothing to be gained in screening diseases whose onset is quite obvious. Detection program should be restricted to those conditions in which the considerable time lag between dis-

然而，表 8-1 中的特点并不是严格和绝对的，有些检测在筛检试验和诊断试验中都是适用的，比如贫血试验和葡萄糖耐量试验，既可以用于人群中的筛检，也可以用于疾病的诊断。筛检试验和诊断试验并不矛盾，只是适用的标准不同。

8.4　"领先时间"的概念

图 8-1 显示了特定疾病发展过程中可能的结果。对于发病很明显的疾病，是没有必要进行筛检的。筛检试验应该在疾病早期进行，即应限于疾病发生到临床期之前的这一时期。在这一时期，通过适当的检测技术，将机体出现的一些异常特

ease onset and the time of diagnosis. In this period, there are usually a number of critical points which determine both the severity of the diseases and the success of any treatment in reversing the disease process. There is clearly little value in detecting disease advance of the usual time of diagnosis unless such detection precedes the final critical point beyond which treatment would be unsuccessful and/or permanent damage would be done. Detection programmes should therefore concentrate on those conditions where the time lag between the disease's onset and its final critical point is sufficiently long to be suitable for population screening.

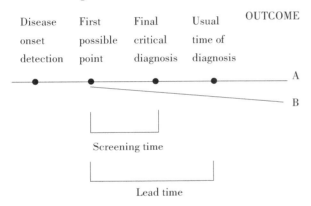

Figure 8-1　Model for early detection programmes

"Lead time" is the advantage gained by screening, i.e., the period between diagnosis by early detection and diagnosis by other means. In Figure 8-1, A is the usual outcome of the disease and B is the outcome to be expected when the disease is detected at the earliest possible moment. The benefits of screening are the early detection of disease. The benefits of the programme must be seen in terms of its outcomes. It is also necessary for the complexities and costs any detection programme to be viewed against the benefits accruing therefrom.

征尽早检测出来，并采取适当治疗，从而提高疾病治愈率，降低死亡风险。在日常的临床诊疗实践中，进行筛检的意义不大。筛检的目的是早发现、早诊断、早治疗，因此筛检应该在疾病早期开展（临床前期），到了临床期，患者已经出现明显的症状和体征，此时进行诊断试验和治疗即可。

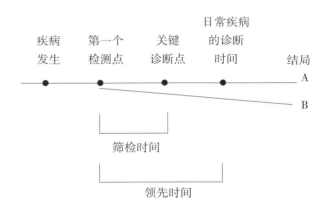

图8-1　筛检程序的模型

"领先时间"是指通过筛检获得的优势，即通过早期筛检发现疾病，到出现明显症状、体征后就诊而确诊疾病之间的时间。图8-1中，A是疾病通常的结局，B是疾病尽可能早被检测到的期望结局。因此，筛检的优势在于早期发现疾病，并由此改善疾病的结局。进行筛检时，不仅要考虑实施的复杂性和成本，还需考虑筛检的益处。

8.5　Aims and Objectives

The basic purpose of screening is to sort out from a large group of apparently healthy persons those likely to have the disease or at increased risk of the disease under study, to bring those who are "apparently abnormal" under medical supervision and treatment (Figure 8-2). Screening is carried out in the hope that earlier diagnosis and subsequent treatment favourably alters the natural history of the disease in a significant proportion of those who are identified as "positive".

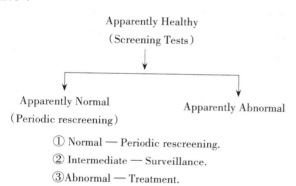

① Normal — Periodic rescreening.
② Intermediate — Surveillance.
③Abnormal — Treatment.

Figure 8-2　Possible outcomes of screening

1.Screening

Strictly speaking, screening is testing for infection or disease in populations or in individuals who are not seeking health care; for example, serological testing for AIDS virus in blood donors, neonatal screening, premarital screening for syphilis.

2. Case-finding

This is use of clinical and/or laboratory tests to detect disease in individuals seeking health care for other reasons; for example, the use of VDRL test is to detect syphilis in pregnant women. Other diseases include pulmonary tuberculosis in chest symptomatics,

8.5　筛检的目的

筛检的基本目的是从大量表面健康的人群中筛选出可能患病的个体或者发现某些疾病的高危个体，并对那些"非正常个体"进行进一步的诊断和治疗（图8-2）。进行筛检的目的，就是希望把结果阳性的人，通过进一步的诊断和治疗改变疾病的自然史，而筛检的疾病应该是当地主要的公共卫生问题，这样筛检出的阳性人数将占很大比例，收益也将更大。

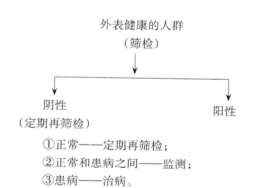

①正常——定期再筛检；
②正常和患病之间——监测；
③患病——治病。

图8-2　筛检的可能结果

以下是几个词语的解释：

1.筛检

严格来说，筛检主要针对人群中的感染者或患有疾病者以及不主动参加医疗保健的个人进行。例如，对献血者进行艾滋病病毒血清学检测，对新生儿进行筛查，婚前进行梅毒筛查等。

2.发现病例

发现病例是指使用其他医疗行为进行临床或实验室检查，以发现病例。比如，使用VDRL检测孕妇梅毒。其他可以检查的疾病还包括肺结核、高血压、宫颈癌、乳腺癌、糖尿病等。

hypertension, cervical cancer, breast cancer, diabetes mellitus, etc.

3. Diagnostic tests

Use of clinical and/or laboratory procedures to confirm or refute the existence of disease or true abnormality in patients with signs and symptoms presumed to be caused by the disease; for example, VDRL testing of patients with lesions suggestive of secondary syphilis; endocervical culture for N. gonorrhoeae.

The distinction between screening, case finding or diagnosis should be clear-cut. Often, however, it is blurred by the multiplicity of tests used and the haphazard nature of diagnostic decision-making. Thus the same test may be used in different contexts for both screening and diagnosis. Each step may involve multiple tests as in the case of syphilis. In evaluating a test, then, one must consider whether it is for screening or diagnosis, alone or in conjunction with other tests.

8.6　Uses of Screening: Four Main Uses have been Described

8.6.1　Case detection

This is also known as "prescriptive screening". It is defined as the presumptive identification of unrecognized disease, which does not arise from a patient's request, e.g, neonatal screening. In other words, people are screened primarily for their own benefit. Specific diseases sought by this method have included bacteriuria in pregnancy, breast cancer, cervical cancer, deafness in children, diabetes mellitus, iron deficiency anaemia, PKU, pulmonary tuberculosis, haemolytic disease of the newborn, etc. Since disease detection is

3.诊断试验

诊断试验是指通过临床症状、体征和实验室检查来确诊或排除疾病。比如，对疑有梅毒病变者进行 VDRL 检查（有损伤提示二期梅毒病变），对疑有宫颈病变的女性进行宫颈淋病奈瑟球菌培养。

筛检、发现病例及诊断试验之间的区别应该是明确的。然而，由于临床实践过程中检测方法的多样性和临床决策的突发性，三者之间并没有清晰的分界线。因此，在不同的情况下，可以使用相同的检测方法进行筛检和诊断。比如梅毒诊断中，每一步可能会涉及多个检测方法。用于筛检或诊断的检测方法需要进行评估，还需评估该检测方法是单独使用，还是要和其他检测方法结合使用。

8.6　筛检的应用：筛检的 四个主要用途

8.6.1　用于发现隐匿的病例

筛检也称为健康筛查，即在表面健康的人群中筛检出可能患病的个体，并进一步诊断和治疗，实现二级预防。此时的检查并不是病人提出的（比如新生儿筛查）。换句话说，筛检是为了进行人群疾病防制。目前，在人群中筛检的疾病包括妊娠菌尿症、乳腺癌、宫颈癌、耳聋、糖尿病、缺铁性贫血、苯丙酮尿症、肺结核及新生儿溶血病等。病例筛检由医务人员和公共卫生从业人员发起，因此他们有责任确保被检者接受进一步诊断和尽早治疗。

initiated by medical and public health personnel, they are under special obligation to make sure that appropriate treatment is started early.

8.6.2 Control of disease

This is also known as "prospective screening". People are examined for the benefit of others, e. g., screening of immigrants from infectious diseases such as tuberculosis and syphilis to protect the home population; and screening for streptococcal infection to prevent rheumatic fever. The screening programme may, by leading to early diagnosis permitmore effective treatment and reduce the spread of infectious disease and/or mortality from the disease.

8.6.3 Research purposes

Screening may sometimes be performed for research purposes. For example, there are many chronic diseases whose natural history is not fully known (e.g., cancer, hypertension). Screening may aid in obtaining more basic knowledge about the natural history of such diseases. As for example, initial screening provides a prevalence estimate and subsequent screening, an incidence figure. Where screening is done for research purposes, the investigator should inform the study participants that no follow-up therapy will be available.

8.6.4 Educational opportunities

Apart from possible benefits to the individual and the acquisition of information of public health relevance screening programmes (as for example, screening for diabetes) provide opportunities for creating public awareness and for educating health professionals.

8.6.2 用于疾病的控制

疾病的控制也被称为"前瞻性的筛检",进行筛检是为了他人的健康利益。例如,对来自肺结核和梅毒等传染病疫区的移民进行筛检,可以保护本国居民免受传染;对链球菌感染者进行筛检,可以预防风湿热。筛检过程中,可以通过早期诊断,进行更有效的治疗,从而降低传染病的传播和疾病的致死率。

8.6.3 用于研究

根据研究目的,有时需要使用筛检。比如,很多慢性病(如癌症、高血压等)的自然史尚不完全清楚,而筛检有助于获得疾病自然史的基本信息。又比如,初步的筛查可以得到疾病的患病率,而之后的筛检又可以得到疾病的发病率。在为了某个研究目的而进行的筛检中,研究人员应该告诉研究参与者没有后续的治疗。

8.6.4 提供人群宣教的机会

筛检可以通过筛查、确诊和治疗给个人带来健康益处,并提供疾病相关信息(比如对糖尿病进行筛查),还可以提高公众健康意识,为教育卫生专业人员提供人群宣教机会,也可以指导有限卫生资源的合理分配。

8.7   Types of Screening

Three types of screening have been described:

8.7.1   Mass screening

Mass screening simply means the screening of a whole population or a subgroup, as for example, all adults to measure blood pressure. It is offered to all, irrespective of the particular risk individual may run of contracting the disease in question.

Mass screening for disease received enthusiastic support in the past. However, when a number of mass screening procedures were subjected to critical review, there appeared to be little justification for their use in many instances. Indiscriminate mass screening, therefore, is not a useful preventive measure unless it is backed up by suitable treatment that will reduce the duration of illness or alter its final outcome.

8.7.2   High risk or selective screening

Screening will be most productive if applied selectively to high - risk groups, the groups defined on the basis of epidemiological research. For example, since cancer cervix tends to occur relatively less often in the upper social groups, screening for cancer cervix in the lower social groups could increase the yield of new cases. One population subgroup where certain diseases（e. g, diabetes, hypertension, breast cancer）tend to be aggregated is the family. By screening the other members of the family（and close relatives）the physician can detect additional cases.

More recently, epidemiologists have extended the concept of screening for disease to screening for "risk factors", as these factors apparently antedate the de-

8.7   筛检的类型

筛检可分为三种类型:

8.7.1   大规模筛检

大规模筛检就是对一定范围内的整个人群或某个团体进行筛检，一般用于发病率较高的情况。比如，针对所有成年人的高血压筛检，即为所有成年人提供血压测量，而不考虑疾病发生的可能性。

过去，大规模筛检获得了广泛的支持。然而，后来研究人员对一些大规模筛检进行严格审查后发现，进行大规模筛检并不是很必要。除非有进一步诊断的方法和适当的治疗，可以缩短病程或者改变疾病的结局，否则，使用大规模筛检是无用的预防措施。

8.7.2   高危人群筛检或选择性筛检

将筛检选择性应用到流行病学研究确定的高危人群中，这时的筛检才是最有成效的。例如，富裕的人群宫颈癌发病率比贫穷的人群低，因此在较贫穷的群体中进行筛检会增加宫颈癌的检出率；某些疾病（如糖尿病、高血压、乳腺癌）呈现家族聚集性，因此通过筛查家族中的其他成员（亲属）会发现更多的病例。

近年来，疾病的筛检已经拓展到对危险因素的筛检上。如果危险因素发生在疾病之前，那么对其进行防制（预防和控制）能够更有效地预防

velopment of actual disease. For example, elevated serum cholesterol is associated with a high risk of developing coronary heart disease. Risk factors, particularly those of a pathophysiological nature such as serum cholesterol and blood pressure are amenable to effective interventions. In this way, preventive measures can be applied before the disease occurs. Besides effectiveness, economical use of resources will also occur if the screening tests are selectively applied to individuals in high risk group.

8.7.3 Multiphase screening

It has been defined as the application of two or more screening tests in combination to a large number of people at one time than to carry out separate screening tests for single diseases. The procedure may also include a health questionnaire, clinical examination and a range of measurements and investigations (e.g., biochemical and haematological tests on blood and urine specimens, lung function assessment, audiometry and measurement of visual acuity). All of which can be performed rapidly with the appropriate staffing organization and equipment.

Multiphasic screening has enjoyed considerable popularity until recently, when evidence from randomized controlled studies in UK and USA suggested that multiphasic screening has not shownany benefit accruing to the population in terms of mortality and morbidity reduction. On the other hand, it has increased the cost of health services without any observable benefit. Furthermore, in multiphasic screening, as currently practised, most of the tests have not been validated. These observations have cast doubts on the utility of multiphasic screening.

疾病。比如，血清胆固醇升高可以增加患冠心病的风险，对其进行筛检和防制，在疾病发生之前就进行干预，能够更有效地预防冠心病。因此，对高危人群进行筛检，不仅可以有效预防疾病，还可以使卫生资源得到经济有效的利用。

8.7.3 多项筛检

多项筛检指同时联合两个或两个以上的方法在人群中进行疾病的筛检。该过程可能包括调查问卷、临床检查和一系列其他检查和调查（如血液和尿液样本的生化和血液学检查、肺功能的评估、听力和视力的检查），可以通过协调组织和设备检测迅速执行。

最近，人们对多项筛检的普及应用有了争议。英国和美国的随机对照研究证据表明，多项筛检在降低疾病的死亡率和发病率方面没有任何作用，还增加了医疗服务的成本，没有带来任何明显的效益。此外，目前应用的多项筛检，大多数没有经过验证。

8.8 Criteria for Screening

Before a screening programme is initiated, a decision should be made whether it is worthwhile, which requires ethical scientific, and, if possible financial justification. Criteria for screening are based on two considerations DISEASE to be screened, and the TEST to be appropriated.

The disease to be screened should fulfil the following criteria before it is considered suitable for screening:

① Condition sought should be an important health problem (in general, prevalence should be high).

② There should be a recognizable latent or an asymptomatic stage.

③ The natural history of the condition, include development from latent to declared disease, should adequately understood (so that we can know at certain stage the process ceases to be reversible).

④ There is a test that can detect the disease prior to onset of signs and symptoms.

⑤ Facilities should be available for confirmation of diagnosis.

⑥ There is an effective treatment.

⑦ There should be an agreed-on policy concerning with to treat as patients (e.g, lower ranges of blood pressure border-line diabetes).

⑧ There is good evidence that early detection treatment reduce morbidity and mortality.

⑨ The expected benefits (e. g, the number of lives saved of early detection exceed the risks and costs).

When the above criteria are satisfied, then only,

8.8 筛检的标准

开始筛检之前，需要评估应用价值、伦理学、科学性和经济合理性。筛检的标准应基于两点考虑，即要筛检的疾病和要采用的筛检方法。

要筛检的疾病应该符合以下标准：

①要筛检的疾病应该是一个重大的公共卫生问题（一般来说，该疾病的患病率较高）。

②该疾病应该有足够长的可识别潜伏期或无症状期。

③对要筛检疾病的自然史要有充分的了解，包括疾病从潜伏期到被发现的发展过程（由此可以知道在疾病发展的某个阶段，该过程是不可逆的）。

④在该疾病的症状和体征出现之前，应该有一种可以检测这种疾病的方法。

⑤应该有可以确认该疾病诊断结果的方法。

⑥应该存在有效的治疗方法。

⑦应该有统一、公认的标准用于疾病的诊断（如低血压的范围及糖尿病的界限）。

⑧应该有充分的证据表明，通过早期发现和治疗可以有效降低疾病的发病率和致死率。

⑨应该有期望的效益（如通过早期发现挽救的生命数量超过了要承担的风险和成本）。

只有当要筛检的疾病满足上述标准，且筛检

it would be appropriate to consider a suitable screening test.

8.9 Screening Test

The test must satisfy the criteria of acceptability and repeatability and validity, besides others such as simplicity, safety, rapidity, ease of administration and operation. Tests most likely to fulfil one condition may however, be more likely to fulfil another — for example, tests with great accuracy may be more expensive and time consuming, the choice of the test must therefore often be based on compromise.

8.9.1 Acceptability

Since a high rate of cooperation is necessary, it's important that the test should be acceptable to the people whom it is aimed. In general, tests that are particular discomforting or embarrassing (e.g., rectal or vagina examinations) are not likely to be acceptable to the population in mass campaigns.

8.9.2 Repeatability

An attribute of an ideal screening test or any measure (e.g., height, weight) is its repeatability (sometimes called reliability, precision or reproducibility). That is, the test will give consistent results when repeated more than once again same individual or material, under the same conditions repeatability of the test depends upon three major facts namely observer variation, biological (or subject) variation and errors relating to technical methods. For example measurement of blood pressure is poorly reproducibility, because it is subjected to all these three major factors.

的方法也适当时，才可以进行人群疾病的筛检。

8.9 筛检试验

用于筛检的方法除了应该简单、安全、易于管理和操作以外，还必须具有可接受性、良好的可重复性和真实性。然而，同时满足以上几个要求比较困难，所以可以根据需要进行取舍。比如高准确度的测试往往更昂贵、更耗时，因此，选择这样的方法进行人群筛检可能不适用。

8.9.1 可接受性

在人群中进行筛检时，筛检的方法必须可接受，这样人们才会有较高的配合度。通常来说，如果筛检的方法使人感到特别不舒服或很尴尬（如直肠或阴道的检查），那么该方法会很难被大众接受。

8.9.2 可重复性

理想的筛检方法或者测量方法（如体重、身高的测量）应该具备可重复性（有时也称为信度、精密度或可靠性），也就是说，相同的个体或物体进行多次检测，所得结果应是一致的。在相同的条件下，筛检方法的可重复性主要取决于三个方面，即观察者产生的偏差、生物学差异和技术方法的误差。例如，血压测量同时受到以上三个因素的影响，所以其可靠性较低。

1. Observer variation

All observations are subjected to variation (or error). These may be of two types.

（1）Intra-observer variation

If a single observer takes two measurements (e.g., blood pressure, chest expansion) in the same subject, at the same time and each time, he obtained a different result, this is termed as intra-observer or within observer variation. This is variation between repeated observations by the same observer on the same subject or material at the same time. Intra-observer variation may often be minimized by taking the average of several replicate measurements at the same time.

（2）Inter-observer variation

This is variation between different observers on the same subject or material, also known as between-observer variation. Inter-observer variation has occurred if one observer examines a blood-smear and finds malaria parasite, while a second observer examines the same slide and finds it normal.

Table 8-2 shows the results when 14 867 chest X-ray films were each read independently by the same eight radiologists.

1. 观察者偏差

所有的观察都有偏差，偏差通常有两种类型：

（1）观察者内的偏差

同一观察者使用同一方法同时进行两次测量（如测量血压、胸部扩张），如果每次测得的结果不同，就称为观察者内的偏差，即同一观察者对同一个体或物体同时重复观察产生的差异。对于观察者内的偏差，通常通过取同时多次重复测量的平均值使其达到最小。

（2）观察者间的偏差

不同的观察者对相同个体或物体进行测量产生的差异，称为观察者间的偏差。例如，甲检查血涂片发现有疟原虫，而乙检查同一张血涂片却发现其正常，这时产生的偏差即观察者间的偏差。

表8-2显示了14 867张胸部X光片的阅读结果，所有X光片均由8位医生单独阅片。

Table 8-2　Showing observer variation among radiologists

"Positive" readings	No. of films	percent/%
0/8	13 560	91.21
1/8	877	5.90
2/8	168	1.13
3/8	66	0.44
4/8	42	0.28
5/8	28	0.19
6/8	23	0.16
7/8	39	0.26
8/8	64	0.43
Total	14 867	100.00

表8-2　放射科医生间的观察者偏差

阅片阳性	X光片的数量	百分比/%
0/8	13 560	91.21
1/8	877	5.90
2/8	168	1.13
3/8	66	0.44
4/8	42	0.28
5/8	28	0.19
6/8	23	0.16
7/8	39	0.26
8/8	64	0.43
总计	14 867	100.00

The results shown in Table 8-2 are sobering and instructive. There was concurrence of all 8 readers that 91.21 percent of the films had one or more positive readings.

Observational errors are common in the interpretation of X-rays, ECG tracings, readings of blood pressure and studies of histopathological specimens. Observer errors can be minimised by: standardization of procedures for obtaining measurements and classifications, intensive training of all the observers and making use of two or more observers for independent assessment, etc. It is probable that these errors can never be eliminated absolutely.

2. Biological (subject) variation

There is a biological variability associated with many physiological variables such as blood pressure, blood glucose, serum cholesterol, etc. The fluctuation in the variate measured in the same individual may be due to:

①Changes in the parameters observed: This is a frequent phenomena in clinical presentation. For example, cervical smears taken from the same woman may be normal one day, and abnormal on another day. Myocardial infarction may occur without pain. Subject variation of blood pressure is a common phenomenon.

② Variations in the way patients perceive their symptoms and answer: This is a common subject variation. There may be errors in recollection of past events when questionnaire is administered. When the subject is aware that he is being probed, he may not give correct replies. In show subject variation can be a potential source of error epidemiological studies.

③ Regression to the mean: Important example of biological variability is regression to the mean. There is a tendency for values at the extremes of distribution,

表8-2清楚显示，8个医生均认为没有阳性的光片占91.21%。

测量误差在X光片、心电图、血压和病理组织切片检测结果的读取中都很常见。观察者偏差可能无法完全消除，但可以通过以下方式减小：采用标准化的方法进行测量和分类；对所有检测人员进行统一的强化培训；对两个或多个检测人员的结果进行一致性评估等。

2.生物学偏差（个体偏差）

很多生理学指标都存在生物学差异，如血压、血糖、血清胆固醇等。同一个体测量值波动的原因可能如下：

①生理学指标的自身变化：这是临床报告中的常见现象。比如，同一女性的宫颈涂片某天检查可能是正常的，而另一天则不正常；并不是所有心肌梗死的发生都有胸痛；血压的自然波动也是一种常见的现象。

②患者发现症状和回答的方式存在差异：这是一种常见的个体差异。在做调查问卷时，被调查者对过去事件的回忆也可能产生差错。当个体意识到他正在被调查时，可能不会给出正确的答案。个体差异可能是流行病学误差的一个潜在来源。

③向均数回归：生物学变异的一个重要现象是向均数回归。变量的分布存在一种趋势——不管是高还是低，在重复测量后，最终都会回归到

either very high or low, to regress toward to mean or average on repeat measurement. Many features disease states vary considerably over time, for example, the pain of rheumatoid arthritis, stool frequency in ulcerative colitis, blood pressure in hypertension or the blood glucose diabetes. This concept is particularly important to remember in evaluating the effects of a specific therapy on a variable. Such as the use of a specific drug reduce blood pressure serum cholesterol.

Whereas observer variation may be checked by repeat measurements at the same time, biological variation is tested by repeat measurements over time. This is due to the facility measurement is done only on a tiny sample of the normal distribution of the physiological variable.

3. Errors relating to technical methods

Lastly, repeatability may be affected by variations inhere in the method, e.g., defective instruments, erroneous calibration, faulty reagents, or the test itself might be inappropriate or unreliable. Where these errors are large repeatability will be reduced, and a single test result may be unreliable.

8.9.3　Validity（accuracy）

The term validity refers to what extent the test accurate measures which it purports to measure. In other word, validity expresses the ability of a test to separate or distinguish those who have the disease from those who do not. For example, glycosuria is a useful screening test for diabetes, but a more valid or accurate test is the glucose tolerance test. Accuracy refers to the closeness with which measured value agree with "true" values.

Validity has two components — sensitivity and

均值或平均值。例如，类风湿性关节炎患者的疼痛次数，溃疡性结肠炎患者的大便次数，高血压患者的血压水平或糖尿病患者的血糖水平。随着时间的推移，疾病特征会发生变化。在评估治疗措施的效果时，需要注意向均数回归对结果的影响，比如评价药物降压或降脂效果时，需要考虑血压和血脂自身的变化。

观察者偏差可通过在同一时间重复测量来评估，生物学偏差则可通过在不同时间重复测量来评估。仪器设备测量偏差可通过对小样本人群正态分布的生理指标进行测量来评估。

3. 检测误差

重复性还可能受检测方法的影响，比如仪器有缺陷，没有进行校准，检测方法不可靠或不准确，由此造成检测值的误差。因此，仅用一次的测量值作为结果不可靠，可以通过重复测量减小检测误差。

8.9.3　真实性（准确度）

真实性是指衡量或测量准确的程度，即利用检测方法将有病的人和无病的人区分开的一种能力。例如，尿糖检测是筛选糖尿病的有效检测方法，但更有效或更准确的检测方法是葡萄糖耐量试验。准确度是指测量值与真值相符的程度。

真实性包括灵敏度和特异度。当评估诊断试

specificity, When assessing the accuracy of a diagnostic test, one must consider both these components. Both measurements and expressed as percentages. Sensitivity and specificity are usually determined by applying the test to one group of persons having the disease, and to a reference group not having the disease (Table 8-3). Sensitivity and specificity together with "predictive accuracy" are inherent properties of a screening test. These are discussed below.

Table 8-3　Screening test result by diagnosis

Screening test results	Diagnosis		Total
	Diseased	Not diseased	
Positive	a(True positive)	b(False positive)	$a+b$
Negative	c(False negative)	d(True negative)	$c+d$
Total	$a+c$	$b+d$	$a+b+c+d$

The letter "a" (Table 8-3) denotes those individual found positive on the test who have the condition or disorder being studied (i. e, true positives). The group labelled "b" includes those who have a positive test result but who do not have the disease (i.e, false positives). The letter "c" includes those with negative test results but who have the disease (i.e, false negatives). Finally, those with negative results who do not have the disease are included in letter "d" (i.e, true negatives).

8.10　Evaluation of a Screening Test

The following measures are used to evaluate a screening test:

① Sensitivity=$a/(a+c)\times100\%$

② Specificity=$d/(b+d)\times100\%$

③ Positive predictive value =$a/(a+b)\times100\%$

④ Negative predictive value=$d/(c+d)\times100\%$

⑤ False negative rate=$c/(a+c)\times100\%$

验的真实性时，必须评价灵敏度和特异度，结果以百分比表示。灵敏度和特异度通过对患有该病的病例组和未患该病的对照组的比较来确定（表8-3）。灵敏度、特异度和"预测准确性"是筛检试验的固有属性。下面将进行详细阐述。

表 8-3　筛检试验评价

筛检试验	诊断结果		合计
	有病	无病	
阳性	a(真阳性)	b(假阳性)	$a+b$
阴性	c(假阴性)	d(真阴性)	$c+d$
合计	$a+c$	$b+d$	$a+b+c+d$

在表8-3中，字母a表示确诊为有病，且筛检结果为阳性的人群（即真阳性）；字母b表示诊断未患该病，但筛检结果为阳性的人群（即假阳性）；字母c表示筛检结果为阴性，但实际确诊为有病的人群（即假阴性）；最后，字母d表示筛检结果为阴性，实际也无疾病的人群（即真阴性）。

8.10　筛检试验的评价

以下为评价筛检试验的指标：

①灵敏度=$a/(a+c)\times100\%$

②特异度=$d/(b+d)\times100\%$

③阳性预测值=$a/(a+b)\times100\%$

④阴性预测值=$d/(c+d)\times100\%$

⑤假阴性率=$c/(a+c)\times100\%$

⑥ False positive rate=$b/(b+d)\times100\%$

The corresponding data are given in Table 8-4, and the above indicators are calculated:

Table 8-4　Screening test result by diagnosis

| Screening test results | Diagnosis | | Total |
	Diseased	Not diseased	
Positive	40	20	60
	(a)	(b)	$(a+b)$
Negative	100	9 840	9940
	(c)	(d)	$(c+d)$
Total	140	9 860	10 000
	$(a+c)$	$(b+d)$	$(a+b+c+d)$

Sensitivity=$(40/140)\times100\%=28.57\%$

（true positive）

Specificity=$(9\ 840/9\ 860)\times100\%=99.79\%$

（true negative）

False negative rate=$(100/140)\times100\%=71.42\%$

False positive rate=$(20/9\ 860)\times100\%=0.20\%$

Positive predictive value=$(40/60)\times100\%=66.66\%$

Negative predictive value=$(9\ 840/9\ 940)\times100\%$ $=98.99\%$

8.10.1　Sensitivity

The term sensitivity was introduced by Yerushalmy in 1940's as a statistical index of diagnostic accuracy. It has been defined as the ability of a test to identify correctly all those who have the disease, which is "true positive". A 90 percent sensitivity means that 90 percent of the diseased people screened by the test will give a "true positive" result and the remaining 10 percent a "false negative" result.

8.10.2　Specificity

It is defined as the ability of a test to identify correctly those who do not have the disease, that is "true negatives". A 90 percent specificity means that 90 per-

⑥假阳性率=$b/(b+d)\times100\%$

表8-4显示了筛检试验评价中各指标的计算：

表8-4　筛检试验的评价

| 筛检 试验 | 诊断结果 | | 合计 |
	有病	无病	
阳性	40	20	60
	(a)	(b)	$(a+b)$
阴性	100	9 840	9940
	(c)	(d)	$(c+d)$
合计	140	9 860	10 000
	$(a+c)$	$(b+d)$	$(a+b+c+d)$

灵敏度=（40/140）$\times100\%=28.57\%$

（真阳性率）

特异度=（9 840/9 860）$\times100\%=99.79\%$

（真阴性率）

假阴性率=（100/140）$\times100\%=71.42\%$

假阳性率=（20/9 860）$\times100\%=0.20\%$

阳性预测值=（40/60）$\times100\%=66.66\%$

阴性预测值=（9 840/9 940）$\times100\%=98.09\%$

8.10.1　灵敏度

20世纪40年代，Yerushalmy 提出将灵敏度作为评价诊断准确性的一个统计学指标。灵敏度是筛检试验正确发现病人的能力，也就是真阳性率。如果灵敏度是90%，意味着90%的患者通过筛检试验可以得到真阳性的结果，剩余10%的患者为假阴性（漏诊率）。

8.10.2　特异度

特异度是通过筛检试验能正确确定非患者的能力，也就是真阴性率。如果特异度是90%，意味着90%的非患者通过筛检试验可以得到真阴性

cent of the non-diseased persons will give "true negative" result, 10 percent of non - diseased people screened by the test will be wrongly classified as "diseased" when they are not.

To illustrate, let us compare the sensitivity and specificity screening for diagnosis of brain tumour (Tables 8-5 and 8-6).

Table 8-5 Diagnosis of brain tumours by EEG

EEG results	Brain tumour	
	Present	Absence
Positive	36	54 000
Negative	4	306 000
Total	40	360 000

Sensitivity=36/40×100%=90%

Specificity=306 000/360 000×100%=85%

Table 8-6 Diagnosis of brain tumors by computer assisted axial tomography

CAT results	Brain tumour	
	Present	Absence
Positive	39	18 000
Negative	1	342 000
Total	40	360 000

Sensitivity=39/40 × 100%=97.5%

Specificity=342 000/360 000×100%=95%

It can be seen from Tables 8-5 and 8-6, the CAT screening test is both more sensitive and more specific than EEG in the diagnosis of brain tumors.

In dealing with diagnostic tests that yield a result (e.g., blood sugar, blood pressure) the situation is different. There will be overlapping of the distribution curve attribute for diseased and non-diseased persons, positives and false negatives comprise the area of the disease. When the distributions overlap, it is not possible to consider assign individuals with these values to either the normal or diseased group on the basis of screening alone.

的结果，而剩余的10%的非患者则会被错误地判定为患者（误诊率）。

现以脑肿瘤筛检试验为例，介绍一下灵敏度和特异度（表8-5和表8-6）。

表8-5　EEG试验筛检脑肿瘤的结果

EEG 结果	脑肿瘤	
	患者	非患者
阳性	36	54 000
阴性	4	306 000
合计	40	360 000

灵敏度=36/40×100%=90%

特异度=306 000/360 000×100%=85%

表8-6　CAT试验筛检脑肿瘤的结果

CAT 结果	脑肿瘤	
	患者	非患者
阳性	39	18 000
阴性	1	342 000
合计	40	360 000

灵敏度=39/40×100%=97.5 %

特异度=342 000/360 000×100%=95%

由表8-5和表8-6可见，CAT筛检脑肿瘤比EEG具有更高的灵敏度和特异度。

定量指标（如血糖、血压）筛检试验结果的评价与定性指标的不同。患者组和非患者组的曲线分布可能会有重叠，真阳性和假阴性组成了疾病的区域。当分布有重叠时，不可能只靠单个筛检试验评价就能将个体分配到对照组或患病组。

For example, if we decide to use the 2-hour post-prandial blood glucose level of 180 mg/100 mL as an index judge presence of diabetes mellitus, the sensitivity and specificity are 50.0 and 99.8 percent respectively (Table 8-7). In other index sensitivity is low, but specificity very high. Further it can be seen from Table 8-7 that sensitivity and specificity are in relation. That is, sensitivity may be increased only expense of specificity and vice versa. An ideal screening should be 100 percent sensitive and 100 percent specificity practice, this seldom occurs.

例如，如果采用餐后2小时血糖180 mg/100 mL作为糖尿病的诊断点，那么灵敏度和特异度分别为50.0%和99.8%（表8-7），其他血糖水平的灵敏度相对较高，但特异度相对较低。此外，从表8-7可以看出，灵敏度和特异度是相关的。也就是说，灵敏度升高，特异度降低，反之亦然。一个理想的筛检试验应该达到100%的灵敏度和100%的特异度，但这种情况很少发生。

Table 8-7   Sensitivity and specificity of a 2-hour postprandial blood test for glucose for 70 true diabetics and 510 true non-diabetics at different levels of blood glucose

Blood glucose level/(mg·100 mL⁻¹)	Sensitivity /%	Specificity /%
80	100.0	1.2
90	98.6	7.3
100	97.1	25.3
110	92.9	48.4
120	88.6	68.2
130	81.4	82.4
140	74.3	91.2
150	64.3	96.1
160	55.7	98.6
170	52.9	99.6
180	50.0	99.8
190	44.3	99.8
200	37.1	100.0

表8-7   餐后2小时血糖水平筛检试验的灵敏度和特异度

血糖水平 /(mg·100 mL⁻¹)	灵敏度 /%	特异度 /%
80	100.0	1.2
90	98.6	7.3
100	97.1	25.3
110	92.9	48.4
120	88.6	68.2
130	81.4	82.4
140	74.3	91.2
150	64.3	96.1
160	55.7	98.6
170	52.9	99.6
180	50.0	99.8
190	44.3	99.8
200	37.1	100.0

注：试验对象为70个糖尿病患者和510个非糖尿病患者。

8.10.3   Predictive accuracy

In addition to sensitivity and specificity, the performance of a screening test is measured by its predictive value, it also reflects the diagnostic power of the test. The predictive accuracy depends upon sensitivity, specificity and disease prevalence. The "predictive value of a positive test" indicates the probability that a

8.10.3   预测值

除了灵敏度和特异度外，预测值也可以反映筛检试验的效果，它也反映了诊断试验的能力。预测值的准确性取决于灵敏度、特异度和疾病流行强度。阳性预测值表示筛检试验阳性者实际患有该病的概率。在特定人群中，疾病的流行强度越高，该筛检试验的阳性预测值就越高。如果患

patient with a positive test result has, in fact, the disease in question. The more prevalent a disease is in a given population, the more accurate will be the predictive positive screening test. The predictive value of a positive result falls as disease prevalence declines.

Table 8-8 shows the predictive value of positive Gram-stained cervical smear test to detect gonorrhoea at prevalence of 5, 15 and 25 percent. In this example, the predictive value of a positive test was calculated to be 21, 47 and 63 percent respectively. Thus in female populations in which the gonorrhoea is low (5 percent prevalence), only 21 percent of patients with positive results really have gonorrhoea; the remaining 79 percent have false-positive results. Furthermore, as the sensitivity of this test is only 50 percent, half of the cases are not detected, which greatly reduces the impact of the detection programme on disease transmission.

病率下降，阳性预测值也会下降。

表8-8显示，革兰染色宫颈涂片检查淋病的试验中，在患病率分别为5%、15%、25%的情况下，阳性预测值发生了变化，分别为21%、47%和63%。因此，在淋病患病率较低的女性（5%）中，只有21%的阳性患者可能患有淋病，其余79%的患者为假阳性。而且，由于这个筛检方法的灵敏度只有50%，因此一半的病例没有被检测到。这些因素在很大程度上降低了筛检试验对疾病传播的影响。

Table 8-8　Predictive value of a positive Gram-stained cervical smear test (with constant sensitivity of 50% and specificity of 90%) at three levels of prevalence

涂片	Prevalence 5%			Prevalence 15%			Prevalence 25%		
	Culture			Culture			Culture		
	+	–	Total	+	–	Total	+	–	Total
+	25	95	120	75	85	160	125	75	200
–	25	855	880	75	765	840	125	675	800
Total	50	950	1 000	150	850	1 000	250	750	1 000
+PV	25/120×100% =21%			75/160×100% =47%			125/200×100% =63%		

Note：+PV is Positive predictive value.

表8-8　三种患病率水平下革兰染色阳性宫颈涂片的预测值

涂片	患病率5%			患病率15%			患病率25%		
	培养			培养			培养		
	+	–	总数	+	–	总数	+	–	总数
+	25	95	120	75	85	160	125	75	200
–	25	855	880	75	765	840	125	675	800
总数	50	950	1 000	150	850	1 000	250	750	1 000
+PV	25/120×100% =21%			75/160×100% =47%			125/200×100% =63%		

注：+PV 值为阳性预测值。

8.10.4   False negatives and positives

Whereas the epidemiologist thinks in terms of sensitivity and specificity, the clinician thinks in terms of false negatives and false positives.

False negatives: The term "false-negative" means that patients who actually have the disease are told that they do not have the disease. It amounts to giving them a "false reassurance". The patient with a "false-negative" test result might ignore the development of signs and symptoms and may postpone the treatment. This could be detrimental if the disease in question is a serious one and the screening test is unlikely to be repeated within a short period of time. A screening test which is very sensitive has few "false negatives". The lower the sensitivity, the larger will be the number of false negatives.

False positives: The term "false-positive" means that patients who do not have the disease are told that they have. In this case, normal healthy people may be subjected to further diagnostic tests, at some inconvenience, discomfort anxiety and expense — until their freedom from disease is established. A screening test with a high specificity will have few false positives. False positives not only burden the diagnostic facilities, but they also bring discredit to screening programmes.

In fact, no screening test is perfect, i.e, 100 percent sensitive and 100 percent specific.

8.10.5   Yield

"Yield" is the amount of previously unrecognized disease that is diagnosed as a result of the screening effort. It depends upon many factors, viz. sensitivity and specificity of the test, prevalence of the disease,

8.10.4   假阴性和假阳性

流行病学关注的是筛检试验的灵敏度和特异度，而临床医学则关注的是假阴性和假阳性。

假阴性指实际患有某疾病的患者被告知未患该病，其实际上是一个错误的报告，属于漏诊。假阴性可能会导致患者忽略症状和体征的发展变化，从而延误疾病的治疗。如果疾病很严重且在短时间内不再做重复的检测，那么假阴性结果对病人是有害的。灵敏度很高的筛检试验很少有假阴性，灵敏度越低，假阴性率（漏诊率）就越高。

假阳性指实际没有患某病的人被告知患有该病。这种情况下，这些实际没患病的人可能会接受进一步的诊断，在疾病没有检查清楚之前，会产生各种问题，比如心理焦虑以及高昂的费用。筛检试验特异度越高，假阳性率（误诊率）就越低。假阳性不仅会加重诊断的负担，也会加重患者的心理负担。

事实上，没有完美的筛检试验，即几乎没有筛检试验可以达到100%的灵敏度和100%的特异度。

8.10.5   收益

收益是指经过筛检而被检测出来的、以前未被识别的疾病数量。它取决于很多因素，包括筛检试验的灵敏度和特异度、疾病的患病率以及参与筛检试验的个体。例如，通过将糖尿病筛检试

the participation of the individuals in the detection programme. For example, by limiting a diabetes screening programme to persons over 40 years, we can increase the yield of the screening test. High risk populations are usually selected for screening, thus increasing yield.

8.10.6　Combination of tests

Two or more tests can be used in combination to enhance the specificity or sensitivity of screening. For example, syphilis screening affords an example whereby all screenees are first evaluated by an RPR test. This test has high sensitivity, yet will yield false positives. However, all those positive to RPR are then submitted to FTA-ABS, which is a more specific test, and the resultant positives now truly have syphilis.

8.10.7　The problem of the borderline

The question arises which of the two qualities (sensitivity or specificity) is more important in screening? No categorical answer can be given. Figure 8-3 illustrates graphically the concepts of sensitivity and specificity.

验限制在40岁以上的人群中进行，可以提高筛检试验的收益。通常选择高风险的患病人群进行筛检，以提高筛检的收益。

8.10.6　联合试验

在进行筛检试验时，可以将两种或两种以上的试验联合进行使用，从而提高筛检的灵敏度或特异度。例如，进行梅毒的筛检时，首先对参与筛检的人进行RPR检测（RPR灵敏度高，但会产生假阳性）；然后，对所有RPR结果阳性的人再做FTA-ABS检测（FTA-ABS有较高的特异度），两种试验的结果均为阳性者就可以诊断为梅毒患者。

8.10.7　诊断点或阈值

筛检试验中，灵敏度高，特异度会降低；灵敏度低，特异度会升高。那么，筛检试验中灵敏度和特异度哪个更重要？这个问题没有绝对的答案。图8-3展示了在不同的分布情况下，利用灵敏度和特异度确定的诊断点或阈值。

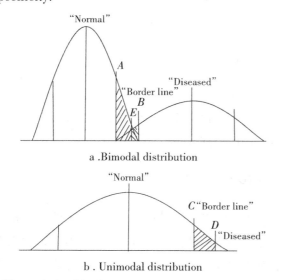

Figure 8-3　Distribution of a variable in a population

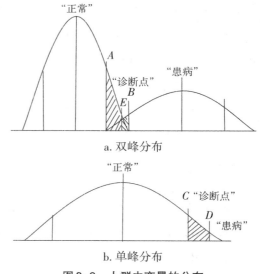

图8-3　人群中变量的分布

Figure 8-3a is a bimodal distribution of a variable in the "normal" and "diseased" populations. Note that the two curves overlap. If the disease is bimodal, as may be expected in certain genetically transmitted characteristics such as phenylketonuria, the shaded area or the border-line group will comprise a mixture of persons with the disease and persons without the disease (i.e, a mixture of false positives and false negatives). The point at which the distributions intersect (i.e., at level E) is frequently used as the cut-off point between the "normal" and "diseased" persons because it will generally minimise the false positives and false negatives.

Figure 8-3b is a unimodal distribution. Many physiological variables such as blood pressure, blood sugar and serum cholesterol show this type of distribution. Their values are continuously distributed around the mean, confirming to a normal or skewed distribution. In these observations, there is no sharp dividing line between the "normal" and "diseased". The "border-line" group (C-D) will comprise a homogeneous sample of persons. The question arises whether the cut-off point between "disease" and "normality" should be set at C or D as in Figure 8-3b. If the cut-off point is set at the level of A or C, it will render the test highly sensitive, missing few cases but yielding many false positives. If the cut-off point is set at B or D, it will increase specificity of the test. Furthermore, in the unimodal distribution, once a cut-off point level has been adopted., all persons above that level (i. e, above level C or D in Figure 8-3b) would be regarded as "diseased".

Taking diabetes as our example, if the cut-off point for blood glucose is lowered to detect diabetes (say less than 120 mg/100 mL), the sensitivity of the

图 8-3a 是变量在正常人群和患者中的双峰分布，需要关注的是这两条曲线的重叠部分。如果某个疾病的筛检结果为双峰，像某些具有遗传特性的疾病（如苯丙酮尿症），那么阴影区或边界线人群将包括病人和非病人（即假阳性和假阴性的混合），两条曲线分布的交点（即点 E）通常被当作"正常"和"患病"的分界点。因为，在这个点上的假阳性率和假阴性率最小。

图 8-3b 是一个单峰分布，许多生理指标（如血压、血糖、血清胆固醇）呈单峰分布。单峰分布是以均值为中心呈连续的正态或偏态分布。在这些观察值中，"正常"和"患病"之间没有明确的界限。"边界线"（C-D）组成了一个同质的样本，问题在于图 8-3b 中"正常"和"患病"的诊断点应设在 C 点还是 D 点。如果诊断点设在 A 点或 C 点，将使灵敏度升高，减少漏诊，但假阳性率会升高；如果诊断点设在 B 点或 D 点，特异度会升高，误诊会减少。对于单峰分布，一旦确定诊断点，所有超过临界点水平（即图 8-3b 中的 C 或 D）的人都会被当作病人。

以糖尿病为例，如果筛检糖尿病的血糖水平降低（低于 120 mg/100 mL），则灵敏度会升高，特异度会降低；如果诊断点升高到 180 mg/100 mL， test is increased at the cost of specificity. If the cut-off point is raised (say to 180 mg/100 mL), the sensitivity is decreased (Table 8-7). In other words, there is no blood sugar level which will ensure the separation of all those with the disease from those without the disease.

In screening for disease, a prior decision is made about the cut-off point, on the basis of which individuals are classified as "normal" or "diseased".

In making this decision, the following factors are taken into consideration:

① Disease prevalence: When the prevalence is high in the community, the screening level is set at a lower level, which will increase sensitivity.

② The disease: If the disease is very lethal (e.g cervical cancer, breast cancer) and early detection markedly improves prognosis, a greater degree of sensitivity, even at the expense of specificity is desired. In these cases, subsequent diagnostic work-up can be relied on to rule out the disease in the false-positives. That is, a proportion of false-positives is tolerable but not false-negatives. On the other hand, in a prevalent disease like diabetes for which treatment does not markedly alter outcome, specificity must be high and early cases may be missed, but false-positives should be limited; otherwise the health system will be overburdened with diagnostic demands on the both true and false. That is, high specificity is necessary when false-positive errors can be avoided.

③ A useful index in making this decision is the predictive value of a positive test. This index measured the percentage of positive results that are true positives; it's function of the sensitivity and specificity as well as frequency of the disease.

There are various other points which must also be

则灵敏度会降低（表8-7）。总之，无法确定一个能够完全将糖尿病病人和血糖正常者区分开的血糖水平。

在人群中进行疾病筛检前，应先确定能将个体区分为"正常"或"病人"的临界点。

选择诊断点时需要注意以下几点：

①疾病的患病率：当社区中某疾病的患病率较高时，在筛检试验中，可以设置较低的临界点，以增加灵敏度，筛检出更多的阳性。

②疾病本身：如果该疾病是致命的（如宫颈癌、乳腺癌），而且早发现可以显著改善预后，那么即使筛检方法的特异度低，也有必要开展筛检，可以通过后续的诊断以及病情的检查排除假阳性的患者。也就是说，这种情况容许适当的假阳性存在，但假阴性不可以。另一方面，像糖尿病等患病率较高的疾病，通过治疗也不能显著改变疾病结局，早期的患者也容易漏诊，这时筛检试验的特异度必须高，假阳性（误诊）应该受到限制，否则，卫生系统会因为过多诊断为阳性的个体而负担过重。也就是说，在假阳性可以避免的情况下，应该尽量提高特异度。

③阳性预测值：选择临界点时，还需考虑阳性预测值。阳性预测值反映了筛检试验阳性的人中患病的人所占的百分比。灵敏度和特异度的分母分别是有病或无病的人数。

开展筛检时还需注意以下几点：首先，应尽

taken into account in screening. First, people who participate in the screening programme may not be those who have more gain from it, as for example, those at greatest risk of cancer the cervix uteri are least likely to attend for cervical cytology. Therefore screening must be applied selectively to people most likely to benefit. Selection might be based on person's age, sex, medical history, occupation, family history or other factors. Secondly, tests with greater accuracy may be more expensive and time-consuming, and the choice of the test therefore often be based on compromise. The screening should not be developed in isolation; it should be integrated into the existing health services. Lastly, the risk as well as the expected benefits must be explained to the people to be screened. These risks include any possible complication of the examination procedures, and the possibility of false-positive and false-negative test results.

Regardless of the approach taken to screening tests, repeatedly patient follow-up visits are important (not to leave out patients high and dry) if effective health and medical care to result from the effort. Garfield has stressed the necessary meet demands for medical care by separating screenees into well, asymptomatic-sick, and sick groups. This separation makes possible the optimal use of health care services.

8.11　Evaluation of Screening Programmes

Many screening tests were introduced in the rough without subjecting them to rigid scrutiny. They were introduced because it was thought a good thing to detect treat cases before they should reach an advanced stage, but modern view is that new screening

量选择可以从筛检中获益的人来开展筛检。例如，利用细胞学检查筛检宫颈癌时，应该选择宫颈癌的高危人群。选择人群时，应考虑到年龄、性别、疾病史、职业、家族史以及其他因素。其次，精确度高的筛检方法可能更昂贵、更耗时，所以在选择筛检方法时通常选择操作简单、廉价的方法。再次，筛检不应单独进行，而应融入到当前的医疗保健体系中，并要有进一步诊断和治疗的方法。最后，应该告知筛检人群参加筛检可能的风险以及预期收益。其中，风险包括检查过程中可能出现的并发症，以及试验结果可能出现的假阴性或假阳性。

只要筛检能够取得有效的医疗保健效果，就应该对筛检出来的患者进行追踪随访（不要让病患感到孤立无援），了解其诊断和治疗的情况。Garfield 等认为有必要根据筛检结果将参加筛检的人员分成确定健康的、表面健康的无症状者和病人群体，不同的群体对医疗保健的需求不同，从而达到最佳的医疗服务利用效果。

8.11　筛检效果的评价

许多筛检试验没有经过严格的审查和评价，就直接被应用，主要是因为用筛检试验早发现疾病有利于改善疾病的预后。但现在，人们认识到只有经过正确的评估，才能实践新的筛检。

programmes should be introduced only after proper evaluation.

8.11.1 Randomized controlled trials

Ideally evaluation should be done by a randomized controlled trial in which one can（randomly selected）receives the screening test, and a control which receives no such test. Ideally RCT should be performed in the setting where the screening programme will be implemented, and should employ the same type of person equipment and procedures that will be used in the programme. If the disease has a low frequency in population, and a long incubation period（e.g, cancer）may require following tens of thousands of people for 10 years with virtually perfect record keeping. The cost logistics are often prohibitive.

8.11.2 Uncontrolled trials

Sometimes uncontrolled trials are used to see if people with disease detected through screening appear to live longer after diagnosis and treatment with patients who were not screened. One such example uncontrolled studies of cervical cancer screening will be indicated that deaths from that disease could be very large reduced if every woman was examined periodically.

8.11.3 Other methods

There are also other methods evaluation such as case control studies and comparison trends between areas with different degrees of screening coverage. Thus it can be determined whether intervention screening is any better than the conventional method managing the disease.

To conclude, the screening concept, filled with

8.11.1 随机对照试验

随机对照试验是理想的评估方法，是指将研究对象随机分为试验组（进行筛检试验）和对照组（不进行筛检试验），再追踪随访两组研究对象的疾病结局。理想的筛检试验研究往往需要庞大的样本量和较长的随访期。在进行整个随机对照试验的过程中，两组的仪器设备和操作要相同，参加试验的研究人员也要相同。需要注意的是，当疾病（如癌症）的发病率较低、潜伏期较长时，需要对很大的基数人群进行长达10年或更久的随访，需要耗费巨大的人力、物力和财力，因此利用随机对照试验对这类疾病进行筛检不可行，往往只能选择近期的效果指标进行评价。

8.11.2 非对照试验

可以利用非对照多中心社区类试验来观察，进行筛检试验后，接受诊断和治疗的病人生存时间是否延长等。例如，一个宫颈癌筛检的非对照试验表明，如果每个妇女定期做检查，那么宫颈癌的致死率将会大大降低。

8.11.3 其他方法

可采用观察性研究方法，进一步验证真实条件下筛查所获得的远期效果和项目的可持续性。比如病例对照研究，可对筛检覆盖度不同的地区进行比较，可以确定干预性筛检试验的效果是否优于常规的治疗方法。

总而言之，要在人群中进行大规模筛检，还

potential has been overburdened with problems, many of which remain unsolved. The construction of accurate tests that are both sensitive and specific is a key obstacle to the wide application of screening. Scientific and technical problem puzzles abound. The common screenings were presented in Table 8-9.

有很多潜在的负担和问题没有解决，导致具有较高灵敏度和特异度的筛检方法无法广泛应用。另外，科学上和技术上也存在很多问题。表8-9列出了现在常用的一些筛检技术。

Table 8-9 Some screening tests

Different people	Some screening tests
Pregnancy	Anaemia、Hypertension toxemia、Rh status、Syphilis（VDRL Test）、Diabetes、Cardiovascular、Neural tube defects、Down's syndrome、HIV
Infancy	LCB、Congenital dislocation of hip、Congenital heart disease、Spina bifida、Cerebral palsy、Hearing defects、Visual defects、Hypothyroidism、Developmental screening tests、Haemoglobinopathies、Sickle cell anaemia、Undescended testis
Middle-aged men and women	Hypertension、Cancer、Diabetes mellitus、Serum cholesterol、Obesity
Elderly	Nutritional disorders、Cancer、Tuberculosis、Chronic bronchitis、Glaucoma、Cataract

表8-9 一些常用的筛检试验

人群	筛查试验
孕妇	贫血、高血压毒血症、Rh血型、梅毒（性病研究试验）、糖尿病、心血管疾病、神经管畸形、唐氏综合征、艾滋病
婴儿	LCB、先天性髋关节脱位、先天性心脏病、脊柱裂、脑瘫、听力障碍、视力障碍、甲状腺功能减退症、发育筛检试验、血红蛋白病、镰状细胞贫血、隐睾
中年人	高血压、癌症、糖尿病、血清胆固醇、肥胖
老年人	营养失调、癌症、肺结核、慢性支气管炎、青光眼、白内障

Chapter 9　Disease Prevention and Control

9.1　Natural History of Disease

Disease results from a complex interaction between an agent（or cause of disease）and the environment. The natural history of disease is a key concept in epidemiology. It signifies the way in which a disease evolves over time from the earliest stage of its prepathogenesis phase to its termination as recovery, disability or death, in the absence of treatment or prevention. Each disease has its unique natural history, which is not necessarily the same in individuals.

The natural history of disease is best established by studies. As these studies are costly laborious, our understanding of the natural history of disease is largely based on other epidemiological studies, such as cross - sectional and retrospective studies, undertaken in different population settings, both national and internal. What the physician sees in the hospital is just an "episode" in the natural history of disease. The epidemiologist, by studying the natural history of disease in the community setting is in a unique position to fill the gaps in our knowledge about the natural history of disease.

A schematic diagram of the natural history of disease is shown in Figure 9-1. It is a necessary framework to understand the pathogenetic chain of events for a particular disease, and for the application of preventive measures. Usually, the natural history of disease includes two phases: Prepathogenesis phase and pathogenesis phase. It is considered the events that take place in the natural history of disease, using infectious disease as aprincipal model.

第9章　疾病的预防和控制

9.1　疾病自然史

疾病是由病原体（或病因）与环境之间复杂的相互作用引起的。疾病自然史是流行病学中的一个重要概念，是指在没有治疗或预防等措施的干预下，从发病前的最早阶段到康复、残疾或死亡等结局出现的疾病发展变化过程。不同疾病的自然史不同。

最好通过研究来确定疾病自然史。前瞻性研究是研究疾病自然史的最佳方法，但其成本高昂，且费时、费力，因此，一般基于其他研究方法认识疾病自然史，比如在不同人群和地区中进行的横断面研究和回顾性研究。医生在医院里看到的只是疾病自然史上的一个"插曲"。流行病学家通过在社区环境中研究疾病的自然史，在填补疾病自然史知识研究方面处于独特地位。

疾病自然史如图9-1所示，认识疾病自然史有利于了解疾病的发病过程以及预防措施的应用。通常将疾病的自然史分为两个阶段：发病前期和发病期。下面以传染病为例，简要阐述疾病自然史。

PERIOD OF PRE-PATHOGENESIS		PERIOD OF PATHOGENESIS		
DISEASE PROCESS	→Before man is involved →	→ The course of the disease in man →		
	Agent　　　Host And **Environment Factors** （known and unknown） Bring agent and host together or produce a disease provoking stimulus	DEATH Chronic state Defect Disability Illness Clinical horizon　Signs&symptoms 　　　　　　　Immunity and resistance Tissue and physiologic changes Stimulus or agent becomes established and increases by multiplication　RECOVERY		
		In the human host　Interaction of host and stimulus → Host reaction →		
		Early pathogeneses → Discernible early lesions → Advanced disease → Convale-scence		
LEVELS OF PREVENTION	PRIMARY PREVENTION	SECONDARY PREVENTION	TERTIARY PREVENTION	
MODES OF INTERVENTION	HEALTH PROMOTION　SPECIFIC PROTECTION	EARLY DIAGNOSIS AND TREATMENT	DISABILITY LIMITATION	REHABILITATION

Figure 9-1　Natural history of disease

（From *Preventive Medicine for the Doctor in His Community*, by Leavell&Clark with permission of McGraw-Hill Book Co.）

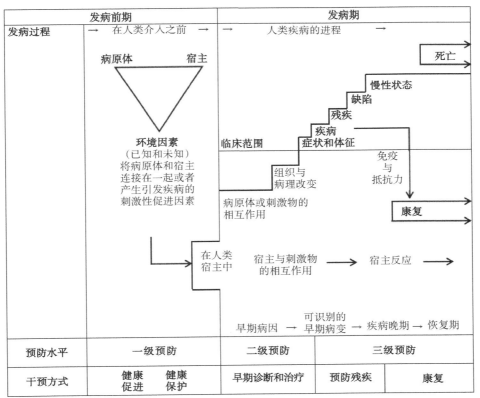

图9-1　疾病自然史

（From *Preventive Medicine for the Doctor in His Community*, by Leavell&Clark with permission of McGraw-Hill Book Co.）

9.1.1 Prepathogenesis phase

This refers to the period preliminary to the onset of disease in man. The disease agent has not yet entered man, but the factors which favour its interaction with the human host already exists in the environment. This situation is frequently referred to as "man in the earlier stage of disease" or "man exposed to the risk of disease". Potentially we are all in the prepathogenesis phase of many diseases, both communicable and non-communicable.

The causative factors of disease may be classified as AGENT, HOST and ENVIRONMENT. These three factors are referred to as epidemiological triad. The mere presence of agent, host and favourable environmental factors in the prepathogenesis period is not sufficient to start the disease in man. What is required is an interaction of these three factors to initiate the disease process in man. The agent, host and environment operating in combination determine not only the onset of disease which may range from a single case to epidemics (as depicted in Figure 9-2's black area) but also the distribution of disease in the community.

9.1.1 发病前期

发病前期指人类发病前的时期。病原体尚未进入人体前，环境中已经存在有利于其与人体宿主相互作用的因素。这种状态下的人被称为"处于疾病前期的人"或"暴露疾病风险的人"，也就是高危人群。现实中，很多人处于疾病前期，包括传染性疾病前期和非传染性疾病前期。

致病因素可分为病原体、宿主和环境，这三个因素被称为"流行病学三角"。在发病前期，仅有病原体、宿主和适合的环境，这三个因素不足以引起疾病。只有三个因素相互作用，才可能启动疾病进程。病原体、宿主和环境的联合作用不仅决定了发病、疾病传播（如图9-2中的黑色区域所示），还决定了社区中疾病的分布。

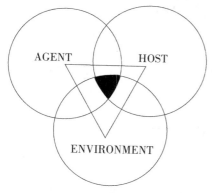

Figure 9-2 Epidemiologic concept of interactions of Agent, Host and Environment

(Adapted from *Health Services Reports*, vol 87, page 672)

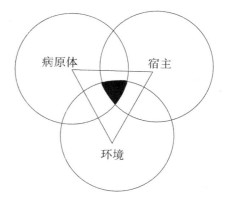

图9-2 病原体、宿主和环境相互作用的流行病学概念

(Adapted from *Health Services Reports*, vol 87, page 672)

9.1.2　Pathogenesis phase

The pathogenesis phase begins with the entry of the disease "agent" in the susceptible human host. The further events in the pathogenesis phase are clear-cut in infection diseases, i.e., the disease agent multiplies and induces tissue and physiological changes, the disease progresses through period of incubation and later through early and late pathogenesis. The final outcome of the disease may be recovery, disability or death. The pathogenesis phase may be modified by intervention measures such as immunization and chemotherapy.

It is useful to remember at this stage that the host's reaction to infection with a disease agent is not predictable. That is, the infection may be clinical or sub - clinical; typical or atypical or the host may become a carrier with or without having developed clinical disease as in the case of diphtheria and poliomyelitis.

In chronic diseases (e.g., coronary heart disease, hypertension, cancer), the early pathogenesis phase is less dramatic. This phase in chronic diseases is referred to as presymptomatic phase. During the presymptomatic stage, there is no manifest disease. The pathological changes are essentially below the level of the "clinical horizon". The clinical stage begins when recognizable signs or symptoms appear. By the time signs and symptoms appear, the disease phase is already well advanced into the late pathogenesis phase. In many chronic diseases, the agent - host - environmental interactions are not yet well understood.

9.1.3　Agent

The first link in the chain of disease transmission

9.1.2　发病期

发病期始于病原体进入易感人群（宿主）体内。传染性疾病的发病和进展是明确的，即病原体在体内繁殖并诱导组织和生理变化，疾病进展包括潜伏期和疾病早期、中期、晚期病理改变。疾病的最终结局可能是康复、残疾或死亡。发病过程可通过免疫和化疗等干预措施得到改善。

在发病期，宿主感染病原体后会有不同的表现。宿主感染后可能是临床的，也可能是亚临床的（如白喉和脊髓灰质炎）；可能是典型的，也可能是非典型的；或者可能成为隐形携带者。

慢性病（如冠心病、高血压、癌症）的早期，没有明显的临床症状和体征，这一阶段称为临床前期，其病理变化基本上低于"临床视野"的水平。当可识别的体征或症状出现时，就意味着进入了临床阶段。往往在出现明显的体征和症状时，疾病已经进入了晚期。在许多慢性疾病中，病原体–宿主–环境的相互作用还没有被人类充分了解。

9.1.3　病原体

疾病传播链中的第一个环节是病原体。疾病

is a disease agent. The disease "agent" is defined as a substance, living or non-living, or a force, tangible or intangible, the excessive presence or relative lack of which may initiate or perpetuate a disease process. A disease may have a single agent, a number of independent alternative agents or a complex of two or more factors whose combined presence is essential for the development of the disease.

Disease agents may be classified broadly into the following groups.

1.Biological agents

These are living agents of disease, e.g., viruses, rickettsia, fungi, bacteria, protozoa and metazoa. These agents exhibit certain "host-related" biological properties such as:

① Infectivity: This is the ability of an infectious agent to invade and multiply (produce infection) in a host.

② Pathogenicity: This is the ability to induce clinically apparent illness.

③ Virulence: This is defined as the proportion of clinical cases resulting in severe clinical manifestations (including sequelae). The case fatality rate is one way of measuring virulence.

2.Nutrient agents

These can be proteins, fats, carbohydrate, vitamins, minerals and water. Any excess or deficiency of the intake of nutritive elements may result in nutritional disorders. Protein energy malnutrition (PEM), anaemia, goitre, obesity and vitamin deficiencies are some of the current vitamin deficiencies are some of the current nutritional problems in many countries.

3.Physical agents

Exposure to excessive heat, cold, humidity, pres-

的病原体被定义为一种物质，不管有生命还是无生命，有形还是无形，可触摸还是不可触摸，过度存在或相对缺乏都将延长疾病病程。疾病可能是一个或多个因素共同作用的结果。

病原体大致可分为以下几类：

1.致病微生物

致病的病原微生物，包括病毒、立克次体、真菌、细菌、单细胞生物和多细胞生物等。致病微生物表现出一定"与宿主相关"的生物学特性，如：

①传染性：指传染性病原体侵入宿主并在体内繁殖（产生感染）的能力。

②致病性：指诱发疾病，使病例呈现出明显临床症状和体征的能力。

③毒性：指在临床病例中，严重临床表现（包括后遗症）病例所占的比例。病死率是衡量毒性的一种方法。

2.营养物质

营养物质可以是蛋白质、脂肪、碳水化合物、维生素、矿物质或水。任何营养元素摄入过量或不足，都可能导致营养失调。蛋白质-能量营养不良（PEM）、贫血、甲状腺肿、肥胖和维生素缺乏是许多国家目前存在的营养问题。

3.物理因素

暴露在过热、过冷、过湿、压力、辐射、电、

sure. radiation, electricity, sound, etc may result in illness.

4.Chemical agents

① Endogenous substances: Some of the chemicals may be produced in the body as a result of derangement of function e.g., urea (ureamia), serum bilirubin (jaundice), ketones (ketosis), uric acid (gout), calcium carbonate (kidney stones),etc.

② Exogenous substances: Agents arising outside of human host, e.g., allergens metals, fumes, dust, gases, insecticides, etc. These may be acquired by inhalation, ingestion or inoculation.

5. Mechanical agents

Exposure to chronic friction and other mechanical forces may result in crushing, tearing, sprains, dislocations and even death.

6.Absence or insufficiency or excess of a factor necessary health

These may be:

① Chemical factors: E.g., hormones, oestrogens, enzymes.

② Nutrient factors: Given above.

③ Lack of structure: E.g., thymus lack of structure, e.g., cardiac defects.

④ Chromosomal disorder: E.g., Trisomy 21 syndrome, turner's syndrome.

⑤ Immune factors: E.g., agammaglobulinaemia.

7.Social agents

It is also necessary to consider social agents of disease. These are poverty, smoking, abuse of drugs and alcohol, unhealthy lifestyles, social isolation, maternal deprivation.

Thus the modern concept of disease "agent" is broad one; it includes both living and non - living agents.

噪音等环境下，都可能导致疾病，这些因素就是物理因素。

4.化学因素

①内源性物质：由于机体功能紊乱而在体内产生的某些化学物质。例如，尿素（与尿毒症相关）、血清胆红素（与黄疸相关）、酮类（与酮症相关）、尿酸（与痛风相关）、碳酸钙（与肾结石相关）等。

②外源性物质：即人体通过吸入、摄入或接种等方式从外界获得的物质。例如，过敏原金属、烟雾、灰尘、气体、杀虫剂等。

5.机械因素

长期接触摩擦或其他机械力，有可能导致挤压、撕裂、扭伤、脱臼甚至死亡。

6.缺乏、不足或过多的健康必要因素

这些因素可能是：

①化学因素：如激素、雌激素、酶。

②营养因素：如上所述。

③结构缺失：如胸腺结构缺失、心脏缺陷。

④染色体疾病：如21-三体综合征、特纳综合征。

⑤免疫因素：如丙种球蛋白血症。

7.社会因素

除了要考虑以上因素外，还要考虑社会因素，如贫穷、吸烟、滥用药物和酒精、不健康的生活方式、社会隔离、母性剥夺等。

因此，在现代概念中，疾病"病原体"的概念是广泛的，它包括有生命的物质和没有生命的致病因素。

9.1.4 Host factors (intrinsic)

In epidemiological terminology, the human host is referred to as "soil" and the disease agent as "seed". In situations, host factors play a major role in determinate outcome of an individual's exposure to infection tuberculosis.

The host factors may be classified as :

①Demographic characteristics such as age, sex, ethnicity.

②Biological characteristics such as genetic factors; biochemical level the blood (e.g., cholesterol); blood groups and cellular constituents of the blood; immunological factors, physiological function of different organ systems of the body (e.g., blood pressure, forced expiratory ventilation).

③Social and economic characteristics such as economic status, education, occupation, stress, marital housing, etc.

④Lifestyle factors such as personal traits, living habits, nutrition, physical exercise, use of drugs and smoking, behavioural patterns, etc. The association of a particular disease with a specific set of host frequently provides an insight into the cause of disease, host factors of importance are further discussed in the later chapters.

9.1.5 Environmental factors (extrinsic)

The study of disease is really the study of man and environment. Hundreds of millions of people are affected preventable diseases originating in the environment in they live. For human beings the environment is not limit it normally is for plants and animals, to a set of factors. For example, for man social and economic conditions are more important than the mean an-

9.1.4 宿主因素（内在）

在流行病学术语中，人类宿主被称为"土壤"，病原体被称为"种子"。在这种情况下，宿主因素在决定个体感染结核病的结局中起着重要作用。

宿主因素可分为：

①人口统计学特征：如年龄、性别、种族。

②生物特性：如遗传因素、血液生化水平（如胆固醇）、血型和血液的细胞成分、免疫因素、身体不同器官与系统的生理功能（如血压、强制呼气通气）。

③社会和经济特征：如经济状况、教育、职业、压力、婚姻住房等。

④生活方式因素：如个人特征、生活习惯、营养、体育锻炼、吸毒和吸烟、行为模式等。部分疾病与宿主的关联为寻找病因提供了线索，宿主因素的重要性将在后面的章节中进一步讨论。

9.1.5 环境因素（外在）

对疾病的研究实际上是对人和环境的研究。由环境引起的、可预防的疾病广泛影响着人类健康。对人类来说，环境并不单纯是植物和动物，还包括一系列与环境相关的因素。例如，社会和经济条件对人类健康的影响可能比年平均温度更大。环境的概念是复杂和全面的。外部或宏观环境被定义为"人体自身外部的，有生命的和无生

nual temperature. The concept of environment is complex and all‑embracing. The external or macro‑environment is defined as "which is external to the individual human host, living, non‑living, and with which he is in constant interaction includes all of man's external surroundings such as air, food, housing, etc".

For descriptive purposes, the environment of man has divided into three components — physical, biological, psychosocial. It should be emphasized that this separation artificial. They are closely related to each other and wide factors.

1.Physical environment

The term "physical environment" is applied to normal things and physical factors (e. g, air, water, soil, climate, geography, heat, light, noise, debris, radiation) with which man is in constant interaction. Man's victory is his physical environment has been responsible for most improvement in health during the past century. In developing countries, defective environment (e.g., in sanitation) continues to be the main heath problem. Man altered practically everything in his physical environment to his advantage. In doing so, he has created for himself a host of new health problems such as air pollution, water pollution, noise pollution, urbanization, radiation hazards, etc. The increasing use of electrical and electronic devices, including the rapid growth of telecommunication system (e. g., satellite systems),radio‑broadcasting, television transmitters and radar installations have increased the possibility of human exposure to electromagnetic energy.

Man is living today in a highly complicated environment which is getting more complicated as man is becoming more ingenious. If these trends continue, it is feared that the very "quality of life" we cherish may soon be in danger.

命的，与人体不断互动的因素，包括人体的所有外部环境，如空气、食物、住房等"。

为了便于描述，人类的环境被人为地分为物理、生物、社会心理三个部分。三者之间密切联系，影响广泛。

1.物理环境

物理环境适用于与人类不断互动的常见物质和物理因素（如空气、水、土壤、气候、地理、热、光、噪声、垃圾、辐射）。在过去的一个世纪里，人类在通过改善物理环境解决健康相关问题方面取得了巨大成就。在发展中国家，不良的环境（如卫生环境）仍然是影响健康的主要问题。人类为了自己的利益几乎改造了一切物理环境，同时也制造出了一些影响健康的新问题，如空气污染、水污染、噪声污染、城市化、辐射危害等。电气和电子设备的使用越来越多，包括电信系统（如卫星系统）、无线电广播、无线通信、电视发射机和雷达装置等，增加了人们接触电磁能的可能性，也由此引发了新的健康问题。

现在，人们生活在一个高度复杂的环境中，随着社会发展，环境变得越来越复杂。如果持续下去，恐怕我们所重视的"生活质量"很快就会面临威胁。

2.Biological environment

The biological environment is the universe of living things which surrounds man, including man himself. The living things are the viruses and other microbial agents, insects, rodents, animals and plants. These are constantly working for their survival, and in this process, some of them act as disease - producing agents, reservoirs of infection, intermediate hosts and vectors of disease. Between the members of the ecological system (which includes man), there is constant adjustment and readjustment. For the most part, the parties manage to effect a harmonious inter - relationship, to achieve a state of peaceful co - existence, even though this may not be always enduring. When for any reason, this harmonious relationship is disturbed, ill health results. In the area of biological environment also, preventive medicine has been highly successful in protecting the health of the individual and of the community.

3.Psychosocial environment

It is difficult to define "psychosocial environment" against the background of the highly varied social, economic and cultural contexts of different countries and their social standards and value systems. It includes a complex of psychosocial factors which are defined as "those factors affecting personal health, health care and community well - being that stem from the psychosocial make-up of individuals and the structure and functions of social groups". They include cultural values, customs, habits, beliefs, attitudes, morals, religion, education, lifestyles, community life, health services, social and political organization.

In addition to this broad aspect of psychosocial environment, man is in constant interaction with that

2.生物环境

生物环境是指围绕着人类的各种生物，包括人类自身。这些生物包括病毒和其他微生物、昆虫、动物和植物。在生存的过程中，一些生物环境充当了病原微生物、感染源、中间宿主和传播媒介。生态系统的成员（包括人）间在不断调整和修正，以实现和谐，但有时也会失衡，这时就会引发疾病等健康问题。在生物环境领域，预防医学在保护个人和社会健康方面也取得了巨大成功。

3.社会心理环境

不同国家的社会、经济、文化、社会标准及价值体系高度不同，很难统一定义"社会心理环境"。社会心理环境是一系列复杂的社会心理因素，这些因素指源于个人的社会心理构成和社会群体的结构和功能，从而影响个人健康、保健和社会福祉的因素，包括文化价值观、习俗、习惯、信仰、态度、道德、宗教、教育、生活方式、社区生活、卫生服务、社会和政治组织。

社会心理环境除了上述概念所包含的范围外，还包括与社会环境不断互动的"人"，人的社会属

part of the social environment known as "people". He is a member of a social group, the member of a family, of a caste, of a community and of a nation. Between an individual and other members of the group, there can be harmony or disharmony, interests and points of view that are shared or that are in conflict. The behavior of one individual can affect others more or less directly; conflict and tension between the individual and the group as a whole or between the individual and other members of the group can yield great distress. The laws of the land, customs, attitudes, beliefs, traditions, all regulate the interactions among groups of individuals and families.

The impact of social environment has both positive and negative aspects on the health of individuals and communities. A favourable social environment can improve health, provide opportunities for man to achieve a sense of fulfilment, and add to the quality of life. Therefore, customs and traditions favouring health must be preserved. Beneficial social behavior（e. g., community participation）should be restored where it has disappeared due to social changes.

Psychosocial factors can also affect negatively man's health and well‐being. For example, poverty, urbanization, migration and exposure to stressful situations such as bereavement desertion, loss of employment, birth of a handicapped child may produce feelings of anxiety, depression, anger, frustration, and so forth; and these feelings may accompanied by physical symptoms such as heartpalpitations and sweating. But these emotional states produce changes in the endocrine, autonomic systems, which, if prolonged and in interaction with personality factors, may lead to structural changes various bodily organs. The resulting from psychosomatic disorders include conditions such

性决定了其是一个团体、家庭、民族、社区和国家的成员。个人和其他成员间可能因为共同的利益冲突产生不和谐，个人的行为也可能影响他人，也可能因为冲突和紧张产生巨大压力。而法律、习俗、态度、信仰、传统都规范着个人和家庭成员间的关系。

社会环境对个人和社区健康既有积极影响，也有消极影响。良好的社会环境可以改善健康，使人们获得满足感，从而提高生活质量。因此，有必要保留有利于健康的习俗和传统，恢复那些因社会发展而逐渐消失的、有益健康的社会行为（如社会参与）。

社会心理因素也会对人的健康和幸福产生负面影响，如因贫困、城市化、移民、失去亲人、失业、出生缺陷等产生的焦虑、抑郁、愤怒、沮丧等情绪。不良情绪可能引起内分泌和自主神经系统失调，从而导致心悸和出汗等症状。如果持续时间过长，可能还会导致器官结构的病理变化，使人出现健康问题，如十二指肠溃疡、支气管哮喘、高血压、冠心病、精神障碍、异常社会行为（如自杀、犯罪、暴力、吸毒）等，其中，与生活方式和心理社会压力相关的冠心病得到了更多关注。另外，交通事故现在已经成为许多国家年轻人的主要死因，这可能与社会心理状态（如无聊、焦虑、沮丧和其他影响注意力的心理问题）有关。

as duodenal ulcer, bronchial asthma, hypertension, coronary heart disease, mental disorders socially deviant behaviour (e.g., suicide, crime, violence, abuse). Most of primary concern is coronary heart disease which may be related to lifestyle and psychosocial stress. In many countries, road accidents are now the principal cause of death in young people. It is related to psychosocial states such boredom, anxiety, frustration and other preoccupations can impair attention.

Man today is viewed as an "agent" of his own diseases; state of health is determined more by what he does to himself than what some outside germ or infectious agent does to him. For example, the medical cause of lung cancer may be chemical substance in cigarettes, but the psychosocial cause behaviour — smoking. From a psychosocial point of view disease may be viewed as a maladjustment of the human organism to his psychosocial environment resulting from misperception, misinterpretation and misbehaviour. The epidemiologists today are as much concerned with psychosocial environment as with physical or biological environment, in search for aetiological causes of disease.

Because of the fact that man exists concurrently in so many environmental contexts, it has become customary to speak man in his "total environment". The social environment is inextricably linked with the physical and biological environments that it is realistic and necessary to view the human environment in to promote health. A stable a harmonious equilibrium between man and his environment needed to reduce man's vulnerability to disease and to permit him to lead a more productive and satisfying life.

现在的观点认为，人类自身就是疾病的病原体。健康状况更多地取决于人类自身做了什么，而不是外部细菌或传染源做了什么。例如，肺癌的医学病因是香烟中的化学物质，但社会心理病因则是吸烟这种行为。从社会心理的角度来看，疾病被视为由误解、曲解和不当行为导致的人体对社会心理环境的不适应。因此，寻找病因时，不仅要关注物理和生物环境，也要关注社会心理环境。

人类生存于环境中，人类是总体环境中的一部分。社会环境与物理和生物环境密不可分，因此，有必要全面了解人类环境，这样才能使人类与环境达到平衡，从而促进健康、减少疾病、提高生活质量。

9.1.6 Risk factors

For many diseases, the disease "agent" is still unidentified, e.g., coronary heart disease, cancer, peptic ulcer, mental illness, etc. Where the disease agent is not firmly established in the aetiology is generally discussed in terms of risk factors.

The term "risk factor" is used by different authors with least 2 meanings:

① An attribute or exposure that is significantly associate with the development of a disease.

② A determinant that can be modified by intervention thereby reducing the possibility of occurrence of disease or other specified outcomes.

Risk factors are often suggestive, but absolute proof of cause and effect between a risk factor and disease is usually lacking. That is, the presence of a risk factor does not imply that the disease will occur, and in its absence, the disease will not occur. The important thing about risk factors is that they are observable or identifiable prior to the event they predict, is also recognized that combination of risk factors in the same individual may be purely additive or synergistic（multiplicative）. For example, smoking and occupational exposure（shoe, leather, rubber, dye and chemical industries）were found to have an additive effect as risk factors for bladder cancer. On the other hand, smoking was found to be synergistic with other risk factors such as hypertension and high blood cholesterol. That is, the effects are more than additiveness.

Risk factors may be truly causative（e.g., smoking for lung cancer）they may be merely contributory to the undesired outcome（e.g., lack of physical exercise is a risk factor for coronary heart disease）, or they may be predictive only in a statistical sense（e.g., illit-

9.1.6 危险因素

目前，许多疾病的病原体仍未确定，如冠心病、癌症、消化性溃疡、精神疾病等。如果疾病的病原体尚未确定，那么通常通过危险因素来讨论病原体。

"危险因素"至少有两种解释：

①与疾病的发展显著相关的特征或暴露。

②通过干预可以改变的因素，改变后，可以降低疾病或其他特定结局发生的可能性。

通常缺乏危险因素与疾病因果关系的绝对证据，危险因素往往只起着提示作用。也就是说，有危险因素的存在并不意味着疾病会发生；但如果没有危险因素，疾病就不会发生。危险因素必须是在疾病之前的、可观察或可识别的因素，多个因素可能存在相加或协同（相乘）作用，比如吸烟和职业接触（如鞋、皮革、橡胶、染料和化学工业）对膀胱癌就具有累加效应。另外，还发现吸烟与其他危险因素（如高血压和高血清胆固醇）在其他疾病中具有协同作用。也就是说，交互效应不仅仅是相加的。

危险因素可能是真正的致病因素（如吸烟会导致肺癌），但也可能只是诱导了不利结局的发生（如缺乏体育锻炼是冠心病的一个危险因素），或者可能仅具有统计学意义上的预测性（如文盲对围产期死亡率的影响）。

eracy for perinatal mortality）.

Some risk factors can be modified, others cannot be modified. The modifiable factors include smoking, hypertension, elevated serum cholesterol, physical activity, obesity, etc. They are amenable to intervention and are useful in the care of the individual. The unmodifiable or immutable risk factors such as age, sex, race, family history and genetic factors are not subject to change. They act more as signals in alerting health professionals and other personnel to the possible outcome.

Risk factors may characterise the individual, the family, the group, the community or the environment. For example, some of the individual risk factors include age, sex, smoking, hypertension, etc. But there are also collective community risks — for example, from the presence of malaria, from air pollution, from substandard housing, or a poor water supply or poor health care services. The degree of risk in these cases is indirectly an expression of need. Therefore it is stated that a risk factor is a proxy for need — indicating the need for promotive and preventive health services.

Epidemiological methods（e.g., case control and cohort studies）are needed to identify risk factors and estimate the degree of risk. These studies are carried out in population groups among whom certain diseases occur much more frequently than other groups. By such comparative studies, epidemiologists have been able to identify smoking as a risk for lung cancer; high serum cholesterol and high blood pressure as risk factors for coronary heart disease. The contribution of epidemiology in the identification of risk factors has been highly significant. Risk factors associated with some major disease groups are as shown in Table 9-1.

有些危险因素可以改变，有些则无法改变。可以改变的因素包括吸烟、高血压、高血清胆固醇、体力活动、肥胖等，这些因素易于干预，有助于个人预防保健。无法改变的危险因素包括年龄、性别、种族、家族史和遗传因素等，这些因素只是对高危人群和医疗保健人员有预警作用。

危险因素可能是个人、家庭、群体、社会或环境的特征，个人危险因素如年龄、性别、吸烟、高血压等，社会危险因素如疟疾、空气污染、住房不达标、水和医疗服务缺乏等。社会危险因素及程度间接地反映了需求，因此，有学者认为危险因素代表了健康促进和预防保健服务的需求。

流行病学研究方法（如病例对照研究和队列研究）可以用来研究危险因素和估计危险度。流行病学研究方法通过比较不同人群疾病的发生率或暴露率，判断暴露因素与疾病之间的关系。目前，已经明确吸烟是肺癌的危险因素，高胆固醇和高血压是冠心病的危险因素。流行病学研究的重要作用就是识别疾病的危险因素。表9-1中列出了一些主要公共卫生问题的危险因素。

Table 9-1 Prominent risk factors

Disease	Risk factors
Heart disease	Smoking, high blood pressure, elevated serum cholesterol, diabetes, obesity, lack of exercise, type A personality
Cancer	Smoking, alcohol, solar radiation, ionizing radiation, work-site hazards, environmental pollution, medications, infectious agents, dietary factors
Stroke	High blood pressure, elevated cholesterol, smoking
Motor vehicle accidents	Alcohol, non-use of seat belts, speed, automobile design, roadway design
Diabetes	Obesity, diet
Cirrhosis of liver	Alcohol

The detection of risk factors should be considered a prelude to prevention or intervention. For each risk factor ascertained, the question has to be asked whether it can be reduced in a cost-effective way and whether its reduction will prevent or delay the unwanted outcome. Since the detection procedure usually involves whole population, it bears some similarity to presymptomatic screening for disease.

9.1.7 Risk groups

Another approach developed and promoted by WHO identify precisely the "risk groups" or "target groups" (e.g., at-risk mothers, at-risk infants, at-risk families, chronic; handicapped, elderly) in the population by certain criteria and direct appropriate action to them first. This is as the "risk approach". It has been summed up as "some for all, but more for those in need — in proportion to the risk". In essence, the risk approach is a managerial device increasing the efficiency of health care services within the of existing re-

表9-1 一些主要公共卫生问题的危险因素

疾病	危险因素
心脏病	吸烟、高血压、高血清胆固醇、糖尿病、肥胖、缺乏锻炼、A型性格
癌症	吸烟、饮酒、太阳辐射、电离辐射、工作场所危害、环境污染、药物、传染源、饮食因素
中风	高血压、高胆固醇、吸烟
机动车事故	饮酒、未使用安全带、车速、汽车设计、道路设计
糖尿病	肥胖、饮食
肝硬化	饮酒

在进行疾病预防和干预前，首先要确定疾病的危险因素。对于每个危险因素，还需确定是否可以通过经济有效的方式减少其暴露，以及减少其暴露后是否可以预防或延缓疾病或不利事件的发生。危险因素的研究往往在人群中进行，需要注意的事项与筛检试验的类似。

9.1.7 高危人群

WHO开发和推广了一种确定高危人群或目标群体（如高危孕妇和婴儿、高危家庭、慢性病高危人群、残障者和老年人）的方法，以便优先对高危人群采取干预措施，预防疾病和促进健康，这种方法被称为风险措施。疾病预防策略包括全人群策略和高危人群策略。本质上，风险措施是一种在现有资源范围内提高医疗服务效率的管理手段。由于医疗资源受限，高危人群策略更符合成本效益原则，因此应用更多，WHO已经在妇幼保健服务中开始使用这种方法（表9-2）。

sources. WHO has been using the approach in MCH services for sometime (Table 9-2).

Table 9-2 Guidelines for defining "at-risk" groups

Guidelines	Examples
Biological situation	age groups, e. g., infants (low birth weight),toddlers;sex, e.g., females in the reproductive age period; physiological state, e.g., pregnancy, cholesterol level, blood pressure;genetic factors, e.g., family history of genetic disorders; other health conditions (disease, physical functioning, unhealthy behaviour)
Physical situation	rural, urban slums; living conditions, overcrowding; environment: water supply, proximity to industries
Sociocultural and cultural situation	social class;ethnic and cultural group; family disruption, education, housing; customs, habits and behaviour (e.g., smoking, lack of exercise, over-eating, drug addicts) ; access to health services;lifestyle and attitudes

表9-2　界定"有风险"群体的准则

准则	举例
生物学特征	年龄组,如婴儿(低出生体重)、幼儿;性别,如育龄期的女性;生理状态,如怀孕、胆固醇水平、血压;遗传因素,如遗传疾病家族史;其他健康状况,如疾病、身体机能、不健康行为
物理环境特征	农村、城市贫民窟;生活条件,如过度拥挤;环境,如供水环境、靠近工厂
社会和文化特征	社会阶层;民族和文化群体;家庭破裂、教育、住房;习俗、习惯和不良行为(如吸烟、缺乏锻炼、过度饮食、吸毒);保健服务;生活方式和态度

9.1.8　Spectrum of disease

The term "spectrum of disease" is a graphic representation of variations in the manifestations of disease. It is akin spectrum of light where the colours vary from one end other but difficult to determine where one colour ends other begins. At one end of the disease spectrum are subclinical infections which are not ordinarily identified and at the other end are fatal illnesses. In the middle of the spectrum lie illnesses ranging in severity from mild to severe different manifestations are simply reflections of different states of immunity and receptivity. Leprosy is an excellent example of the spectral concept of disease. For almost every disease there exists a spectrum of severity, with few exceptions such as rabies. In infectious disease spectrum of disease is also referred to as the "gradient

9.1.8　疾病谱

疾病谱指表示疾病变化过程的图形,类似光谱,用不同颜色的谱阶表示疾病的变化,各谱阶间没有明显的界线,相互交错。疾病谱的一端是无明显症状和体征的亚临床状态,另一端是致命的疾病,中间范围为疾病从轻微到严重的不同程度(病情反映了机体免疫力和抵抗力的不同状态)。麻风病就有典型的疾病谱,几乎每种疾病都有一个严重程度的谱系,只有狂犬病等少数疾病除外。传染病的疾病谱也被称为感染梯度。

of infection".

The sequence of events in the spectrum of disease interrupted by early diagnosis and treatment or by preventing measures which if introduced at a particular point will accelerate or retard the further development of the disease. The spectrum of disease provides for inclusion of all subclinical and clinical, in the study of disease.

A concept closely related to the spectrum of disease is the concept of the iceberg phenomenon of disease. According to this concept, disease in a community may be compared with an iceberg (Figure 9-3). The floating tip of the iceberg represents what the physician sees in the community, i.e., clinical cases. The vast submerged portion of the iceberg represents the hidden mass of disease, i.e., latent, inapparent, presymptomatic and undiagnosed cases and carriers in the community. The "waterline" represents the demarcation between apparent and inapparent disease.

In some diseases (e. g., hypertension, diabetes, anaemia, malnutrition, mental illness) the unknown morbidity (i.e., the submerged portion of the iceberg) far exceeds the known morbidity. The hidden part of the iceberg thus constitutes an important, undiagnosed reservoir of infection or disease in the community, and its detection and control is a challenge to modern techniques in preventive medicine. One of the major deterrents in the study of chronic diseases of unknown aetiology is the absence of methods to detect the subclinical state — the bottom of the iceberg.

一级预防和"三早"的二级预防会中断疾病谱(包括亚临床和临床期),如果在某个特定点采取措施,将会加速或延缓疾病的发展。

疾病的冰山现象与疾病谱密切相关。如果将社区中所有存在的疾病比作冰山(图9-3),漂浮的冰山一角就代表具有明显症状和体征而被识别的临床病例,冰山巨大的水下部分就代表大量的隐藏疾病,即潜在的、不明显的、临床前期和未诊断的病例及携带者,"水线"代表显性疾病和隐性疾病之间的界限。

某些疾病(如高血压、糖尿病、贫血、营养不良、精神疾病)的未知病例(即冰山的水下部分)所占的比例远远超过已知病例。因此,冰山的隐藏部分是未被诊断或未被社区监测发现的感染或疾病的"蓄水池",其检测和控制是对现代预防医学技术的挑战。研究病因不明的慢性病的主要障碍之一是缺乏检测亚临床状态(即冰山一角)的方法。

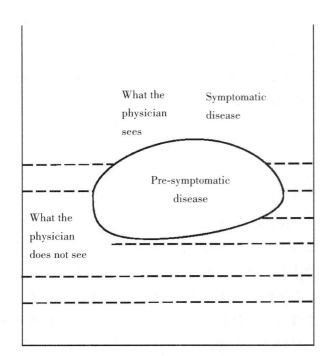

Figure 9-3　The Iceberg of Disease

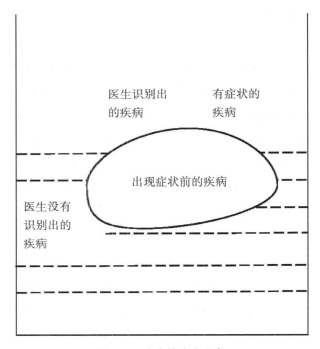

图 9-3　疾病的冰山现象

9.2　Strategies for Disease Prevention and Control

A "strategy", is an essential principle to guide overall situations. It is a concept that is developed from concrete situations and addresses problems from a macro perspective. In contrast, a "measure" entails the application of actual methods, steps and plans that are used to realize goals. Methods are based on analyses of problems from a microperspective and are established in a local context. A disease control strategy and its associated measures supplement each other. The established prevention goal can be reached only under the guidance of correct strategies and reasonable measures that are adopted at the same time. Alternatively, without considering the feasibility of the planned measures, a disease prevention strategy cannot be put into practice, and the expectant targets cannot be reached. The effect of prevention measures will be minimized, because they are only based on local ex-

9.2　疾病的预防和控制策略

"策略"是指导全局的基本原则，它是一个从具体情况发展而来的概念，从宏观角度解决问题。"措施"是为了实现目标所采取的具体方法、步骤和计划，是局部的、要结合当地情况制定的具体防制手段。疾病的控制策略与其相关措施密切相关，相互影响。只有采取正确的策略和合理的措施，才能实现预期的预防目标。如果不考虑措施的可行性和有效性而制定策略，那么很难实现预期的目标。如果没有健全的策略指导，只是根据当地经验制定，措施的效果也会大打折扣。因此，必须同时考虑策略和措施，这样才能以最少的成本获得最大的收益。

periences and do not have the benefit of a sound strategy. Therefore, it is important to consider both strategies and measures together, so that the largest beneficial effects can be achieved with the least investment.

9.3 Establishment of a Prevention Strategy

In practice that the most effective strategies for disease prevention and control are constituted in view of the epidemic backgrounds and characteristics of diseases in a particular area, the specific situation and needs of this area, and the human and organizational resources that are available. An effective disease prevention strategy should significantly change the environment that causes people to be prone to the disease. The strategy may be global, national or regional, and it may focus on multiple diseases and health problems in the whole population or on a single disease. The following four factors must be considered when developing a disease prevention strategy: ①evidence for the effectiveness of relevant measures; ② availability of resources;③the population's health needs; ④the population's value orientation.Hence, when we develop the disease prevention strategy, we first must do situation analysis, then coping analysis, and finally we should design a plan.

Situation analysis involves the study of the epidemic status of diseases according to the social, economic and cultural situation in a country or a region. It provides essential background data for establishing a plan, including demographic and geographic information, data on the natural environment, health care patterns and resources, characteristics of the social environment, behavioral features of the population, political considerations, economical and legal challenges,

9.3 制定预防策略

疾病的预防策略往往是根据特定地区疾病的流行特征、该地区的具体情况和需求、可利用的人力和物力等资源而制定的。有效的疾病预防策略可以在很大程度上改善容易使人患病的环境。策略可以是全球性的、国家性的或区域性的指导思想、行动方针，它既可以侧重于人群中的多种疾病和健康问题，也可以侧重于某一疾病。在制定疾病的预防策略时，必须考虑以下4个因素：①相关措施的有效性证据；②资源的可用性；③人群的健康需求；④人群的价值取向。因此，制定疾病预防策略时，首先必须进行形势分析，然后进行应对分析，最后制定策略。

形势分析是指根据一个国家或地区的社会、经济和文化状况去研究疾病的流行状况，为制订计划提供必要的基础数据，包括人口学和地理信息、自然环境、医疗模式和资源、社会环境特征、人群行为特征、政治因素、经济和法律规范及社会服务资源等数据。

social service resources, etc.

Coping analysis is mainly focused on the practical aspects of disease control. It involves consideration of the whole strategy for disease prevention and control in a country or a region with an emphasis on the fields that play important roles in the epidemiology of diseases and their influences. It further entails evaluation and analysis of the relevant publications and reports of prior activities in these fields. Coping analysis mainly answers the following questions:

① What are the essential aspects of disease prevention and control in this population?

② What measures have been carried out, which of them have been effective or not, and what factors caused them to be effective or ineffective?

③ Are disease prevention and control activities suitable for the current situation, what are their expected effects, and are they scientifically based, reasonable and sustainable? Which current methods should be terminated, which should be promoted, and what new work should be carried out?

Establishing a strategy leads to development of guidelines for managing the entire project. The guidelines are based on both the results of situation analysis and coping analysis, and on integrating the results to fit local situations. When developing the strategy for disease prevention and control, the following principles should be followed:

① Methods should be evidence-based.

② They should adaptable to rapid changes in the epidemiology of the disease.

③ They should be consistent with a macro view of the society's health.

④ They should be based on macro-epidemiological thinking.

应对分析主要集中在疾病控制的实践方面，涉及对一个国家或地区整体疾病防制战略的考虑，重点在流行病学及其应用发挥重要作用的领域。应对分析还需对这些领域的相关出版物和活动报告进行评估和分析。应对分析主要回答以下问题：

①人群疾病防制的基础是什么？

②采取了哪些措施？哪些措施有效，哪些方法无效？哪些因素影响了措施的效果？

③疾病防制的措施是否符合当前形势？预期效果如何？是否科学、合理、可持续？哪些方法应该终止，哪些方法应该继续推广？还需开展哪些新的工作？

策略是在形势分析和应对分析的结果及与当地情况的适用性的基础上，制定的管理整个项目的指导方针。在制定疾病预防和控制策略时，应遵循以下原则：

①方法应该以证据为基础。
②应该适应疾病流行病学的快速变化。

③应该与社会健康的宏观观点一致。

④应该基于宏观流行病学的思维。

⑤ They require objective consideration of available resources.

⑥ They should employ these resources reasonably and effectively.

⑤需要客观评价可利用资源。

⑥能合理有效地利用资源。

9.4　Health Care

9.4　卫生保健

Health care is an expression of concern for fellow beings. It is defined as a "multitude of services rendered to individuals, families or communities by the agents of the health services or professions, for the purpose of promoting, maintaining, monitoring or restoring health". Such services might be staffed, organized, admininstered and financed in every imaginable way, but they all have on in common: People are being "served" that is diagnosed, helped, cured, educated and rehabilitated by health personnel. In many countries, health care is completely or largely parts of government function.

卫生保健被定义为"卫生服务机构或专业人员为促进、维持、监测或恢复健康，而向个人、家庭或社会提供的多种服务"。服务的人员、组织、管理和经费可能有各种形式，但它们都有一个共同点：由医务人员向人群提供诊断、帮助、教育和康复等服务。在许多国家，卫生保健完全或在很大程度上是政府的职能。

Health care includes "medical care". Many mistakenly believe that both are synonymous. Medical care is a subset of a health care system. The term "medical care（which ranges from domiciliary care to resident hospital）refers chiefly to those personal services that are provided directly by physicians or rendered as a result of the physiological instructions".

许多人错误地认为卫生保健和医疗护理是相同的。其实，卫生保健包括医疗护理，医疗护理是卫生保健系统的子系统。医疗护理（范围从辅助性保健到医院）主要指由医生直接提供或根据生理指示提供的个人服务。

Health care has many characteristics; they include:

医疗保健有以下几个特点：

① Appropriateness（relevance）,i.e., whether the service is needed at all in relation to essential human needs, priorities and policies.

①适当性（相关性），即就人类的基本需求、优先事项和政策而言，是否需要该服务。

② Comprehensiveness, i.e., whether there is an optimum mix of preventive, curative and promotional services.

②全面性，即预防、治疗和健康促进服务是否有一个最佳组合。

③ Adequacy, i.e., if the service is proportionate

③充分性，即服务是否与需求相称。

to requirement.

④ Availability, i.e., ratio between the population of an administrative unit and the health facility (e.g., population per centre; doctor-population ratio).

⑤ Accessibility, i.e., this may be geographic accessibility, economic accessibility or cultural accessibility.

⑥ Affordability, i.e., the cost of health care should be within the means of the individual and the state.

⑦ Feasibility, i.e., operational efficiency of certain procedures, logistic support, manpower and material resources.

9.4.1 Health system

The "health system" is intended to deliver health services; in other words, it constitutes the management sector and involves organizational matters, e.g., planning, determining priorities, mobilizing and allocating resources, translating policies into services, evaluation and health education.

The components of the health system include: concepts (e.g., health and disease); ideas (e.g., equity, coverage, effectiveness, efficiency, impact); objects (e.g., hospitals, health centres, health programmes) and persons (e.g., providers and consumers). Together, these form a whole in which all the components interact to support or control one another. The aim of a health system is health development — a process of continuous and progressive improvement of the health status of a population. The goal of the health system had been to achieve "Health for all by the year 2000" which was put forward by the WHO in 1981.

④可用性，即行政区域内的人口与医疗机构的比例（如中心服务的人群比、人均医护比）。

⑤可及性，即地理可及性、经济可及性或文化可及性。

⑥可负担性，即医疗费用应在个人和国家的承受范围之内。

⑦可行性，即实施过程、后勤支持、人力和物力的运行效率。

9.4.1 卫生系统

卫生系统旨在提供卫生服务，它是管理部门的一部分，涉及组织事项，如规划、确定优先事项、调动和分配资源、将政策转化为服务、健康教育和健康评价等。

卫生系统的组成部分包括概念（如健康和疾病）、理念（如公平性、覆盖面、效果、效率、影响）、对象（如医院、健康中心、健康计划）和人员（如提供者和消费者），各组成部分相互作用、相互支持、相互限制，共同组成了卫生系统。卫生系统的目标是健康发展，健康发展是一个持续和逐步改善人群健康状况的过程。1981年，WHO提出了到2000年实现"人人享有健康"（简称HFA）的战略目标。为了积极应对我国主要健康问题和挑战，推动卫生事业全面协调可持续发展，我国先后启动了"健康中国2020"和"健康中国2030"等系列"健康中国"计划。

9.4.2 Levels of health care

Health services are usually organized at three levels, each level supported by a higher level to which the patient is referred. These levels are:

1.Primary health care

This is the first level of contact between the individual and the health system where "essential" health care (primary health care) is provided. A majority of prevailing health complaints and problems can be satisfactorily dealt with at this level. This level of care is closest to the people. In the Chinese context, this care is provided by the community health centres and their subcentres, with community participation.

Disease prevention and control strategies are best integrated with other health services, and they are especially well suited for primary health care (PHC) programs. The key features of PHC were described by the Alma Ata Conference organized by the WHO in 1978.

（1）Definition

The concept of primary health care came into limelight in 1978 following an international conference in Alma - Ata USSR. It has been defined as: "Essential health care based on practical, scientifically sound and socially acceptable methods and technology made universally accessible to individuals and families in the community through their full participation and at a cost that the community and the country can afford to maintain at every stage of their development in the spirit of self reliance and self determination."

The primary health care approach is based on principles of social equity, nation-wide coverage, self-reliance, intersectoral coordination, and people's in-

9.4.2 卫生保健的级别

卫生保健通常分为三级，每个级别都应为患者转诊到更高级别提供支持。三级卫生保健分别是：

1.初级卫生保健

初级卫生保健（PHC）是社区内的个人和家庭能够普遍获得的基本卫生保健（初级保健）。普遍存在的大部分健康问题都可以通过初级卫生保健得到解决。初级卫生保健是实现全民健康覆盖最有效的方式，是人人都能得到的卫生服务。在我国，初级卫生保健由社区卫生服务中心及卫生服务站提供，是个人、家庭、社区与国家卫生系统接触的第一环，是卫生保健持续进程中的初始一级。

疾病的预防和控制策略最好与其他卫生服务相结合，尤其是适合初级卫生保健的项目。初级卫生保健的概念由WHO于1978年在阿拉木图会议上正式提出。

（1）定义

1978年，在苏联阿拉木图举行的国际会议上，初级卫生保健概念的提出成为众人瞩目的焦点。它被定义为："基于实用的、科学的和社会可接受的方法和技术，通过社区内个人和家庭的充分参与，以社区和国家能够负担得起的费用，本着自力更生和自我决定的精神，在发展的每个阶段普遍提供给群众的基本卫生保健。"

初级卫生保健基于社会公平、全国覆盖、自力更生、部门间协调以及全民参与卫生方案的规划和实施，目的是实现共同的健康目标。共同的

volvement in the planning and implementation of health programmes in pursuit of common health goals. This approach has been described as "Health by the people" and "placing people's health in people's hands". Primary health care was accepted by the Member Countries of WHO as the key to achieving the goal of HFA by the year 2000 AD.

（2）Principles

There are five principles in PHC as follows: rational distribution, community participation, prevention first, suitable techniques, and comprehensive utilization.

（3）Contents

According to "Declaration of Alma-Ata" in 1978, PHC contains four aspects and nine contents. The four aspects include: promoting health; preventing disease; rational treatment; and community rehabilitation. The nine contents include: Health education on current major health problems and their prevention and control measures; improvement of food supply and rational nutrition; provision of adequate safe water and essential environmental health mechanisms; maternal and child health care and family planning; prophylactic vaccination for major communicable diseases; prevention and control of endemic disease; rational treatment of common diseases and injuries; provision of basic medicines; and prevention and control of non-communicable disease and promotion of mental health.

The concept of primary health care involves a concerted effort to provide the rural population of developing countries with at least the bare minimum of health services. The list can be modified to fit local circumstances. For example, some countries have specifically included mental health, physical handicaps, and the health and social care of the elderly. The primary

健康目标也被称为"人民的健康"和"将人民的健康掌握在人民手中"。WHO成员国将初级卫生保健视作实现"2000年人人享有健康"这一目标的关键。

（2）原则

初级卫生保健有5个原则：合理布局、社区参与、预防为主、适宜技术、综合利用。

（3）内容

根据1978年颁布的《阿拉木图宣言》，初级卫生保健包含4个方面、9项内容。这4个方面包括：健康促进、预防疾病、合理治疗、社区康复。9项内容包括：对当前主要卫生问题及其防制措施的健康教育、改善食品供应和合理营养、保障足够安全用水和基本卫生环境、妇幼保健和计划生育、主要传染病的预防接种、地方病的防治、常见疾病和外伤的合理治疗、提供基本药物、预防和控制非传染病和促进心理健康。

初级卫生保健需要全社会共同参与，其概念涉及为发展中国家的农村人群提供最低限度的卫生服务。初级卫生保健的内容可根据当地情况进行调整。例如，一些国家专门将心理健康、身体残疾、老年人的健康和社会关怀列入在内。作为《阿拉木图宣言》的签署国，我国政府承诺提供初级卫生保健。在我国，实施初级卫生保健的障碍

health care approach integrates at the community level all the factors required for improving the health status of the population. As a signatory to the Alma Ata Declaration, the government of China has pledged itself to provide primary health care. Obstacles to the implementation of primary health care in China include shortage of health manpower, entrenchment of a curative culture within the existing health system, and a high concentration of health services and health personnel in urban areas.

（4）Traits

① Social goals: Health is defined by the WHO as a state of complete physical, mental and social well being, not merely the absence of disease or infirmity. Health is the basic right of everyone, and an important society target is to make all people reach higher states of health as soon as possible.

② Participation goals: PHC is directed at all residents in an area. PHC involves every individual, family, and community. Therefore, it has extensive popular appeal. Residents not only have the right to be served, but also have an obligation to take part in and conduct PHC.

③ Difficulties in reaching goals: The unsolved health problems around the world and the current health conditions in China illustrate that the task of PHC is very difficult. There are some major challenges in China, such as: our country's levels of wealth and education are less than those of the world's highest income countries; The development of health projects is not tightly linked to development of the economy; Investment in PHC requires more manpower and development of new and feasible technique. Hence, health care services can not yet meet all of the increased needs of the people, especially the rapidly aged popu-

包括卫生从业人员短缺、现有卫生系统中固有的医疗文化，以及卫生服务和卫生人员高度集中在城市地区所造成的卫生资源不平衡等。

（4）特点

①社会性：WHO将健康定义为躯体、心理和社会适应都处于良好健康状态，而不仅仅是没有疾病或虚弱。健康是人的基本权利，一个重要的社会目标是使所有人尽快达到更高的健康状态。

②群众参与性：初级卫生保健针对一个地区的所有居民，包括个人、家庭和社区，具有广泛的群众性。居民不仅有权利得到服务，而且有义务参与和实施初级卫生保健。

③艰巨性：无论从全球亟待解决的卫生问题来看，还是从我国的卫生状况来分析，初级卫生保健的任务都是相当艰巨的。我国面临着一些重大挑战，比如经济和教育水平低于发达国家，卫生项目的发展与经济发展没有紧密联系，初级卫生保健缺乏适宜的人才和适宜的、新的可行技术等。因此，初级卫生保健服务还不能满足人们日益增长的需求，特别是我国人口迅速老龄化，以及慢性病和残疾带来的巨大的疾病负担。

lation and the huge burden of chronic diseases and disability in China.

④ Time investment: Humans pursue good health throughout their lives. Only "Health for all" can help people to do this. Therefore, PHC is a long-term project.

（5）Significance

① Fully enjoying the right of health: PHC stands for all the world's people and thus reflects social justice and people's rights to health. However, there are huge disparities between developing and developed countries in terms of people's health, provision of health resources, and the level of health care services. Similar difference may also exist between urban and rural areas within a country. Fortunately, PHC can effectively eliminate these disparities in health services and health status.

② Promoting economic development: On the one hand, PHC depends on the development of a social economy, and on the other hand, it can help every person to achieve a satisfactorily healthy state and thereby protect the labor force and increase manpower resources. Because people's health states are very important to the development of a productive workforce, PHC can promote the development of the economy and of the whole society.

③ Improving everyone's health levels: People are gradually realizing that PHC plays a major role in helping people to benefit from disease prevention and health promotion measures provided by the society.

④ Improving the level of civility in society: There are two aspects to improving civility. One is ideological and moral development, and the other is the development of education, science, culture and health. Provision of high quality PHC can change the quality

④长期性：全生命周期健康是人类一生的追求。只有全民健康，才能帮助人们实现这一追求。随着时间推移、经济发展，初级卫生保健不断扩展。因此，初级卫生保健是一个长期项目。

（5）意义

①使人们充分享受健康权。初级卫生保健是全世界人民最基本的需要和权利，反映了社会公平和人民的健康权。然而，发展中国家和发达国家在健康水平、卫生资源和卫生保健服务水平方面存在着巨大差距，同一个国家的城市和农村地区之间也存在着差异。初级卫生保健可以有效消除医疗服务和健康状况方面的差异。

②促进经济发展。一方面，初级卫生保健有赖于社会经济的发展；另一方面，初级卫生保健有助于人们达到健康状态，从而保护劳动力，增加人力资源。由于健康状况对生产力的发展非常重要，因此初级卫生保健可以促进经济和整个社会的发展。

③提高每个人的健康水平。初级卫生保健在帮助人们受益于社会提供的疾病预防和健康促进措施方面发挥着重要作用。

④提高社会文明水平。社会文明有两个方面，一是思想道德建设，二是教育、科学、文化、卫生建设。提供高质量的初级卫生保健，可以改变人们的生活环境质量，提高人们保护公共卫生的意识，为我国构建和谐社会树立榜样。

of people's living environments, improve people's willingness to protect public health, and serve as a model for building a harmonious society in our country.

2.Secondary health care

At this level, more complex problems are dealt with. This care comprises essentially curative services and is provided by the district hospitals and community health centres. This level serves as the first referral level in the health system.

3.Tertiary health care

This level offers super - specialist care. This care is provided by the regional/central level institutions. These institutions provide not only highly specialized care, but also planning and managerial skills and teaching for specialized staff. In addition, the tertiary level supports and complements the actions carried out at the primary level.

9.4.3　Health team concept

It is recognized that physician of today is overworked professionally. It is also recognized that many of the function of the physician can be performed by auxiliaries, given suitable training. An auxiliary worker has been defined as one "who has less than full professional qualifications in particular field and is supervised by a professional worker". The WHO no longer uses the term "paramedical" for the various health professions allied with medicine.

The practice of modern medicine has become a joint effort of many groups of workers, both medical and non - medical, viz. physicians, nurses, social workers, health assistants, trained village health guides and a host of others. The composition of the team varies. The hospital team is different from the team that works

2.中级卫生保健

这一层次解决的是更复杂的问题。中级卫生保健主要由地区医院和社区卫生服务中心提供治疗服务，是卫生系统中第一个接受转诊的层次。

3.高级卫生保健

高级卫生保健由省级或中央级别的卫生机构提供高级专家医疗服务。高级医疗机构不仅提供高度专业化的医疗服务，还为下级医院提供专业的技术指导和管理培训。此外，高级医疗机构还会给予初级医疗机构一定的医疗服务支持和补充。

9.4.3　健康团队的概念

医生工作强度大，长期超负荷工作。如果有适当的培训，医生的许多工作就可以由辅助人员来完成。医辅人员被定义为"在特定领域不具备完整的职业资格，需在专业人员的监督下辅助完成专业工作的人"。WHO不再用"医辅人员"一词来表示与医学相关的各种卫生职业。

现代医学实践由医务工作者和非医务工作者共同完成，包括医生、护士、社会工作者、健康助理、经过培训的村医和其他人等。不同的健康团队，其组成各不相同（比如医院团队不同于社会团队），但每个团队成员都应该有特定且公认的职能，并能自由发挥其技能。健康团队被定义为

in the community. Whether it is hospital team or community health work team, it is important for each team member to have a specific and recognized function in the team and to have freedom to exercise his or her particular skills. In this context, a health team has been defined as "a group of persons who share a common health goal and common objectives, determined by community needs and toward the achievement of which each member in the team contributes in accordance with her/his competence and skills, and respecting the functions of the other". The auxiliary is an essential member of the team. The team must have a leader. The leader should be able to evaluate the team adequately and should know the motivations of each member in order to stimulate and enhance their potentialities. The health team concept has taken a firm root in the delivery of health services both in the developed and developing countries. The health team approach aims to produce the right "mix" of health personnel for providing full health coverage of the entire population. The mere presence of variety of health professionals is not sufficient to establish teamwork; it is the proper division and combination of the operations from which the benefits of divided labour will be derived.

9.4.4 Health for all

After three decades of trial and error and dissatisfaction in meeting people's basic health needs, the World Health Assembly, in May 1977, decided that the main social goal on governments and WHO in the coming years should be the "attainment by all the people of the world by the year 2000 AD of a level of health that will permit them to lead a socially and economically productive life". This goal has come to be popularly known as "Health for All by the year 2000"

"一个拥有共同健康目标和目的的团体，根据社会需求决定团队组成，每个成员根据自己的知识和技能为实现这些目标做出贡献，并尊重其他人的职能"。医辅人员是健康团队的重要成员。团队必须有一名领导者，领导者应能够充分评估团队，了解每个成员的目的，以激发和增强成员的潜力。在发达国家和发展中国家，健康团队在提供健康服务的过程中发挥着重要作用。健康团队旨在产生正确的"组合"，为整个人群提供全面的健康服务。健康团队不仅需要各种各样的卫生专业人员，还需要团队中的成员合理分工和协调合作。

9.4.4 全民健康

经过30年的试验，仍无法满足人民的基本健康需求后，1977年5月，经WHO倡议，WHO成员国一致通过了一项全球性战略目标："到2000年使世界所有公民在社会和经济方面达到生活得有成效的那种健康水平"。这一目标普遍被称为"到2000年人人享有健康"（HFA）。这个"新"思想产生的背景是世界上大多数人（尤其是农村贫困地区的居民）处于恶劣的健康状态，国家之间和国家内部的贫富差距带来的巨大健康差距，以

（HFA）. The background to this "new" philosophy was the growing concern about the unacceptably low levels of health status of the majority of the world's population especially the rural poor and the gross disparities in health between the rich and poor, urban and rural population, both between and within countries. The essential principle of HFA is the concept of "equity in health", that is, all people should have an opportunity to enjoy good health.

9.4.5 Millennium development goals

In the *Millennium Declaration* of September 2000, Member States of the United Nations made a most passionate commitment to address the crippling poverty and multiplying misery that grip many areas of the world. Governments set a date of 2015 by which they would meet the Millennium Development Goals: Eradicate extreme poverty and hunger, achieve universal primary education, promote gender equality and empower women, reduce child mortality, improve maternal health, combat HIV/AIDS, malaria and other diseases, ensure environmental sustainability and develop a global partnership development.

9.4.6 Health policy

Policies are general statements based on human aspirations, set of values, commitments, assessment of current situation and an image of a desired future situation. A national health policy is an expression of goals for improving the health situation, the priorities among these goals, and the main directions for attaining them. Health policy is often defined at the national level.

Each country will have to develop a health policy of its own aimed at defined goals, for improving the

及城市和农村存在的巨大健康差距。HFA的基本原则是"健康公平"，也就是说，所有人都应该有机会享受健康。

9.4.5 千年发展目标

2000年9月，联合国成员国共同签署了《千年宣言》，共同承诺要解决困扰世界许多地区的严重贫困问题和日益增加的苦难问题，2015年作为目标完成的期限。具体目标包括：消除极端贫困和饥饿，普及初等教育，促进男女平等并赋予妇女权力，降低儿童死亡率，改善产妇健康，防治艾滋病、疟疾和其他疾病，确保环境的可持续发展，建立全球发展伙伴关系。

9.4.6 卫生政策

政策是基于人类愿望、价值观、承诺、对当前形势的评估和对未来形势预测的一般性声明。一个国家的卫生政策体现了改善健康状况的目标、这些目标中的优先事项以及实现这些目标的主要方向。卫生政策通常由国家政府部门制定。

每个国家都必须根据其自身存在的问题、特定的环境、社会和经济结构以及政治和行政机制，

people's health, in the light of its own problems, particular circumstances, social and economic structures, and political and administrative mechanisms. Among the crucial factors affecting realization of these goals are: a political commitment; financial implications; administrative region community participation and basic legislation.

A landmark in the development of health policy is world - wide adoption of the goal of HFA by 2000. And further landmark was the *Alma - Ata Declaration* (1978) on all governments to develop and implement primary care strategies to attain the target of HFA by 2000. And more recently, Millennium Development Goals.

9.4.7 Health services research

Health research has several ramifications. It may have:

① Biomedical research, to elucidate outstanding problems and develop new or better ways of dealing them.

② Intersectoral research, for which relation would have to be established with the institutions combine with the other sectors.

③ Health services research, health practice research (now called "health research").

The concept of health services research (HSR) developed during 1981-1982. It has been defined as the systematic study of the means by which biomedical and other relevant knowledge is brought to bear on the health of individuals and communities under a given set of conditions. HSR is wide in scope. It deals with all management of health services, viz. prioritization of problems, planning, management, logistics and deliver health care services. It deals with such topics as many

制定符合其目标的卫生政策，改善人民健康。影响目标实现的关键因素包括：政治因素、经济发展因素、公众参与因素和合法性。

卫生政策发展史上的一个里程碑是全球达成了"到2000年人人享有健康"的共识，另一个里程碑是《阿拉木图宣言》（1978年）正式提出初级卫生保健是实现"到2000年人人享有健康"战略目标的基本策略和关键途径，以及后续提出的"千年发展目标"。

9.4.7 卫生服务研究

卫生服务研究包括：

①生物医学研究：阐明突出的生物医学问题，并研究新的或更好的方法解决问题。

②交叉研究：建立多学科、多部门的联系，进行跨领域、跨学科、多学科交叉的科学研究、技术研究和应用研究。

③卫生服务研究、卫生实践研究（即现在狭义的"卫生研究"）。

卫生服务研究（HSR）的概念是1981—1982年发展形成的。它是指利用生物医学和其他相关知识，系统研究特定条件对个人和社区健康产生的影响。卫生服务研究涉及的范围广，包括所有与卫生服务相关的管理，即确定需优先解决的健康问题、规划、组织管理、后勤保障和要提供的卫生保健服务，还包括与其他组织机构的协调、设施利用、护理质量和成本效益等。

organizations, the utilization of facilities, the quality of care, cost-benefit and cost-effectiveness.

Thousands of people suffer morbidity, mortality disability not because of deficiencies in biomedical knowledge but as a result of the failure to apply this knowledge effectively. Health services research aims to correct this. The concept of HSR is holistic and multidisciplinary prime purpose of HSR is to improve the health of the human through improvement not only of conventional health service but also of other services that have a bearing on health is essential for the continuous evolution and refinement health services.

9.5 Prevention and Control of Chronic Non-communicable Diseases

Chronic non-communicable diseases, or simply chronic diseases, are prolonged conditions that often have a sub-clinical onset, tend to worsen over time and are rarely cured completely. Their causes are usually complicated and uncertain, and they often have a close relationship with psychosocial factors and life styles; they are therefore also called "life-style diseases".

Chronic disease prevention is accomplished by choosing strategies and measures that have been proven to be effective and be consistent with scientific evidence regarding disease etiology, physiological functions, and the natural history of disease. The aims of prevention are to prevent the occurrence, development or deterioration of disease and to improve patients' and disabled persons' quality of life. Chronic diseases have multiple causes, including genetic, environmental and psychosocial factors. All of these factors depend on and interact with each other. They also are related to demographic characteristics, cultural systems, personal preferences, mental state, ecological balance

很多疾病、死亡和残疾的发生，不是因为人们缺乏生物医学知识，而是因为人们未能有效应用知识。卫生服务研究的目的就是改善这一状况。卫生服务研究的概念是全面和多学科的，主要目的是通过改善传统的卫生服务和对健康有影响的其他服务来改善人们的健康。卫生服务研究是卫生服务持续发展和完善所必不可少的。

9.5 慢性非传染病的预防和控制

慢性非传染病，简称"慢性病"，是一类起病隐匿、病程长、病情迁延不愈、病因复杂的疾病。慢性病通常与心理社会因素和生活方式密切相关，因此，慢性病也被称为生活方式疾病。

慢性病的预防是通过选择已被证明有效且与疾病病因、生理功能和疾病自然史相关的科学证据一致的策略和措施来实现的。预防的目的是防止疾病的发生、发展或恶化，提高患者和残疾者的生活质量。慢性病的病因包括遗传因素、环境因素和心理社会因素，这些因素相互依赖、相互影响。慢性病的发生还与人口学特征、文化背景、个人偏好、心理状态、生态平衡和自然资源有关。因此，慢性病的预防不仅要依靠生物医学方法，还必须注意心理社会因素。人体在生态系统中生存，生态系统的内部和外部环境因素相互联系、相互作用，因此，有必要全面、多角度地研究医学和健康。

and natural resources. Preventing chronic disease cannot just depend on biomedical methods, and psychosocial factors must also be paid attention to. The human body can be viewed as functioning within an ecological system in which both internal and external environmental factors mutually connect and interact. People can thus regard both medicine and health through holistic and multiple stratum views.

When strategies and measures for preventing and controlling chronic disease are established, the following principles should be considered:

① Prevention comes first and should be combined with comprehensive measures including both prevention and treatment.

② Community-based health promotion strategies should be used.

③ Primary prevention, followed by secondary prevention and tertiary prevention should be employed.

④ The focus of chronic disease control should shift from scientific research to health services, from hospitals to patients and even healthy persons, and from passive clinical services to comprehensive services including active continuous preventive health care, rehabilitation and health education.

⑤ Prevention begins with children and emphasizes continuous health management throughout life.

⑥ Both a whole population strategy and a high-risk population strategy should be used as appropriate.

制定慢性病的防制策略和措施时，应注意以下原则：

①预防为主，防治结合。

②应采用以社区为基础的健康促进策略。

③应采用疾病的三级预防策略。

④慢性病防制的重点应从科学研究转向卫生服务，从医院转向患者甚至健康人，从被动的临床服务转向积极的综合服务（包括预防保健、康复和健康教育）。

⑤预防应从儿童开始，强调全生命周期的健康管理。

⑥应适当采用全人群策略和高危人群策略。

9.6 Three Levels of Preventive Measures for Chronic Disease

9.6.1 Primary prevention

Primary prevention is also called causal prophylaxis, and it is a measure mainly aimed at the causation (or risk factors) of disease. Primary prevention is an essential measure that aims to prevent the occurrence of disease and reduce its incidence. Primary prevention activities fall into two major categories: health promotion and health protection. Health promotion includes establishing a healthy environment in which people may avoid or decrease exposure to etiological factors (or risk factors). It also includes reinforcing the body's resistance to disease. Health protection means providing special measures to protect high-risk populations from disease.

1.Health promotion

Health promotion is a social strategy that uses administrative and organizational means to mobilize and harmonize all relevant elements of society at the community, family and individual level to meet obligations for maintaining and promoting health. The WHO indicates that health promotion mainly involves five domains:

① Establishing policies that are beneficial to health.

② Changing the direction of health services.

③ Improving individuals' and populations' health knowledge and skills.

④ Creating a good physical and natural environment.

9.6 慢性病的三级预防措施

9.6.1 一级预防

一级预防也称为病因预防，是在疾病尚未发生前，主要针对病因（或危险因素）采取的措施，目的是预防疾病的发生、降低发病率。一级预防措施包括健康促进和健康保护。健康促进不仅包括加强个体行为和生活技能的健康教育、提高个体对疾病的抵抗力，还包括建立健康的环境，避免或减少对致病因素（或危险因素）的接触。健康保护是指提供特殊措施，保护高危人群免受疾病威胁。

1.健康促进

健康促进是一个社会策略，是指通过行政和组织手段，动员和协调个人、家庭和社区等社会各方面共同履行维护和促进健康义务的过程。WHO指出，健康促进主要涉及以下5个领域：

①制定有利于健康的政策。

② 改变卫生服务的方向。

③ 提高个人和人群的健康知识和技能。

④创造良好的物质和自然环境。

⑤ Developing communities' abilities to promote health.

2.Health protection

Health protection entails measures for preventing a particular disease or health condition, or preventing diseases in a specified high - risk population, through targeted preventive methods that eliminate the effects of the causes of disease.

3. The whole population strategy and the high-risk population strategy

The focus of the whole population strategy is all the people in a society or community, and this strategy may be realized through health education, media programs and detailed guidelines. The objective of the whole population strategy is to reduce or control the risk factors for disease in a population by changing people's unhealthy lifestyles and behavioral factors, as well as other social, economic and environmental factors. A high - risk population strategy provides prevention targeted at people with specific risk factors of disease. This strategy usually addresses high-risk individuals first and provides them with special preventive measures.

Primary prevention is a desirable goal. It is worthwhile to recall the fact that the industrialized countries succeeded in eliminating a number of communicable diseases like cholera, typhoid and dysentery and controlling several others like plague, leprosy and tuberculosis, not by medical interventions but mainly by raising the standard of living (primary prevention). And much of this success came even before immunization became universal routine. The application of primary prevention to the prevention of chronic disease is a recent development. To have an impact on the popula-

⑤ 发展社区健康促进的能力。

2.健康保护

健康保护指采取有针对性的措施，保护个体或高危人群免受病因影响，从而预防疾病，改善健康状况。

3.全人群策略和高危人群策略

全人群策略针对的是全社会或社区的所有人，是指利用健康教育、媒体节目和指南等进行信息传播和行为干预，以改善人群不健康的生活方式和行为因素，以及其他社会、经济和环境有害因素，减少或控制人群疾病危险因素。高危人群策略针对具有特定疾病危险因素的人群（即高危人群）提供预防措施，从而降低危险暴露水平和发病风险。

一级预防是最佳的预防，是指疾病尚未发生前的病因预防。发达国家已经成功消灭了霍乱、伤寒和痢疾等传染病，并控制了鼠疫、麻风病和肺结核等传染病，这些成果不是医疗干预的结果，而是通过改善生活水平（一级预防）得以实现的，这些措施在免疫接种前就已经取得了效果。现在利用一级预防措施进行慢性病的防制已经取得了很大进展，为了更好地在人群中产生影响，应该联合使用以上三种方法。

tion, all the above three approaches should be implemented as they are usually complementary.

In summary, primary prevention is a "holistic" approach. It relies on measures designed to promote health or to protect against specific disease "agents" and hazards in the environment. It utilizes knowledge of the prepathogenesis phase of disease, embracing the agent, host and environment. The safety and low cost of primary prevention justifies its wider application. Primary prevention has become increasingly identified with "health education" and the concept of individual and community responsibility for health.

9.6.2 Secondary prevention

Secondary prevention refers to early detection, timely diagnosis and prompt treatment of disease. With such measures it is sometimes possible to cure disease or slow its progression and minimize its severity. At present, the causation of many chronic diseases is uncertain, and the efficacy of many primary prevention strategies remains unproven. However, chronic diseases often develop slowly, with a long latent period; therefore, early detection, timely diagnosis and prompt treatment offer good prospects for reducing disease burdens.

Secondary prevention is largely the domain of clinical medicine. The health programmes initiated by governments are usually at the level of secondary prevention. The drawback of secondary prevention is that the patient has already been subject to mental anguish, physical pain; and community to loss of productivity. These situations sometimes are encountered in primary prevention.

Screening involves using relatively simple tests to identify potentially diseased, but asymptomatic, indi-

总之，一级预防是利用健康促进或降低病原体和环境中危险暴露水平的措施进行全面的疾病预防的方法。它利用了疾病发病前关于病原体、宿主和环境的知识，采取多种措施，通过健康教育及个人和社会的力量，降低有害暴露水平，提高个体对抗有害暴露的能力，从而预防疾病的发生。一级预防因其安全性和低成本而被广泛应用。

9.6.2 二级预防

二级预防是指疾病的早期发现、早期诊断和早期治疗，也称为"三早"预防。患者在疾病早期尚无明显的症状、体征，此时通过及早发现并诊断疾病，及时给予适当治疗，可以治愈疾病或减缓疾病进展，将严重程度降至最低。目前，许多慢性病的病因尚不完全清楚，一级预防的有效性尚未全部得到证实，而慢性病发展缓慢、潜伏期长，因此，二级预防为降低疾病负担创造了良好前景。

二级预防主要涉及临床医学领域。政府发起的健康计划大多是二级预防。二级预防的缺点是，疾病已经发生，患者已经遭受了生理和心理上的痛苦，社会也已经损失了劳动力。这些情况有时在有些疾病的一级预防中也会遇到。

疾病的早发现可以通过筛检实现，对筛检阳性的人群可以进行进一步的诊断和治疗。筛检应

viduals who then undergo more specific diagnostic testing and treatment. Before screening is conducted, the following requirements should be met:

① The target disease must be an important public health problem in the area at this time.

② Further diagnostic and treatment services must be available to those identified by screening.

③ The natural history of the screened disease is understood.

④ The test used for screening is innocuous, rapid, inexpensive, effective and acceptable to people.

⑤ Cost-effectiveness analyses of the program, including screening, diagnosis and treatment aspects, are favorable.

Secondary prevention is an imperfect tool in the control of transmission of disease. It is often more expensive and less effective than primary prevention. In the long run, human health, happiness and useful longevity will be achieved at far less expense with less suffering through primary prevention than through secondary prevention.

9.6.3　Tertiary prevention

Tertiary prevention is also called "clinical prevention". Its aim is to prevent disability, improve function, promote quality of life, prolong life and reduce mortality when disease has already occurred. Its major measures include relief of symptoms and rehabilitation.

Symptomatic relief can alleviate suffering, decrease adverse effects, prevent disease progression and complications, and limit disability. Rehabilitation attempts to restore an affected individual to a useful, satisfying, and self-sufficient role in society. Its major theme is maximal utilization of the individual's residu-

满足以下要求：

①筛检的疾病必须是当地目前重要的公共卫生问题。

②必须有进一步诊断和治疗的方法。

③了解筛检疾病的自然史。

④筛检的方法应安全、简单、经济、准确，且易被受检者接受。

⑤筛检项目（包括筛检、诊断和治疗）的成本效益分析评估是有卫生经济学价值的。

二级预防通常比一级预防花费高、效果差，因此并不是控制疾病传播的完美方法。从长远看，一级预防才应该是消除疾病的根本措施。

9.6.3　三级预防

三级预防也称为临床预防。其目的是预防残疾，改善功能，提高生活质量，延长寿命，降低死亡率。其主要措施包括缓解症状和康复治疗。

缓解症状可以减轻痛苦，减少不良反应，防止疾病恶化，预防并发症和残疾的发生。康复治疗是指最大限度地恢复个体的机体功能和社会功能，其主要作用是最大限度地利用机体的剩余功能，强调的是剩余功能而不是损失。康复治疗包括功能康复、心理康复、社会康复和职业康复。

al capacities, with emphasis on remaining abilities rather than on losses. Rehabilitative treatment includes functional rehabilitation, psychological rehabilitation, social rehabilitation and occupational rehabilitation.

9.7 Concepts of Disease Control

9.7.1 Disease control

The term "disease control" describes (ongoing) operations aimed at reducing:

① The incidence of disease.

② The duration of disease, and consequently the risk of transmission.

③ The effects of infection, including both the physical and psychosocial complications.

④ The financial burden to the community.

Control activities may focus on primary prevention or secondary prevention, and most control programmes combine the two. The concept of tertiary prevention is comparatively less relevant to control efforts.

In disease control, the disease "agent" is not permitted to persist in exist in the community at a level where it ceases to be a public health problem according to the tolerance of the local population. A state of equilibrium becomes established between the disease agent, host and environment components of the disease process. An excellent embodiment of this concept is malaria control, which is distinct from malaria eradication.

9.7.2 Disease elimination

Between control and eradication, an intermediate goal has been described, called "regional elimina-

9.7 疾病控制的概念

9.7.1 疾病控制

疾病控制描述的是旨在减少以下指标的（持续）行动：
①发病率。
②病程及传播风险。

③患病的影响，包括躯体和心理的不适及其并发症。
④社会经济负担。

疾病控制侧重于一级预防或二级预防，大多数情况是二者结合。三级预防与疾病控制的相关性相对较小。

当病原体已经不是威胁健康的重要的公共卫生问题时，依据当地居民的耐受性，病原体可以在社区持续存在，此时病原体、宿主和环境之间处于一种平衡状态。这也充分体现了控制疟疾和根除疟疾二者的区别。

9.7.2 疾病消除

在控制和根除之间，有一个中间目标，即"区域消除"。"消除"一词用于描述疾病传播的中

tion". The term "elimination" is used to describe interruption of transmission of disease, as for example, elimination of measles, polio and diphtheria from large geographic regions or areas . Regional elimination is now seen as an important precursor eradication.

9.7.3 Disease eradication

Eradication literally means to "tear out by roots". Eradication of disease implies termination of all transmission of infection by extermination of the infectious agent. As the name implies, eradication is an absolute process, not a relative goal. It is "all or none phenomenon". The world eradication is reserved to cessation of infection and disease from the whole world.

Today, smallpox is the only disease that has been eradicated. So far next strategy for global eradication of poliomyelitis has been developed and achievement will be in sight. Even disease like every human being is unique with its own epidemiological characteristics and specific strategies control, eradication is tough.

During recent years, three diseases have been serious advanced as candidates for global eradication within forseeable future: polio, measles and dracunculiasis. The feasibility of eradicating polio appears to be greater than them of others.

Experience gained from eradication programmes (e.g., malaria, yaws) has shown that once the morbidity of a disease reaches a very low level, a "residual" infection usually persistent in the population leading to a state of equilibrium between the agent, host and environmental components of the disease process. In this situation, there are always hidden infections, unrecognized methods of transmission, resistance the vector or organism, all of which may again flare up where the agent - host - environment equilibrium is dis-

断，比如在大的地理区域或地区内消灭麻疹、脊髓灰质炎和白喉。区域消除被视为根除的重要前提。

9.7.3 疾病根除

"根除"的字面意思是"连根拔起"。根除疾病是指通过消灭传染源，终止所有感染的传播。根除是一个绝对的过程，不是一个相对的目标，是"全或无"的现象。世界疾病根除行动就是在全球范围内消灭感染和疾病。

目前，天花是唯一在全球范围内被根除的疾病。脊髓灰质炎是全球下一个计划要根除的疾病，相关的策略已经制定，将很快实现。即使每个疾病都有其独特的流行病学特征和具体防控措施，但疾病的根除依然很艰难。

近年来，可预见未来将会在全球根除的三种疾病是脊髓灰质炎、麻疹和睑腺炎。其中，根除脊髓灰质炎的可行性似乎更大。

从疾病（如疟疾、雅司病）根除项目中获得的经验发现，一旦疾病的发病率降到非常低的水平，通常就会在人群中持续存在"残留"感染，导致病原体、宿主和环境之间处于平衡状态。当平衡被打破时，隐性感染、未被识别的传播方式、机体对媒介或致病微生物的抵抗力降低会导致疾病的再次暴发，这也是对疟疾、鼠疫、黑热病和黄热病等的根除计划失败的原因。

turbed. Failure to understand this led to disappointment in the eradication programmes mounted against malaria, plague, kala-azar and yellow fever.

9.8　Disease Surveillance

9.8.1　Definition

Disease surveillance is a long - term, continuous and systematic process of collection, analysis, interpretation, and dissemination of data on dynamic trends of disease and of factors that influence disease incidence. Results of analyses of disease surveillance data are reported to individuals and organizations that are responsible for preventing and controlling disease so that they can intervene in a timely manner and evaluate the effects of their programs.

The above definition reflects the four essential characteristics of disease surveillance:

① Only continuously and systematically collected data can uncover the distribution, characteristics, and trends in occurrence of a disease or problem.

② To meet medical and public health needs, surveillance must cover a range of factors that are relevant to disease and health, not just the rates of disease occurrence and death.

③ Original data reflecting public health problems must be coordinated, analyzed and explained in order to have value.

④ The objectives of surveillance can be achieved only after health information is returned to the responsible departments and persons and appropriately applied.

9.8　疾病监测

9.8.1　定义

疾病监测是指长期、连续和系统地收集、分析、解释和反馈有关疾病的动态变化趋势及其影响因素数据信息的过程。疾病监测数据的分析结果将报告给负责疾病预防和控制的个人和机构，用以指导、完善和评价干预措施的效果与策略。

根据定义，疾病监测有4个基本特征：

①只有持续、系统地收集数据，才能揭示疾病或健康问题的分布、特征和变化趋势。

②为了满足医疗和公共卫生需求，监测必须涵盖与疾病和健康相关的系列因素，而不仅仅是发病率和死亡率。

③反映公共卫生问题的原始数据必须经过整理、分析和解释，才能转化为有价值的、重要的公共卫生信息。

④只有将健康信息及时反馈给责任部门和人员并充分合理利用，才能实现监测目标。

9.8.2 Categories of surveillance

1.Communicable disease surveillance

Malaria, influenza, polio, epidemic typhus and relapsing fever are designated by the WHO as internationally monitored communicable diseases, and dengue fever is added as an internationally monitored communicable disease in China according to the local situation. Because of increased communication with other countries, and to prevent the spread of AIDS in China, AIDS also is quarantined at the borders of China before 2010. According to the Law of the People's Republic of China on Prevention and Control of Communicable Diseases, legally reported communicable diseases are divided into three categories and 39 species. Any communicable disease case occurring and causing death in China must be reported to local and national Centers for Disease Control and should be prevented by persons responsible for preventing controlling disease. In addition, dengue fever is defined as a legally reported communicable disease in both Guangdong and Hainan province.

2.Non-communicable disease surveillance

Due to the changing nature of the disease spectrum, some countries have expanded the scope of disease surveillance to cover non-communicable diseases including malignant tumors, cerebrovascular disease, diabetes mellitus, birth defects, occupational diseases, etc. The National Cancer Institute (NCI) of the United States began to monitor cancer incidence and survival beginning in the 1970's and now provides detailed information on cancer occurrence and death. The Centers for Disease Control (CDC) of the United States launched a health promotion program for pre-

9.8.2 监测类别

1.传染病监测

WHO将疟疾、流感、脊髓灰质炎、流行性斑疹伤寒和回归热列为国际监测传染病，我国根据实际情况将登革热也列为国际监测传染病。随着与其他国家交流的增加，为了防止艾滋病在我国的传播，2010年前我国也限制艾滋病感染者入境。根据《中华人民共和国传染病防治法》，法定报告的传染病分为三类39种。在我国境内发生并导致死亡的任何传染病病例都必须向当地和国家疾病预防控制中心报告，并由负责疾病预防控制的人员采取防控措施。此外，在广东省和海南省，登革热也是法定报告的传染病。

2.非传染病监测

随着疾病谱的改变，一些国家已将疾病监测的范围扩大到非传染病（包括恶性肿瘤、脑血管疾病、糖尿病、出生缺陷、职业病等）。20世纪70年代，美国国家癌症研究所（NCI）开始监测癌症的发病率和生存率，并提供相关的详细信息。20世纪80年代，美国疾病控制中心（CDC）启动了一项关于慢性病防制的健康促进计划，主要针对10种可预防的慢性病，如冠心病、糖尿病、肝硬化与酒精中毒等。由WHO资助的MONICA（心血管疾病趋势和决定因素多国监测）项目旨在监测心血管疾病的发病率和病死率，以及相关的危

venting and controlling chronic disease beginning in the 1980's. In this process, ten preventable chronic diseases, such as coronary heart disease, diabetes, cirrhosis and alcoholism, were initially monitored through surveillance efforts. The MONICA (multinational monitoring of trends and determinants in cardiovascular diseases) project supported by WHO is designed to monitor incidence and mortality from cardiovascular diseases as well as the association of these diseases with relevant risk factors. The goals of the project include improvement of health care services and social economic development, so that effective intervention measures can be conducted to decrease the number of deaths from cardiovascular disease. In some areas of China, health authorities have launched programs of surveillance of non - communicable diseases, including malignant tumors, cardiovascular disease, birth defect, etc. For example, malignant tumors, coronary heart disease, stroke and hypertension have been monitored in Tianjin.

With the development of the economy, aging of the population, and the change in life styles, chronic diseases, injuries and sexually transmitted diseases (STDs) have become major public health problems affecting human health. All of these diseases are closely associated with personal behaviors, and the main measures for preventing and controlling these diseases therefore include promoting behavior change at the individual level. An increasing number of countries have realized the importance of behavioral surveillance surveys (BSS), and have set up the monitoring system of behavioral risk factors. Behavioral surveillance can be used for both communicable diseases and non - communicable diseases. In the former, the main indices of surveillance are various behaviors that can foster trans-

险因素、卫生服务和社会经济发展的变化，以便采取有效的干预措施，减少心血管病的死亡。在我国的一些地区，卫生部门已经启动了非传染病的监测项目，包括恶性肿瘤、心血管病、出生缺陷等。例如，天津已经对恶性肿瘤、冠心病、中风和高血压等进行了监测。

随着经济的发展、人口的老龄化和生活方式的改变，慢性病、伤残和性传播疾病（STD）已成为影响人类健康的主要公共卫生问题。这些疾病都与个人行为密切相关，因此疾病防制的主要措施应包括改善个人行为。越来越多的国家已认识到行为监测的重要性，并建立了行为风险因素监测体系。行为监测可用于预防传染病和非传染病。在传染病中，行为监测主要针对可能促进传播的各种行为，比如共用注射器和有多个性伴侣是传播艾滋病的行为。对于非传染病，行为监测主要针对不健康的生活方式，如吸烟、饮酒、营养缺乏或过剩、缺乏体育锻炼等。

mission, for example, sharing syringes and having multiple sexual partners are examples of behaviors that spread AIDS. For non - communicable diseases, the main behavioral indices to monitor are unhealthy life styles, such as smoking, excess alcohol drinking, nutritional deficiency. or surplus, physical inactivity, etc.

9.8.3 Terms of disease surveillance

1. Passive surveillance and active surveillance

Passive surveillance refers to the reporting of surveillance data by lower level units, such as doctors and health care facilities, to superior level units, such as regional health authorities. It typically relies on standardized reporting forms that are completed and returned to health authorities whenever a case of a reportable disease is detected. The activity is passive in that health authorities do not act until report forms are received; however, the process requires active participation by doctors and others who must complete the forms. Active surveillance entails outreach by health authorities and may involve activities such as regular contacts by telephone or in person to encourage reporting of diseases by doctors and facilities.

2. Routine reports and sentinel surveillance

Routine reporting is a national or local reporting system that functions continuously. Sentinel surveillance is defined as disease screening or case reporting in a certain time and in a certain area; the goals are to decrease costs and increase efficiency relative to routine reporting systems.

3. Direct indicators and indirect indicators

The numbers of cases, deaths, incidence rates, mortality, etc. are direct indicators of a disease. How-

9.8.3 疾病监测相关术语

1. 被动监测和主动监测

被动监测是指下级单位（如医院和医疗机构）常规向上级单位（如区域卫健局）报告监测到的数据。被动监测主要依据相关的法律法规要求进行，一旦发现需要上报的疾病，必须及时填报标准化的信息报告系统。上级单位被动接受信息，在收到报告之前不采取行动；整个过程需要医生和下级单位相关人员积极参与。主动监测需要卫生当局外联，通过电话或定期接触等活动，鼓励下级单位的医生和医疗机构及时上报疾病信息。

2. 常规报告和哨点监测

常规报告是一种持续运行的国家或地方报告系统，是针对卫生行政部门规定的疾病或健康相关问题进行常规监测。哨点监测是指在特定时间和区域内进行疾病筛查或病例报告，目的是减少常规报告的成本，并提高效率。

3. 疾病监测的直接指标和间接指标

病例数、死亡数、发病率、死亡率等是疾病监测的直接指标。因为需要明确疾病的诊断，所

ever, it is not feasible to monitor direct indicators for some conditions and authorities must rely on indicators of disease. For example, it is difficult to diagnose each case of influenza and to distinguish between deaths caused by influenza and those due to other respiratory diseases. In this situation, the weekly total of all deaths attributed to both influenza and pneumonia has been used in the US as an indirect indicator of the extent of epidemic influenza activity.

4.Symptom-based surveillance

Symptom - based surveillance is a continuous and systematic process for collecting and analyzing data on a certain group of symptoms, with the goal of rapidly detecting and predicting the occurrence of a disease so that authorities can mount a quick response.

9.8.4　Content and method

The process of disease surveillance involves collecting a great quantity of population — based health and disease data through routine reports, laboratory tests, population - based statistical investigations and field surveys. It allows authorities to describe and analyze disease patterns with a population perspective so that disease can be prevented and controlled. The relevant activities of surveillance thus include collecting data, analyzing data, disseminating information and utilizing information.

9.8.5　Data collection

Based on a normative schedule, information related to diseases is collected and managed with uniform criteria and methods using an effective information system. Data content includes demographic information, morbidity reports, death registration, laboratory

以有时很难获得疾病监测的直接指标。例如，很难诊断每一例流感病例，也很难区分流感引起的死亡和其他呼吸道疾病引起的死亡。为此，美国采用流感监测的间接指标——每周流感和肺炎引起的死亡总数，来反映流感疫情的活动程度。

4.基于症状的监测

基于症状的监测是连续、系统地收集和分析某一组症状的数据，目的是快速监测和预测疾病的发生，以便相关机构能够做出快速反应。

9.8.4　内容和方法

疾病监测过程通过常规报告、实验室检测、人群调查和现场调查等收集大量人群的健康和疾病数据，分析描述人群的疾病模式，从而预防和控制疾病。因此，疾病监测包括收集数据、分析数据、反馈信息和利用信息。

9.8.5　数据收集

数据收集是指根据疾病监测的时间要求，利用疾病监测上报信息系统，以统一的标准和方法收集和管理与疾病相关的信息，包括人口学信息、发病率报告、死亡登记、实验室数据（如抗体检测、水质监测）、危险因素调查（如吸烟、职业暴

data (e. g. , antibody tests, water quality monitoring), risk factor surveys (e.g. , smoking, occupational exposure, etc.), records of intervening measures (e.g., dispensing vaccine, supplying iodized salt), special surveys (e.g., outbreak investigations, case surveys), and other relevant data (e.g., sociological, demographic, meteorological, biological).

露等)、干预措施记录(如分发疫苗、供应碘盐)、专项调查(如疫情调查、病例调查)和其他相关数据(如社会学、人口统计学、气象学、生物学)。

9.8.6　Data analysis

Original data on disease surveillance are comprehensively analyzed and summarized into reports. The process of data analysis involves the following steps:

① Carefully checking and cleaning original data and documenting their sources and collection methods.

② Transforming reported data into relevant indices using statistical methods.

③ Explaining the connotation of these indexes. In the process of data analysis, the influence of various factors on the results of disease surveillance must be considered so that correct and reasonable explanations can be arrived at.

9.8.6　数据分析

数据分析是指对疾病监测的原始数据进行综合分析,并汇总成报告。数据分析的过程包括以下几个步骤:

①核查和清理原始数据,记录数据来源和收集方法。

②使用统计方法计算疾病监测的相关指标。

③解释结果。在数据分析过程中,必须考虑各种因素对疾病监测结果的影响,以便得出正确合理的解释。

9.8.7　Information dissemination

Information dissemination is a bridge linking disease surveillance and intervention. The "Epidemic Weekly Report" published by the WHO, the "Morbidity and Mortality Weekly Report" by the United States CDC, and "Disease Surveillance" by the China CDC all serve as access points for disseminating information on disease surveillance — information from disease surveillance activities must be distributed in a timely fashion to all relevant organizations and to individuals responsible for preventing and controlling disease, so that they may rapidly respond to health prob-

9.8.7　信息反馈

信息反馈是连接疾病监测和干预的桥梁。WHO发布的疫情周报、美国疾控中心发布的发病率和死亡率周报、我国疾控中心发布的疾病监测都是疾病监测信息反馈的接受点——疾病监测信息必须及时反馈给所有相关机构和个人,以便迅速应对。信息反馈分为纵向和横向两个方面,纵向指向上反馈给卫生行政部门及其领导,向下反馈给下级监测机构及其工作人员;横向指反馈给有关的医疗卫生机构及其专家,以及相关社区及其居民。信息反馈的内容和方式应视对象不同而异。

lems. The surveillance information can be disseminated in both vertical and horizontal directions. The vertical direction refers to reporting the surveillance information to higher - level health administrative departments and managers. The horizontal direction refers to transmitting the surveillance information to relevant medical and health care institutes and experts as well as communities and residents. Different surveillance information is provided to individuals and organizations, depending on their objectives.

9.8.8　Information utilization

Information from disease surveillance can be used to understand the characteristics of disease distribution, to confirm the occurrence of an epidemic, to predict the epidemiological trend of disease, to evaluate the effect of an intervention, and to provide evidence for developing strategies and measures for disease prevention and control.

9.8.9　System of disease surveillance

Systems of organizationally planned surveillance of disease or public health problems can be divided into three categories.

① Population - based surveillance systems: The work of this kind of disease surveillance is mainly carried out among populations in a community. Examples in China are the Legal Communicable Disease Report System and the Comprehensive Disease Monitoring Net.

② Hospital - based surveillance systems: This type of system mainly monitors hospital infections, pathogenic bacterial drug resistance, and birth defects in hospitals.

③ Laboratory - based surveillance systems: This

9.8.8　信息利用

疾病监测信息可用于了解疾病的分布特征，确认流行的存在，预测疾病的流行趋势，评估干预的效果，为制定疾病防制的措施和策略提供依据。

9.8.9　疾病监测系统

对疾病或公共卫生问题进行有组织、有计划的监测的系统可分为三类：

①以人群为基础的监测系统：主要在社区人群中进行监测。我国主要有法定传染病报告系统和疾病监测网。

②以医院为基础的监测系统：主要监测院内感染、病原体耐药性和出生缺陷等。

③以实验室为基础的监测系统：主要指利用

type of system mainly monitors pathogens or other etiological factors using laboratory tests. For example, the influenza surveillance system in China not only tests for influenza viruses, but also disseminates surveillance information.

实验室方法对病原体或其他致病因素开展监测。例如，我国的流感监测系统不仅监测流感病毒，而且反馈监测信息。

9.8.10 Assessment

Disease surveillance programs can be evaluated in terms of a number of important characteristics.

1.Sensitivity

To what extent does the system identify all of the events in the target population? This assessment involves comparing the proportion of cases reported by the system to the number real cases, and it affects the system's ability to detect when an outbreak or epidemic of disease has occurred.

2.Timeliness

This attribute refers to the time from information collection to relevant departments receiving a report. It reflects the speed of information dissemination and is an important aspect of acute communicable diseases surveillance that may directly affect intervention efforts.

3.Representativeness

To what extent do events detected through the surveillance system represent persons with conditions of interest in the target population? A lack of representativeness may lead to misallocation of health resources.

4.Simplicity

Are forms easy to complete? Are procedures unobtrusive? Is software "user-friendly"? Is data collection kept to a necessary minimum?

9.8.10 评估

疾病监测系统的质量可以从以下几个特征进行评价：

1.敏感性

敏感性是指监测系统发现和确认目标人群中公共卫生问题的能力，包括监测系统报告的监测病例占实际病例的比例，监测系统判断疾病或其他公共卫生事件暴发或流行的能力。

2.及时性

及时性指从信息收集到相关部门收到报告的时间间隔。它反映了信息上报和反馈的速度，对急性传染病暴发和突发公共卫生事件尤为重要，将直接影响到干预的效果和效率。

3.代表性

代表性指监测系统发现的公共卫生问题能在多大程度上代表目标人群的实际发生情况。缺乏代表性可能会导致卫生决策失误和卫生资源分配不当。

4.简单性

简单性指监测系统的资料收集、监测方法和系统运作简便易行，具有较高的工作效率，省时且节约卫生资源。例如，表格容易填写吗？软件是否"用户友好"？数据收集是否保持在必要的最低限度？

5.Flexibility

Can the system change to address new question? Can it adapt to evolving standards of diagnosis or medical care?

6.Acceptability

To what extent are the participants in a surveillance system enthusiastic about the system? Do they report cases, welcome staff into their hospitals or offices, complete forms, etc.? Does the effort they invest yield useful information?

7.Positive predictive value

To what extent are reported cases really cases? To what extent are measured changes in trends truly reflective of events in the community?

8.Accuracy and completeness of descriptive information

Forms for reporting health events often include descriptive personal information, such as demographic characteristics, clinical patterns of disease, or potential exposures. To what extent are these sections of forms completed? Is the information sufficiently reliable?

9.9　Modes of Intervention

"Intervention" can be defined as any attempt to intervene or interrupt the usual sequence in the development of disease in man. This may be by the provision of treatment, education help or social support. Five modes of intervention have been described which form a continuum corresponding to the natural history of any disease. These levels are related agent, host and environment.

5.灵活性

灵活性指监测系统针对新的公共卫生问题、操作程序或技术要求能进行及时调整或改变的能力，以适应新需要。

6.可接受性

例如，使用监控系统的工作人员对该系统是否满意？通过病例报告、填写数据等是否会产生有用的信息？

7.阳性预测值

报告的病例在多大程度上是真实病例？趋势变化在多大程度上真正反映了社区事件？

8.准确性和完整性

准确性和完整性即监测内容或指标的多样性，包括报告哨点与监测形式的完整性、病例报告的完整性和监测数据的完整性，通常应该包括个人信息（人口学特征、疾病模式或潜在暴露等）。需要注意的问题是，信息填写是否完整？信息是否可靠？

9.9　干预方式

干预指任何试图干预或中断疾病自然进展的行为，可以通过提供治疗、教育帮助或社会支持来实现。下面根据疾病自然史，介绍5种与病原体、宿主和环境相关的干预方式。

9.9.1 Health promotion

Health promotion is "the process of enabling people to increase control over, and to improve, their health". It is not directed against any particular disease, but is intended to strengthen the host through a variety of approaches (interventions). The well - known interventions in this area are:

1.Health education

This is one of the most cost effective interventions. A large number of diseases could be prevented with little or no medical intervention if people were adequately informed about them and if they were encouraged to take necessary precautions in time. Recognizing this truth the WHO's constitution states that "the extension to all people of the benefits of medical, psychological and related knowledge is essential to the fullest attainment of health". The targets for educational efforts may include the general public patients, priority groups, health providers, community leaders and decision-makers.

2.Environmental modifications

A comprehensive approach to health promotion requires environmental modifications, such as provision of safe water; installation of sanitary latrines; control of insects and rodents; improvement of hosing, etc. The history of medicine has shown that many infectious diseases have been successfully controlled in western countries through environmental modifications, even prior to the development of specific vaccines or chemotherapeutic drugs. Environmental interventions are non- clinical and do not involve the physician.

9.9.1 健康促进

健康促进是指增强人们控制影响健康的因素，改善自身健康能力的过程。它并不针对任何特定的疾病，而是旨在通过各种方法（干预措施）促进宿主健康。具体干预措施有：

1.健康教育

健康教育是最具成本效益的干预措施之一。它是指帮助群体或个体掌握卫生保健知识，鼓励实施改善健康的行为和生活方式等必要的预防措施，只需很少或根本不需要进行医疗干预，就可以预防大量疾病。为此，WHO指出，"将医疗、心理和相关知识的惠益扩大到所有人是实现全面健康的必要条件"。健康教育在三级预防中都可以发挥作用，对象包括普通群众、患者、高危人群、健康提供者、社区领导和决策者。

2.环境改造

环境改造是健康促进的综合方法，例如，提供安全用水、安装卫生的厕所、控制昆虫和啮齿动物、改善水管等。医学史表明，早在疫苗和化疗药物出现前，西方国家就已经通过环境改造成功控制了许多传染病。环境改造不是临床措施，也不需要医生。

3.Nutritional interventions

These comprise food distribution and nutrition improvement of vulnerable groups; child feeding programmes; food fortification; nutrition education, etc.

4.Lifestyle and behavioural changes

The conventional public health measures or interventions have not been successful in making inroads into lifestyle reforms. The action of prevention in this case, is one of individual and community responsibility for health, the physician and in fact each health worker acting as an educator than a therapist. Health education is a basic element of all health activity. It is of paramount importance in changing the views, behaviour and habits of people.

Since health promotion comprises a broad spectrum of activities, a well - conceived health promotion programme would first attempt to identify the "target groups" or at - risk individuals in a population and then direct more appropriate message to them. Goals must be defined. Means and alternative means of accomplishing them must be explored. It involves "organizational, political, social and economic interventions designed to facilitate environmental and behavioural adaptations that will improve or protect health".

9.9.2 Specific protection

To avoid disease altogether is the ideal but this is possible only in a limited number of cases. The following are some of the currently available interventions aimed at specific protection:

① Immunization.

② Use of specific nutrients.

③ Chemoprophylaxis.

④ Protection against occupational hazards.

3.营养干预

营养干预包括食物分配和改善弱势群体的营养状况、改善儿童喂养方案、食品强化、营养宣教等。

4.生活方式和行为改变

传统的公共卫生措施或干预措施未能成功地推进生活方式改革。因此，个人和社区都应该积极为改变生活方式和行为负责，医生和其他卫生工作者作为健康教育者，也应该采取行动。健康教育是所有健康活动的基本要素，对改变人们的观点、行为和习惯至关重要。

健康促进是一个综合活动过程，首先要确定目标群体或高危人群，然后向他们提供适合的健康信息。必须明确健康促进的目标，也必须探索实现目标的方法和替代方法，包括"通过组织、政治、社会和经济手段，改善环境和行为，以提高或保护健康"。

9.9.2 健康保护

只有在少数情况下才可以完全预防疾病，以下是目前常见的针对性保护措施：

①免疫接种。

②使用特殊营养素。

③预防性用药。

⑤ Protection against accidents.

⑥ Protection from carcinogens.

⑦ Avoidance of allergens.

⑧ The control of specific hazards in the general environment, e.g., air pollution, noise control.

⑨ Control of consumer product quality and safety of foods, drugs, cosmetics.

The term "health protection" which is quite often used is not synonymous with specific protection. Health protection is defined as "the provision of conditions for normal mental and physical functioning of the human being individually and in the group. It includes the promotion of health, the prevention of sickness and curative and restorative medicine in all its aspects". In fact, health protection is conceived as an integral part of an overall community development programme, associated with activities such as literacy campaigns, education and food production. Thus health protection covers a much wider field of health activities than specific protection.

9.9.3 Early diagnosis and treatment

A WHO Expert Committee defined early detection of health impairment as "the detection of disturbances of homeostatic and compensatory mechanism while biochemical, morphological, and functional changes are still reversible". Thus, in order to prevent overt disease or disablement, the criteria of diagnosis should, if possible, be based on early biochemical, morphological and functional changes that precede the occurrence of manifest signs and symptoms. This is of particular importance in diseases.

Early detection and treatment are the main intervention of disease control. The earlier a disease is diagnosed and treated the better it is from the point of

④防止职业危害。

⑤防止意外事故。

⑥采取防癌措施。

⑦避免接触过敏原。

⑧保护环境卫生，如空气污染和噪声的控制。

⑨保障食品卫生、药品和化妆品安全等。

"健康保护" 并不是 "特殊保护" 的同义词，健康保护是指采取有针对性的措施维持个体或群体正常的心理和生理功能，免受外界有害物质对健康的威胁，包括健康促进、疾病防治和康复等各方面。事实上，健康保护被视为整个社会发展的组成部分，与扫盲运动、教育和食品生产等相关。因此，健康保护涵盖的范围比具体保护更广。许多健康保护措施是个体能力所不及的，也非医疗卫生部门可单独实施的，而是需要政府和社会的共同努力。

9.9.3 早诊断和早治疗

WHO专家委员会将健康损害的早期检测定义为 "在生化、形态和功能变化仍然可逆的情况下，检测到机体稳态和代偿机制的紊乱"。因此，为了预防疾病进展和残疾，应尽可能地在出现明显症状和体征之前，利用疾病早期的生化、形态和功能变化进行诊断。

早发现和早治疗是控制疾病的主要干预措施。为了有良好的预后并预防疾病恶化（继发症）或

view of prognosis and preventing the occurrence of further cases（secondary）or any long‐term disability. It is like stamping out the "spark" rather than calling the fire brigade to put out the fire.

Strictly speaking, early diagnosis and treatment can not called prevention because the disease has commenced in the host. However, since early diagnosis and treatment intercepts the disease process, it has been included in the schema of prevention, called as secondary prevention, in as much as the goal of prevention is "to oppose or intercept a cause to prevent or dissipate its effect".

Early diagnosis and treatment though is not as effective economical as "primary prevention" may be important in reducing the high morbidity and mortality certain diseases such as essential hypertension, cancer and breast cancer. For many others such as tuberculosis leprosy and STD, early diagnosis and treatment are effective mode of intervention. Early effective therapy made it possible to shorten considerably the communicability and reduce the mortality from communicable diseases.

A mass treatment approach is use control of certain diseases, viz. yaws, pinta, nonvenereal syphilis and malaria. The rationale for a mass treatment programs the existence of at least 4-5 cases of latent infection and clinical case of active disease in the community. Patients in a latent（incubating）infection may develop disease during specified time. In such cases, mass treatment is a critical factor interruption of disease transmission. There are many of mass treatment — total mass treatment, juvenile mass treatment, selective mass treatment, depending upon nature and prevalence of disease in the community.

残疾的发生，应争取早发现、早诊断和早治疗。好比发现起火时应及时扑灭火花，而不是等着消防员来灭火。

严格来说，疾病已经在宿主体内存在，早诊断和早治疗不算预防。然而，预防的目标是消除或控制病因，以预防或消除其影响，早诊断和早治疗阻断了疾病的进程，所以也被纳入预防的范围内，为二级预防。

二级预防虽然不如一级预防经济有效，但对阻止和延缓高发病率和高死亡率的慢性病（如原发性高血压、癌症和乳腺癌）的进展很重要；早诊断和早治疗也可以缩短很多传染病（如肺结核、麻风病和性病）的流行过程，降低其致死率，是有效的干预模式。

群体治疗方法主要用于控制某些疾病，如雅司病、品他病、非传染性梅毒和疟疾。采取群体治疗方法的前提是社区中至少有4～5例潜伏期病例和活动期临床病例。具有传染性的潜伏期患者可能在一定时间内发病，群体治疗是阻断疾病传播的关键。根据疾病的性质和流行程度不同，群体治疗的方法也不同，如全面群体治疗、青少年群体治疗、选择性群体治疗等。

9.9.4 Prevent disability

When a patient reports late in the pathogenesis phase the mode of intervention is to prevent disability. The objective this intervention is to prevent or halt the transition of the disease process from impairment to handicap.

1.Concept of disability

The sequence of events leading to disability and have been stated as follows:

Disease → impairment → disability → handicap

The WHO has defined these terms as follow

①Impairment: An impairment is defined as "any loss or abnormality of psychological, physiological or anatomical structure or function", e.g., loss of foot, defective mental retardation. An impairment may be visible or temporary or permanent, progressive or regressive one impairment may lead to the development of "secondary" impairments as in the case of leprosy where damage (primary impairment) may lead to plantar ulcers (secondary impairment).

②Disability : Because of an impairment, the person may be unable to carry out certain considered normal for his age, sex, etc. This inability to perform out certain activities is termed "disability". A disability is been defined as "any restriction or lack of ability to perform an activity in the manner or within the range considered normal for a human being".

③Handicap: As a result of disability, the person experiences certain disadvantages in life and is not able to discharge the obligations required of him and play the role expected of him in society. This is termed "handicap", and is defined as "a disadvantage for a countries. Primary prevention is given individual, re-

9.9.4 伤残预防

疾病后期，干预是为了预防伤残，阻止疾病从病理损害向残疾进展。

1.残疾的概念
导致残疾的系列事件的顺序如下：

疾病→ 损害→ 残疾→ 残障
WHO定义如下：

①损害：损害被定义为"心理、生理、解剖结构或功能的任何损失或异常"，如手足缺失、先天智力发育迟缓。损害可以是可见的、暂时的或永久的、进行性的或退行性的一种损害，也可发展为继发性的损害。例如，麻风病自身的损害（原发性损害）就可能导致足底溃疡（继发性损害）。

②残疾：由于身体受到损害，特定个体无法进行与其年龄、性别相符的正常活动，被称为残疾。残疾的定义为"人类正常方式或范围的活动受到任何限制或能力缺乏"。

③残障：由于残疾，特定个体在生活中处于某些不利地位，无法履行其义务，也无法在社会中发挥期望的作用，被称为残障。残障的定义为"损害或残疾对特定个体造成缺陷，限制或妨碍其履行正常职能（取决于年龄、性别、社会和文化因素）"。

sulting from an impairment or a disability, that limits or prevents the fulfillment of a role that is normal (depending on age, sex, and social and cultural factors) for that individual".

Taking accidents as an example, the above terms can be explained further as follows:

Accident — Disease(or disorder)

Loss of foot — Impairment (extrinsic or intrinsic)

Cannot walk — Disability (objectified)

Unemployed — Handicap(socialized)

Figure 9-4　Concept of disability

The intervention in disability will often be social or environmental as well as medical. While impairment which is the earliest stage has a large medical component, disability and handicap which are later stages have large social and environmental components in terms of dependence and social cost.

2.Disability prevention

Another concept is "disability prevention". It relates to all the levels of prevention:

① Reducing the occurrence of impairment, viz. immunization against polio (primary prevention).

② Disability limitation by appropriate treatment (secondary prevention).

③ Preventing the transition of disability into handicap (tertiary prevention).

The major causes of disabling impairments in the developing countries are communicable diseases, malnutrition, low quality of perinatal care and accidents. These are responsible for about 70 percent of cases of disability in developing the most effective way of dealing with the disability problem in developing countries.

以交通事故为例，图9-4中进一步解释上述术语：

事故——疾病（或紊乱）

缺失手足——损害（外在或内在）

不能走路——残疾（客观化）

失业——残障（社会化）

图9-4　残疾的概念解释

对残疾的干预通常综合医疗、社会或环境等多方面。残疾的早期阶段主要依靠医疗干预，后期残疾和残障很大程度上需要社会和经济支持，也就是说，社会和环境发挥着很重要的作用。

2.残疾的预防

残疾的预防涉及所有级别的预防：

①减少损害的发生，如脊髓灰质炎免疫接种（一级预防）。

② 通过早期的适当治疗控制残疾的发展（二级预防）。

③防止残疾转变为残障（三级预防）。

发展中国家致残的原因70%是传染病、营养不良、围产期护理质量低下和意外事故。一级预防是发展中国家预防残疾的最有效方法。

9.9.5 Rehabilitation

Rehabilitation has been defined as "the combined and coordinated use of medical, social, educational and vocational measures for training and retraining the individual to the highest possible level of functional ability". It includes all measures aimed at reducing the impact of disabling and handicapping conditions and at enabling the disabled and handicapped to achieve social integration. Social integration has been defined as the active participation of disabled and handicapped people in the mainstream of community life.

Rehabilitation medicine has emerged in recent years as a medical speciality. It involves disciplines such as physical medicine or physiotherapy, occupational therapy, speech therapy, audiology, psychology, education, social work, vocational guidance and placement services. The following areas of concern in rehabilitation have been identified:

① Medical rehabilitation — restoration of function.

② Vocational rehabilitation — restoration of the capacity to earn a livelihood.

③ Social rehabilitation — restoration of family and social relationships.

④ Psychological rehabilitation — restoration of personal dignity and confidence.

Rehabilitation is no longer looked upon as an extracurricular activity of the physician. The current is view that the responsibility of the doctor does not end when the "temperature touches normal and stitches are removed". The patient must be restored and retained "to live and work within the limits of his disability but to the hilt of his capacity". As such medical re-

9.9.5　康复

康复指联合和协调使用医疗、社会、教育和职业措施，通过培训和再培训，使患病个体达到尽可能高的功能水平。康复旨在减少残疾和残障影响，使残疾/残障者恢复社会功能。恢复社会功能指残疾/残障者能够积极参与社区主流生活。

康复医学是近年来兴起的一门医学专业。它涉及物理医学或物理治疗、职业治疗、言语治疗、听力学、心理学、教育、社会工作、职业指导和安置服务等学科。康复医学关注的领域如下：

①医疗康复——功能恢复。

② 职业康复——恢复谋生能力。

③社会康复——恢复家庭和社会关系。

④心理康复——恢复个人尊严和信心。

康复不再被视为医生的课外活动。目前的观点认为，医生的责任不是在"体温达到正常水平，缝线被拆掉"时就结束了，而是必须恢复和维持患者"在其残疾范围内，尽其所能地生活和工作"。因此，康复应在医疗过程中尽早开始。

habilitation should start very early in the process of medical treatment.

Examples of rehabilitation are: establishing schools for the blind, provision of aids for the crippled, reconstructive surgery in leprosy, muscle re‐education and graded exercises in neurological disorders like po‐lio, change of profession for a more suitable one and modification of life in general in the case of tuberculo‐sis, cardiac patients and others. The purpose of reha‐bilitation is to make productive people out of non‐pro‐ductive people. Health for All by 2000 AD aims at pro‐viding "rehabilitation for all".

It is now recognized that rehabilitation is a diffi‐cult and demanding task that seldom gives totally satis‐factory results; but needs enthusiastic cooperation from different segments of society as well as expertise, equipment and funds not readily available for this pur‐pose even in affluent societies. It is further recognized that interventions at earlier stages are more feasible, will yield results and are less demanding of scarce re‐sources.

9.10　Changing Pattern of Disease

Although diseases have not changed significantly through human history, their patterns have. It is said that every decade produces its own pattern of disease. The truth of this will be obvious when one compares the leading causes of death in the developed countries at the beginning of this century and now (Table 9‐3).

康复的实例如建立盲人学校，为残疾人提供辅助工具，麻风病患者的重建手术，肌肉训练，神经系统的分级训练，更换合适的职业，肺结核、心脏病等患者改善生活方式等。康复的目的是将不具有生产能力的人转变成具备生产能力的人。"到2000年人人享有健康"的目标是提供"人人康复"。

现在人们已认识到，康复是一项困难而艰巨的任务，需要全社会协调合作，即使在富裕的社会中也会受到专业知识、仪器设备和经费的限制，很少能达到完全令人满意的结果。因此，疾病早期阶段的干预措施更可行，也更有效，对稀缺资源的要求也较低。

9.10　疾病模式的变化

虽然疾病在人类历史上没有发生重大变化，但其模式已经改变。据说，每十年都会产生新的疾病模式。比较20世纪初和20世纪末发达国家的主要死因时，可以明显看到疾病模式的改变（表9‐3）。

Table 9-3　Leading causes of death in the United States 1900 and 1994

Cause of death	Percent of deaths From all causes/%
1900	
Pneumonia and influenza	11.8
Tuberculosis	11.3
Diarrhoea and enteritis	8.3
Heart disease	8.0
Cerebrovascular disease	6.2
Chronic nephritis	4.7
Accidents	4.2
Cancer	3.7
Certain disease of infancy	3.6
Diphtheria	2.3
1994	
Heart disease	32.1
Cancer	23.5
Cerebrovascular disease	6.8
Accidents	3.9
Chronic obstructive pulmonary disease	4.5
Pneumonia and influenza	3.6
Diabetes	2.4
Suicide	1.4
Chronic liver diseases and cirrhosis	1.1
HIV infection	1.8
All other causes	18.9

表9-3　1990年和1994年美国的主要死因

主要死因	死因构成比 /%
1900年	
肺炎和流感	11.8
肺结核	11.3
腹泻和肠炎	8.3
心脏病	8.0
脑血管病	6.2
慢性肾炎	4.7
事故	4.2
癌症	3.7
某些婴儿疾病	3.6
白喉	2.3
1994年	
心脏病	32.1
癌症	23.5
脑血管病	6.8
事故	3.9
慢性阻塞性肺疾病	4.5
肺炎和流感	3.6
糖尿病	2.4
自杀	1.4
慢性肝病与肝硬化	1.1
艾滋病感染	1.8
其他	18.9

9.10.1　Developed countries

Table 9-3 shows that during the past 90 years, the developed world has experienced a dramatic change in the pattern of disease. By far the greatest part of this development has the decline in many of the infectious diseases (e. g., tuberculosis, typhoid fever, polio, diphtheria). Whereas in 1900, out of the 10 leading causes of death 3 were primarily of infectious nature, in 1994 only two were primarily communicable diseases. However problems of a different nature have achieved ascendancy, e.g., coronary heart disease, cancer and accident, as can be seen from Table 9-3.

9.10.1　发达国家的疾病模式

如表9-3显示，在20世纪初到20世纪末的90多年中，发达国家的疾病模式发生了巨大变化。其中，变化最大的是由传染病（如肺结核、伤寒、脊髓灰质炎、白喉）引起的死亡减少。1900年，10个主要死因中有3个是传染病，且前2位都是传染病。1994年，10个主要死因中虽然有2个是传染病，但慢性病和其他性质疾病占主导地位，如冠心病、癌症和事故。

Heart disease is the leading cause of death in United States, being responsible for almost 32.1 percent of all mortality (Table 9-3). Second and third are cancer and cerebrovascular diseases which account for 23.5 per cent and 6.8 per cent of deaths respectively. Heart disease, cancer and cerebrovascular disease cause almost 62 per cent of deaths in the United States. The picture is more or less similar in other developed countries. In short, the chronic noncommunicable diseases and conditions have now supplanted acute infections as the major cause of illness.

The morbidity pattern has also changed. In recent years, there has been a steady increase in mental disorders. Alzheimer's disease described as the "silent epidemic" of the century is an important cause of morbidity and mortality. There has been a steady increase in social pathology due to alcohol and drug abuse. Lung cancer as well as other chronic lung diseases due to smoking, and obesity due to overeating have become common. Environmental health problems connected with toxic, carcinogenic and mutagenic material in the external environment due to industrialization and growing urbanization are assuming growing importance.

As Dubos has pointed out, the microbial diseases that are now becoming prominent are often caused by organisms previously regarded as being innocuous such as the coliforms and the other gram-negative bacilli, the non-haemolytic streptococci, campylobacters, legionella, chalmydia, rotaviruses and the newly identified delta hepatitis virus and AIDS virus.

9.10.2 Developing countries

The pattern of diseases in developing countries is very different. In a typical developing country, about 40 percent of deaths are from infectious, parasitic and

心脏病是美国的主要死因，几乎占全部死因的32.1%（表9-3）；第二和第三位是癌症和脑血管疾病，分别占全部死因的23.5%和6.8%。在美国，心脏病、癌症和脑血管疾病造成的死亡人数几乎占62%。其他发达国家的情况与此相似。简而言之，慢性非传染病现在已经取代急性传染病成了发达国家的主要死因。

除了疾病模式，发病模式也发生了变化。近年来，精神障碍的发病率稳步上升。阿尔茨海默病被称为20世纪的"无声流行病"，是发病和死亡的一个重要原因。酗酒和药物滥用等导致的社会病态在持续增长，吸烟导致的肺癌和其他慢性肺病以及暴饮暴食导致的肥胖症已经变得很普遍。随着工业化和城市化的进展，源于环境的毒物、致癌物和致突变物的健康问题逐渐增多。

正如Dubos所指出的，现在日益突出的微生物疾病通常是由以前认为无害的微生物所引起的，如大肠菌群和其他革兰阴性杆菌、非溶血性链球菌、弯曲杆菌、军团菌、查氏菌、轮状病毒、新发现的三角洲肝炎病毒和艾滋病病毒。

9.10.2 发展中国家的疾病模式

发展中国家的疾病模式与发达国家大不相同。在典型的发展中国家，约40%的死亡是由传染病、寄生虫病和呼吸道疾病造成的，而发达国家的这

respiratory diseases, compared with about 8 percent in developed countries.

In India, as in other developing countries, most deaths result from infectious and parasitic diseases, abetted by malnutrition. Diarrhoeal diseases are widespread. Cholera has shown a declining trend. Malaria and black fever which showed a decline in the 1960's have staged a comeback. In China, chronic noncommunicable diseases have shown an increasing trend. Some new infectious diseases emerge and spread as "new" health problems such as SARS, COVID, and Avian Influenza.

The factors which play a role in the changing patterns of disease are multiple. They include changing lifestyles and living standards, demographic factors, urbanization and industrialization, medical interventions, maintenance of people with transmissible genetic defects, and the widespread effects of technology on ecology.

The changing pattern of disease in both developed and developing countries and the emergence of new problems emphasize the needfor forward - looking approaches in the planning and management.

9.11　Population Medicine

Knowledge about human health and disease is sum of contributions of a large number of disciplines, classified into basic sciences, clinical sciences, and population medicine. The basic sciences (e. g., biochemistry, physiology, microbiology) are primarily sited in laboratories; clinical activities are carried out in hospitals, and population medicine in the community. Tuberculosis provides a good illustration the three different approaches to the same disease. The basic sci-

一比例约为8%。

与其他发展中国家一样，印度的大多数死亡是由营养不良助长的传染病和寄生虫病造成的，腹泻病很普遍，霍乱呈下降趋势，疟疾和黑热病在20世纪60年代有所下降，在20世纪末又卷土重来。我国慢性非传染病呈上升趋势，新的传染病出现，如SARS、新冠和禽流感等。

很多因素在疾病模式变化中发挥着作用，包括生活方式和生活水平的改变、人口学因素、城市化和工业化、医学干预、对遗传性基因缺陷者的资助和科技对生态的广泛影响。

发达国家和发展中国家疾病模式的变化和新健康问题的出现，都说明了加强远期规划和管理的必要性。

9.11　群体医学

人类健康和疾病的知识是多学科的结合，包括基础医学、临床医学和群体医学。基础医学（如生物化学、生理学、微生物学）主要在实验室进行，临床医学主要在医院进行，群体医学主要在社区进行。现以结核病为例，说明三者在结核治疗中发挥的作用：基础医学发现结核病与结核分枝杆菌有关；临床医学采用个体化治疗方案治疗结核病患者；群体医学在社区中进行结核病的预防和控制。由此可见，三者高度相关，紧密

ences are concerned with tubercle bacilli; the clinical sciences with the treatment of tuberculosis in the individuality and population medicine with prevention and control tuberculosis in the community. All these approaches highly interrelated.

In different settings, population medicine is referred as hygiene, public health, preventive medicine, social medicine or community medicine. All these share common ground in their concern for promotion of health and prevention of disease. Each has originated at a different time and each has introduced a new direction or emphasis. There should be little expectation that definitions can be opened than arbitrary and imprecise. It has been truly said every definition is dangerous.

9.11.1　Hygiene

The word "hygiene" is derived from Hygeia, the goddess of health in Greek mythology. She is represented a beautiful woman holding in her hand a bowl from which a serpent is drinking. In Greek mythology, the serpent testifies the art of healing which symbol is retained even to Hygiene is defined as "is the science of health and embraces factors which contribute to healthful living".

9.11.2　Public health

The term "public health" came into general use arose 1840. It arose from the need to protect "the public" from spread of communicable diseases. Later, it appeared in the name of a law, the *Public Health Act* in England crystallise the efforts organized by society to protect, promote and restore the people's health.

In 1920, C.E.A. Winslow, a former professor of public health at Yale University, gave the often-quot-

联系。

群体医学被称为卫生学、公共卫生学、预防医学、社会医学或社区医学，每个定义源于不同的时代背景，也引入了不同的研究方向或重点，但它们的共同点都是健康促进和疾病预防。每个定义都存在过于绝对的问题和不准确的风险，但定义也是在不断发展和进步的。

9.11.1　卫生

"卫生"（hygiene）一词来源于希腊神话中的健康女神Hygeia。传说中她是一个美丽的女人，手里拿着一个碗，一条蛇正在从碗里喝水。在希腊神话中，蛇具有治疗的功效，这一标志在医学界延用至今。

9.11.2　公共卫生

"公共卫生"一词于1840年开始普遍使用，因保护公众免受传染病传播的需要而产生。后来，又以法律的形式出现，如英国的《公共卫生法》明确了公共卫生是社会组织为保护、促进和恢复人民健康而做出的努力。

1920年，耶鲁大学的公共卫生学专业教授C.E.A.温斯洛给出了后来经常被引用的公共卫生定

ed definition in public health. The WHO Expert Committee on Public Health Administration, adapting Winslow's earlier definition, defined it as: "The science and art of preventing disease, prolonging life and promoting health and efficiency through organized community efforts for the sanitation of the environment, the control of community infections, the education of the individual in personal hygiene, the organization medical and nursing services for early diagnosis and preventive treatment of disease, and the development of the social machinery to ensure for every individual a standard of living adequate for the maintenance of health and organizing these benefits as to enable every citizen to realize his birthright of health and longevity".

Whereas in developing countries such as India, public health has not made much headway in terms of sanitary reforms and control of communicable diseases, it has tremendous strides in the industrialized western countries resulting in longer expectation of life and significant decline in deathrates. As a result of improvements in public health during the past decades years, public health in the developed countries has moved from sanitation and control communicable diseases (which have been largely controlled) to preventive, therapeutic and rehabilitative aspects of chronic diseases and behavioural disorders.

A EURO symposium in 1966 suggested that the definition of public health should be expanded to include the organization of medical care services. This was endorsed by another Expert Committee of WHO in 1973. Thus modern public health also includes organization of medical care, as a means of protecting and improving the health of people. Since the organization of public health tends to be determined by cultural,

义。WHO公共卫生管理专家委员会根据温斯洛的定义,将其补充为:"通过有组织的社区环境卫生工作、社区感染控制、个人卫生教育、早期诊断和预防性医疗和护理服务、社会机制的发展等,来预防疾病、延长寿命、促进健康、提高健康服务效率的科学和技术,以确保每个人的生活水平足以维持健康,使每个公民能够实现与生俱来的健康和长寿权利"。

在印度等发展中国家,公共卫生在卫生改革和传染病控制方面并没有取得多大进展,而在工业化的西方国家,公共卫生取得了巨大进步,使人们的预期寿命延长,死亡率显著下降。发达国家通过几十年的努力,主要公共卫生问题已从改善卫生环境和控制传染病(基本上已得到控制)方面转向慢性病和行为紊乱的预防、治疗和康复方面。

1966年的一次欧洲研讨会建议,将公共卫生的范围扩大到包括医疗保健服务在内的组织。1973年,WHO的另一个专家委员会认可了这一点。因此,现代公共卫生也包括医疗保健的组织,将其作为保护和改善人民健康的一种手段。各国的公共卫生组织往往因文化、政治和管理模式的不同而不同,因此有着各种各样的组织安排。

political and administrative patterns of the countries, there is a wide mosaic of organizational arrangements.

Public health, in its present form, is a combination of scientific disciplines (e.g., epidemiology, biostatistics, laboratory sciences, social sciences, demography) and skills and strategies (e.g., epidemiological investigations, planning and management, interventions, surveillance, evaluation) that are directed to the maintenance and improvement of the health of the people.

With the adoption of the goal of "Health for All" which was proposed by WHO as a global strategic initiative in Almaty in 1977, a new public health is now evident wold-wide, which may be defined as: the organized application of local, state, national and international resources to achieve "Health for All", i.e., attainment by all people of the world of a level of health that will permit them to lead a socially and economically productive life.

Although the term "public health" has lost its original meaning, the term is still widely used. Terms like preventive medicine, social medicine and community medicine are used as synonyms for public health. Public health is not only a discipline but has become a "social institution" created and maintained by society to do something about the death rate and sanitary conditions and many other matters relating to life and death. In this sense public health is both a body of knowledge and also a means to apply that knowledge.

9.11.3 Preventive medicine

Preventive medicine developed as a branch of medicine distinct from public health, based on aetiology. It is, by definition, applied to "healthy" people. It scored several successes in the prevention of commu-

目前的公共卫生是科学学科的知识（如流行病学、生物统计学、实验室科学、社会科学、人口学）、技术和策略（如流行病学调查、规划和管理、干预、监测、评估）的综合，其目的是维护和改善人民的健康。

随着WHO于1977年在阿拉木图大会上提出的"人人享有健康"的全球战略倡议达成共识，公共卫生有了新的定义：有组织地运用地方、州、国家和国际资源，从而实现"人人享有健康"，即全世界所有人都达到健康水平，能够过上社会和经济上富足的生活。

虽然"公共卫生"一词已经失去了它原来的含义，但目前仍被广泛使用。预防医学、社会医学和社区医学等也曾被视作公共卫生的同义词。公共卫生不仅是一门学科，也是一个由社会创建和维护的"社会机构"，用来解决与生活和死亡相关问题，如降低死亡率和改善卫生条件。从某种意义上来说，公共卫生既是一个知识体系，也是一种应用知识的手段。

9.11.3 预防医学

预防医学是不同于公共卫生的医学分支，它是以病因学为基础发展起来的。根据定义，它适用于健康的人。预防医学利用免疫在传染病预防方面取得了成功，以至于早期，预防医学曾等同

nicable diseases based on immunization, so much so, in its early years, preventive medicine was equated with the control of infectious diseases.

As concepts of the aetiology of disease changed through time, so too have the techniques and activities of preventive medicine. Preventive medicine is no longer concerned, as it used to be, with immunization, important though it may be. The concept of preventive medicine has broadened to Include health promotion, treatment, and prevention of disability as well as specific protection. Preventive medicine has thus come to include both specific medical measures (e.g., immunization), as well as general health promotional measures (e.g., health education). Within this change in the definition and scope of preventive medicine, it has become clear that promoting health and preventing illness involve responsibilities and decisions at many levels - individual, public and private; and that these efforts are applied to whole population or to segments. In this, preventive medicine has become akin to public health.

Preventive medicine has become a growing point in medicine. It has branched into newer areas such as screening for disease, population control, environmental control, genetic counselling and prevention of chronic diseases. Community prevention and primordial prevention are relatively new concepts which are being applied in the community control of coronary heart disease hypertension and cancer with palpable success. The emergence of preventive paediatrics, preventive geriatrics and preventive cardiology are relatively new dimensions prevention.

Since preventive medicine has increasingly tended to applied to the organized health activities of the community, the term "preventive medicine" is regard-

于传染病的防控。

随着时间的推移，病因的概念发生了变化，预防医学的技术和活动也发生了变化。预防医学不再像过去那样只关注免疫，而是已经扩大到健康促进、治疗、残疾预防以及特殊保护等方面。因此，预防医学既包括具体的医疗措施（如免疫），也包括一般的健康促进措施（如健康教育）。在预防医学定义和范围的变化中，促进健康和预防疾病显然涉及许多层面的责任和决定——个人、公共和私人，需要整个人群或部分人群共同努力。在这一点上，预防医学已类似于公共卫生。

预防医学在医学领域越来越受到重视，也已经扩展到新领域，如疾病筛查、人口控制、环境保护、遗传咨询和慢性病预防。社区预防和初级预防是相对较新的概念，在社区控制冠心病、高血压和癌症方面取得了明显的成功。预防性儿科、预防性老年医学和预防性心脏病学是相对较新的预防分支。

由于预防医学越来越倾向于应用社区有组织的健康活动，因此"预防医学"被认为是"公共卫生"的同义词。这两个术语经常组合出现（例

ed as synonymous with public health. Both terms often appear combination（e.g., Maxcy‐Rosenau Textbook of "Public Health and Preventive Medicine"）.

Associated with the concept of public health, preventive medicine has been defined as meaning "not only the organized activities of the community to prevent occurrence as well as progression of disease and disability of mental and physical, but also the timely application of all means promote the health of individuals, and of the community as whole, including prophylaxis, health education and similar work done by a good doctor in looking after individuals and families". In this the goals of preventive medicine and public health have become identical, i.e., Health for All. line with this extension of the scope of preventive medicine, is now customary to speak of primary, secondary and tertiary levels of prevention. The cornerstone of preventive medicine is, however, "primary prevention".

9.11.4　Community health

The term "community health" has replaced in some countries, the terms public health, preventive medicine and social medicine. A EURO symposium in 1966 defined community health as including "all the personal health and environmental services in any human community, irrespective of whether such services were public or private ones". In some instances, community health is used as a synonym for "environmental health". It is also used to refer to "community health care". Therefore, a WHO Expert Committee in 1973 observed that without further qualification, the term "community health" is ambiguous, and suggested caution the use of the term.

如，Maxcy‐Rosenau 主编的书 *Public Health and Preventive Medicine*）。

与公共卫生的概念相关，预防医学被定义为"不仅是社区有组织的活动，而且还包括及时应用各种方法（包括预防、健康教育和医护工作等），以防止疾病的发生和发展，预防精神和身体的残疾，从而促进个体和社区的整体健康"。可见，预防医学和公共卫生的目标已变得相同，即"人人享有健康"。随着预防医学范围的扩大，现在人们习惯上谈论一级预防、二级预防和三级预防。预防医学的基石是一级预防。

9.11.4　社区卫生

在一些国家，"社区卫生"一词已取代公共卫生、预防医学和社会医学。1966年欧洲研讨会将社区卫生定义为"人类社区中的所有个人卫生和环境服务，无论这些服务是公共的还是私人的"。在某些情况下，社区卫生被当作"环境卫生"的同义词，也被指代"社区卫生保健"。因此，WHO的一个专家委员会在1973年指出，如果没有进一步的限定，"社区卫生"的定义是模糊的，并建议谨慎使用。

9.11.5　Social medicine

The term "social medicine" was first introduced by Jules Guerin, a French physician in 1848. In 1911, the concept social medicine was revived by Alfred Grotjahn of Berlin which stressed the importance of social factors as determinants health and disease. These ideas of social medicine spread throughout Europe and England after the First World War.

By derivation, social medicine is "the study of man as social being in his total environment". It is concerned with the factors affecting the distribution of health and illhealth population, including the use of health services. Social medicine is not a new branch of medicine, but rather an extension of the public health idea reflecting the strong relationship between medicine and social sciences.

Professor Crew of Edinburgh University defined social medicine follows: "Social medicine stands upon two pillars, medicine and sociology. Social medicine, by derivation is concerned with the health of groups, health of individuals with these groups with a view to create, promote, preserve, and maintain optimum health. The laboratory to practice social medicine is the whole community; the tools for diagnosing community ills are epidemiology and biostatistics; and social therapy does not consist in administration of drugs but social and political action for the betterment of conditions of life man. Social medicine is one more link in the chain of social organizations of a civilized community." Terms such as social anatomy, social physiology, social pathology and social therapy came into vogue to describe the various aspects aspects of social medicine.

9.11.5　社会医学

"社会医学"一词于 1848 年由法国医生 Jules Guerin 首次提出。1911 年，柏林的 Alfred Grotjahn 重新提出了社会医学的概念，强调社会因素作为健康和疾病的决定因素的重要性。第一次世界大战后，这些社会医学思想传遍了欧洲（包括英国）。

派生出来的社会医学的定义为"研究人类在其整体环境中的社会存在"。它关注影响健康和不健康人群分布的因素，包括卫生服务的使用。社会医学不是医学的一个新分支，而是公共卫生理念的延伸，反映了医学与社会科学之间的密切关系。

爱丁堡大学的 Crew 教授对社会医学的定义如下："社会医学建立在医学和社会学两大支柱上。社会医学关注的是个体和群体的健康，以期创造、促进、维护和保持最佳健康。社会医学实践的实验室是整个社区；诊断社区疾病的工具是流行病学和生物统计学；社会疗法不包括药物治疗，而是为改善人类生活条件而采取的社会和政治行动。社会医学是文明社会组织链中的又一个环节。"目前，社会解剖学、社会生理学、社会病理学和社会治疗等也已涌现出来，以描述社会医学的各层面。

Although the term "social medicine" was introduced more than 180 years ago, the characteristic aspect was its repeated advent and disappearance. It never came to be generally accepted. There was no unanimity in its objectives or subject matter. This is reflected in more than 50 definitions given to social medicine.

Social medicine had achieved academic respectability in England when John Ryle was appointed as professor of social medicine at Oxford, and Crew at Edinburgh. The post‐war period (1945-1967) saw considerable expansion of social medicine as an academic discipline.

With the development of epidemiology as a new discipline and a practical tool in the planning, provision and evaluation of health services, interest in social medicine began to wane. In 1968, the Report of the Royal Commission on Medical Education (Todd Report) for the first time referred to "community medicine" instead of social medicine, and defined it in terms which embraced social medicine, but went beyond it, by giving greater emphasis to the organizational and administrative aspects than had academic social medicine in the past. This gave a blow to the further development of social medicine which had tended in many countries to be displaced by the newer term "community medicine".

9.11.6　Community medicine

The term "community medicine" is a newcomer. It is the successor of what has been previously known as public health, preventive medicine, social medicine and community health. Since community medicine is a recent introduction, it has borrowed heavily from the concepts, approaches and methods of public health,

虽然"社会医学"一词在180多年前就已被提出，但其特点是反复出现和消失，它从未被普遍接受。关于社会医学的50多个定义说明其目标和主题一直没有达成共识。

在John Ryle担任牛津大学和爱丁堡大学的社会医学教授时，社会医学在英国学术界获得了认可。第二次世界大战后（1945—1967年），社会医学作为一门学术学科得到了很大发展。

随着流行病学作为一门新学科和规划、提供、评估卫生服务的实用工具的发展，人们对社会医学的关注开始减弱。1968年，皇家医学教育委员会的报告（Todd报告）第一次提到"社区医学"而不是"社会医学"，并将其定义为包含社会医学，但又超越社会医学，更加强调组织和行政方面。这给社会医学的发展带来了打击，在许多国家，"社会医学"被"社区医学"所取代。

9.11.6　社区医学

"社区医学"是一个新的术语，它从公共卫生、预防医学、社会医学和社区卫生发展而来，大量借鉴了公共卫生、预防医学和社会医学的概念、方法和手段。

preventive medicine and social medicine.

The history of community medicine in England is interesting. It was instituted by Ordinance and by Act of Parliament. The Todd Commission (1968) forcibly recommended that every medical school in England should have a department of community medicine. The Royal College of Physicians of Edinburgh and London and the Royal College of Physicians and Surgeons of Glasgow established the Faculty of community medicine, which came into being in March 1972 as the central body with a responsibility of setting standards and overseeing the quality of postgraduate education and training in the field. On the night of 31 March 1974, the traditional medical officer of health passed into the pages of the history book, and was thereafter designated as the "community physician".

The term community medicine means different things in different countries. For example, in most European countries various aspects of community medicine are taught at medical universities, though under different names, such a general practice, family medicine, community medicine or social medicine. Even in the same country and region, the variation in the amount and range of teaching remains remarkable. These variations are reflected in the definitions quoted below.

1.definition

①The field concerned with the study of health and disease in the population of a defined community or group. Its goal is to identify the health problems and needs of defined population (community diagnosis) and to plan, implement and evaluate the extent to which health measures effectively meet these needs.

②The practice of medicine concerned with group population rather than with individual patients. And

英国社区医学的历史很有趣,它是根据法令和议会法案建立的。托德委员会(Todd Commission, 1968年)强烈建议英国的医学院都应该有一个社区医学系。伦敦皇家医学院和格拉斯哥皇家医学院于1972年3月成立了社区医学系,它是负责制定标准和监督研究生教培质量的中央机构。1974年3月31日晚,传统的卫生官员成为了历史,此后被称为"社区医生"。

在不同的国家,"社区医学"的含义不同。例如,在大多数欧洲国家的医学院,尽管专业的名称不同,如全科医学、家庭医学、社区医学或社会医学,但这些专业都教授社区医学。即使在同一个国家和地区,教学内容和范围也有很大差异,这些差异反映在下面的定义中。

1.定义

①研究特定社区或人群的健康和疾病的领域。目的是确定特定人群的健康问题和需求(社区诊断),并规划、实施和评估健康措施有效满足这些需求的程度。

②与群体而非个体患者相关的医学实践,包括定义①中列出的内容,以及社区或群体层面的

includes the elements listed in definition ①, together with the organization and provision of health care community or group level.

③The term is also used to describe the practice of medicine in the community, e.g., by a family physician. Some writers equate the terms "family medicine" "community medicine"; others confine its use to public health practice.

④Primary health care of individuals in the community. In this of practice, the community practitioner or community health team has responsibility for health care community or at an individual level.

It will be seen that a common thread runs through a above definitions. Diagnosis of the state of health community is an important foundation of community medicine. As used in the present context, community medicine is a practice which focuses on the health needs the community as a whole. The combination of community medicine with "primary health care" extends the function of both elements to a health care system which aims to change the state of health of the community by intervention both the individual and group level. The foundations of community medicine are in no way different from those of modern public health and social medicine, viz. epidemiology, biostatistics, social sciences and organization of health care which includes planning, implementation and evaluation.

It is anomalous that in England and United States the term community medicine is not freely used, their standard textbooks on the subject are still titled Public Health. e.g., Oxford "Textbook of Public Heath", Maxcy - Rosenau "Public Health and Preventive Medicine".

医疗保健组织和提供的服务。

③也用于描述社区中的医疗实践，比如由家庭医生进行的医疗实践。有人将"家庭医学"等同于"社区医学"，也有人将其应用局限于公共卫生实践。

④以社区为导向的初级卫生保健是社区医学与初级卫生保健的结合。在实践中，社区从业人员或社区卫生团队负责社区或个人层面的医疗保健。

可以看出，一个共同的主线贯穿了上述定义。社区诊断是社区医学的重要基础。在目前的情况下，社区医学是一种专注于整个社区健康需求的实践。社区医学与"初级卫生保健"的结合，将两个要素的功能扩展到卫生保健系统，旨在通过个体和群体的干预来改变社区健康状况。社区医学的基础与现代公共卫生和社会医学的基础相同，即流行病学、生物统计学、社会科学，以及具有规划、实施和评估职能的医疗保健组织。

反常的是，在英国和美国，"社区医学"这个词并没有被随意使用，他们关于这个主题的标准教科书仍然以"公共卫生"为标题。例如，牛津大学的《公共卫生教材》，Maxcy-Rosenau的《公共卫生和预防医学》）。

2.Hospitals and community

The hospital is a unique institution of man. A WHO Expert Committee in 1963 proposed the following word definition of a hospital: "A hospital is a resident establishment which provides short-term and long-term medical care consisting of observational, diagnosis therapeutic and rehabilitative services for persons suffering suspected to be suffering from a disease or injury and parturients. It may or may not also provide service for ambulatory patients on an out-patient basis."

The criticism leveled against the hospital is that it exists in splendid isolation in the community, acquiring the euphemism "an ivory tower of disease"; it absorbsa vast proportion (50%-80%) of health budget; it is not people-oriented; its procedures and styles are inflexible; it overlooks the cultural aspects of illness (treating the disease without treating the patient); the treatment is expensive; it is intrinsically resistant to change, and so on. The relative isolation of hospitals from the broader health problems of the community which has its roots in the historical development of health services, has contributed to the dominance of hospital model of health care.

In 1957, an Expert Committee of WHO emphasized that the general hospital cannot work in isolation; it must part of a social and medical system that provides community health care for the population. Subsequent years witness the efforts of WHO, UNICEF and non-governmental age to involve hospitals in providing basic and referral services. The establishment of primary health centres was a forward to integrate preventive and curative services.

The community hospital should be a flexible institution, capable of adapting its resources to the total

2.医院与社区

医院是一个独特的机构。1963年，WHO专家委员会将医院定义为："医院是为居民提供短期和长期医疗护理的机构，包括观察、诊断、治疗和康复服务，为可疑患者、伤员和产妇提供服务。"

医院也存在一定的弊端，如占据的卫生预算大（50%～80%）、缺乏人文关怀、流程和风格死板、忽视疾病文化（治病而不治人）、费用昂贵、机制体制陈旧等，医院又因与社区及社区广泛的健康问题不融合，而被称为"疾病的象牙塔"。其根源在于医疗服务的历史发展，这促成了医院医疗模式的主导地位。

1957年，WHO的一个专家委员会强调，综合医院不能孤立地工作，它必须是社区和医疗体系的一部分，能为民众提供社区保健。随后几年，WHO、儿童基金会和非政府组织努力让医院参与提供基本医保服务和转诊服务。建立初级保健中心是整合预防和治疗服务的进步。

社区医院应该是一个灵活的机构，能够根据社区的总体医疗保健需求调整其资源。这种调整

health care needs of the community. This Rene Sand adaptation requires hospital administration that is both a science and art. Dr. Rene Sand has said that the right patient should receive the right care at the right time in the right place at the right cost. This ideal, seemingly simple, is perhaps never achieved, like all other ideals because of a complex set of interacting and often conflicting social forces operating both within and outside the hospital system.

With the acceptance of the goal of "Health for All", the involvement of hospitals in primary health care activities is being discussed. Member countries of WHO have enunciated in their national policies to re-orient and restructure their health care systems on the basis of primary health care. Primary health care cannot work unless there is effective hospital support to deal with referred patients, and to refer patients who do not require hospital attention to one of the other primary health care services. Without hospital support primary health care could not achieve its full potential. The trend is now set to redefine the role of the hospital as a community - health oriented institution, which means that it is not only disease oriented but has responsibilities in the field of preventive medicine and health promotion.

3.Functions of a physician

The object of medical education is to prepare a doctor (physician) for the tasks he is likely to given. In view of the fact that there is no internationally accepted definition of the word "physician", the WHO has adopted the following definition.

"A physician is a person who, having been regularly admitted to a medical school, duly recognized in the country in which it is located has successfully completed the prescribed courses of studies in medicine

要求医院管理既是一门科学，又是一门艺术。Rene Sand博士说过，患者应该在正确的时间和地点，花费合适的成本，接受正确的治疗。这个看似简单的理想可能永远无法实现，就像其他理想一样，因为在医院系统内外都有一组复杂的相互影响、相互矛盾的社会力量在运行。

随着"人人享有健康"的目标被广泛接受，医院参与初级卫生保健的计划被提上日程。WHO成员国已在其国家政策中阐明，要在初级卫生保健的基础上调整和重组卫生保健系统。前提是，需要医院有效支持转诊患者，并将不需要医院照顾的病人转到其他初级卫生保健服务机构，否则初级卫生保健无法发挥作用。也就是说，如果没有医院的支持，初级卫生保健就无法发挥其全部潜力。医院被重新定义为一个以社区健康为导向的机构，这意味着它不仅是以疾病为导向，而且在预防医学和健康促进领域也负有责任。

3. 医生的职能

医学教育的目的是使医生（医师）为可能承担的任务做好准备。鉴于"医生"一词没有国际公认的定义，WHO采用了以下定义：

"医生是指被所在国正式承认的医学院正常录取，成功完成规定的医学课程，并获得合法行医资格（包括预防、诊断、治疗和康复），可以独立作出有助于促进社区和个人健康判断的人。"

and has acquired the requisite qualification to be legally licensed to practise medicine (comprising prevention, diagnosis, treatment and rehabilitation) using an independent judgement to promote community and individual health".

4.Community diagnosis

The diagnosis of disease in an individual patient is fundamental idea in medicine. It is based on signs and symptoms and the making of inferences from them. When this is applied to a community, it is known as community diagnosis. The community diagnosis may be defined as the pattern of disease in a community described in terms of the important factors which influence this pattern.

The community diagnosis is based on collection and interpretation of the relevant data such as: ① the age and sex distribution of a population; the distribution of population based social groups; ② vital statistical rates such as the birth rate and the death rate; ③ the incidence and prevalence of the important diseases of the area. In addition, a doctor must be able to find information on a wide variety of social and economic factors that may assist him in making a community diagnosis. The focus is on the identification of the basic health needs and health problems of the community. The needs all felt by the community (some of which may have no connection at all with health) should be next investigated and listed according to priority for community treatment.

5.Community treatment

Community treatment or community health action is the sum of steps decided upon to meet the health needs of the community taking into account the resources available and the wishes of the people, as re-

4.社区诊断

个体化诊断和治疗是临床医学的基本理念，临床诊断是基于个体的症状和体征做出推断。借用临床诊断的概念，社区诊断可定义为通过一定的方式和收集必要的资料，通过科学、客观的方法确定，并得到社区人群认可的该社区主要的公共卫生问题及其影响因素的一种调查研究方法。

社区诊断基于相关数据的收集和分析，如人群的年龄和性别分布、基于社会群体的人口学特征、出生率和死亡率等重要统计指标、该地区重要疾病的发病率和患病率，以及社会和经济等影响因素的信息，帮助做出社区诊断，重点是确定社区的基本卫生需求和健康问题。社区卫生需求（有些可能与健康有关）应根据社区治疗的优先次序进行调查，并列出清单。

5.社区治疗

社区治疗或社区健康行动是为满足社区卫生需求，同时考虑社区诊断确定的卫生资源和人民意愿，而进行的决策和干预。例如，改善供水、免疫接种、健康教育、控制特定疾病、卫生立法

vealed by community diagnosis. Improvement of water supplies, immunization, health education, control of specific diseases, health legislation and examples of community health action or interventions as actions may be taken at three levels: at the level of the individual, at the level of the family and at the level of the community.

A programme of community action must have the following characteristics: ① It must effectively utilize all the available resources; ② It must coordinate the efforts of all other agencies in community, now termed a "intersectoral coordination"; ③ It must encourage the full participation of the community in the programme. These are the principles on which primary health care, as defined in the Alma - Ata Declaration, is based. This approach is a significant departure from the earlier basic services approach.

9.12   Disease Classification

There is a wide variation among countries in the criteria and standards adopted for diagnosis of diseases and their notification, making it difficult to compare national statistics. A system of classification was needed whereby diseases could be grouped according to certain common characteristics, that would facilitate the statistical study of disease phenomena. Over the years, many approaches were tried to classify diseases. John Graunt in the 17th century in his study of *Bills of Mortality*, arranged diseases in an alphabetical order. Later, a more scientific approach was adopted in classifying diseases according to certain characteristics of the disease or injuries such as the part of the body affected, the aetiologic agent ,the kind of morbid change produced by the disease, and the kind of disturbance

和社区健康行动或干预。社区治疗可以从三个层面采取行动，即个人层面、家庭层面和社区层面。

社区行动方案必须具有以下特点：①必须有效利用所有可用资源；②必须协调其他部门的工作，即"跨部门合作"；③必须鼓励社区全员参与。这些是《阿拉木图宣言》中定义初级卫生保健所依据的原则，与早期的基本卫生服务不同。

9.12   疾病分类

各国疾病诊断和报告的标准和规范存在很大差异，所以很难比较各国的统计数据。因此需要一个能根据共同特征将疾病进行分组的分类系统，以便对疾病进行统计研究。多年来，人们尝试了许多方法。17世纪，John Graunt 在《死亡清单》（*Bills of Mortality*）中按照字母顺序排列疾病。后来，人们采用了一种更科学的方法，根据疾病或伤害的某些特征进行分类，如受影响的身体部位、病原体、疾病引起的病变种类，以及疾病或伤害引起的功能紊乱种类。因此，疾病有许多分类标准，可以根据研究目的选择不同的标准。

of function produced by the disease or injury. Thus there are many axes of classification, and the particular axis selected will depend on the interest of the investigator.

9.12.1　International classification of diseases

All the above criteria formed the basis of the *International Classification of Diseases*（ICD）produced by WHO and accepted for national and international use. Since its inception, ICD has been revised about once every 10 years; the last revision, the 10th revision, came into effect on January 1, 1993. Earlier, the scope of ICD was expanded in the sixth revision in 1948 to cover morbidity from illness and injury. The ICD also provides a basis that can be adapted for use in other fields e.g., dentistry, oncology and ophthalmology.

As in previous revisions, the ICD-10 is arranged in 21 major chapters.

Ⅰ. Certain infectious and parasitic diseases（A00-B99）

Ⅱ. Neoplasms（C00-D48）

Ⅲ. Diseases of the blood and blood forming organs and certain disorders involving the immune mechanism（D50-D89）

Ⅳ. Endocrine, nutritional and metabolic diseases（E00-E90）

Ⅴ. Mental and behavioural disorders（F00-F99）

Ⅵ. Diseases of the nervous system（G00-G99）

Ⅶ. Diseases of the eye and annexes（H00-H59）

Ⅷ. Diseases of the ear and mastoid process（H60-H95）

Ⅸ. Diseases of the circulatory system（100-199）

Ⅹ. Diseases of the respiratory system（J00-J99）

Ⅺ. Diseases of the digestive system（K00-K93）

9.12.1　国际疾病分类

上述标准构成了WHO编制的《国际疾病分类》（ICD）的基础，被许多国家和国际社会采用。自成立以来，ICD大约每10年修订一次，第10次修订于1993年1月1日生效。1948年的第6次修订，将ICD的范围扩大到涵盖所有疾病和伤害。ICD也为其他领域的使用提供了基础，如口腔科学、肿瘤学和眼科学领域。

与以前的修订一样，ICD-10分为21个主要分类章节。

Ⅰ.传染病和寄生虫病（A00—B99）

Ⅱ.肿瘤（C00—D48）

Ⅲ.血液、造血器官疾病及免疫疾病（D50—D89）

Ⅳ.内分泌、营养和代谢疾病（E00—E90）

Ⅴ.精神和行为障碍（F00—F99）

Ⅵ.神经系统疾病（G00—G99）

Ⅶ.眼睛和附器疾病（H00—H59）

Ⅷ.耳和乳突疾病（H60—H95）

Ⅸ.循环系统疾病（100—199）

Ⅹ.呼吸系统疾病（J00—J99）

Ⅺ.消化系统疾病（K00—K99）

ⅫⅠ.Diseases of the skin and subcutaneous tissue（L00-L99）

Ⅷ.Diseases of the musculoskeletal system and connective tissue（M00-M99）

ⅩⅣ.Diseases of the genitourinary system（N00-N99）

ⅩⅤ.Pregnancy, childbirth and puerperium（O00-O99）

ⅩⅥ.Certain conditions originating in perinatal period（P00-P96）

ⅩⅦ.Congenital malformations, deformations and chromosomal abnormalities（Q00-Q99）

ⅩⅧ.Symptoms, signs and abnormal clinical and laboratory findings, not elsewhere classified（R00-R99）

ⅩⅨ.Injury, poisoning and certain other consequences of external causes（S00-T98）

ⅩⅩ.External causes of morbidity and mortality（V01-Y98）

ⅩⅪ.Factors influencing health status and contact with health services（Z00-Z99）

9.12.2　The coding system

The first character of the ICD-10 code is a letter and each letter is associated with a particular chapter, except for the letter D, which is used in chapter II and chapter III, and letter H which is used in chapter VII and chapter VIII. Chapter I,II. XIX and XX use more than one letter in the first position of their codes.

Each chapter contains sufficient three - character categories to cover its contents. Not all the available codes are allowing space for future revision and expansion. The rather categories is given in parentheses after each block title.

Ⅻ.皮肤和皮下组织疾病（L00—L99）

Ⅷ.肌肉骨骼和结缔组织疾病（M00—M99）

ⅩⅣ.泌尿生殖系统疾病（N00—N99）

ⅩⅤ.妊娠、分娩和产褥期（O00—O99）

ⅩⅥ.源自围产期的某些情况（P00—P96）

ⅩⅦ.先天性畸形、变形和染色体异常（Q00—Q99）

ⅩⅧ.症状、体征、异常的临床与实验室结果，无法归于其他类的（R00—R99）

ⅩⅨ.伤害、中毒和外因所致的某些后果（S00—T98）

ⅩⅩ.疾病和死亡的外部原因（V01—Y98）

ⅩⅪ.影响健康状况和获得卫生服务的原因（Z00—Z99）

9.12.2　编码系统

ICD-10编码的第一个字符是字母，每个字母都与特定章节相关，但字母D（用于第二章和第三章）和字母H（用于第七章和第八章）除外。第一、第二、第十九、第二十章在其代码的第一位置使用了多个字母。

每章都有足够的三字分类涵盖其内容。但不是所有可用代码都为将来的修订和扩展留出了空间。每个标题后面的括号中给出了对应的类别。

Although not mandatory for reporting at the internal level, most of the three - character categories are subdivided by means of a fourth numeric character after a decimal allowing up to 10 subcategories. Where a three - character category is not subdivided, it is recommended that the "X" be used to fill the fourth position so that the codes are standard length for data - processing.

Examples :

Chapter XXI　Factors influencing health status and contact with health services （Z00-Z99）

　　Z72　Problems relating to lifestyle

　　　Z 72.0　Tobacco use

　　　Z 72.1　Alcohol use

　　　Z 72.2　Drug use

　　　Z 72.3　Lack of physical exercise(S00-T98)

　　　Z 72.4　Inappropriate diet and eating habits

　　　Z 72.5　High-risk sexual behaviour

The unused "U" code: Codes U00-U49 are to be for provisional assignment of new diseases of uncertain aetiology. Codes U50-U99 may be used in research when testing an alternative subclassification for a special project.

ICD-10 consists of three volumes. Volume 1 contains the report of the International conference for the Tenth Revision, the classification itself at the three- and four-character levels, the classification of the morphology of neoplasms, special tabulation lists for mortality and morbidity, definitions and the nomenclature regulations. Volume 2 is instruction manual and volume 3 contains alphabetical index.

The ultimate purpose of ICD is to contribute to a unfixed classification that can be used throughout the world to accurate comparisons of morbidity and mortality dared decision-making in prevention, in manage-

尽管在内部报告中没有强制要求，但大多数三字类别在小数点后的第4个数字字符进行细分，最多允许10个子类别。如果一个三字类别没有被细分，建议用"X"来填补第4个位置，这样代码就会成为数据处理的标准长度。

示例：

第二十一章　影响健康状况和获得卫生服务的原因（Z00-Z99）

　　Z72　与生活方式有关的问题

　　　Z 72.0　吸烟

　　　Z 72.1　饮酒

　　　Z 72.2　滥用药物

　　　Z 72.3　缺乏体育锻炼（S00—T98）

　　　Z 72.4　不良的饮食和饮食习惯

　　　Z 72.5　高危性行为

未使用的"U"代码：代码U00—U49用于临时分配不确定病因的新疾病。代码U50—U99可以在研究中用于测试一个特殊项目的替代亚分类。

ICD-10由三卷组成。第一卷包括第10次修订的会议报告、三字和四字分类本身、肿瘤的形态分类、死亡率和发病率特别报表、定义和命名规则；第二卷是使用手册；第三卷包含字母索引。

ICD的最终目的是建立一个不固定的分类，可以在全世界范围内使用，以准确比较发病率和死亡率，从而在预防、健康管理和健康促进的研究方面做出决策。读者可参阅ICD第10次修订版，

ment of health and in facilitating research on particular health problems. For reader is referred to the Tenth Revision of the ICD for getting principles and description of the ICD classification.

了解ICD分类的原则和说明。

9.13 Hospital Infection and Its Prevention and Control

9.13 医院感染及其防制

9.13.1 Definition

9.13.1 定义

Hospital infection (HI), or nosocomial infection (NI), or hospital acquired infection (HAD), refers to the acquisition by in patients of an infection in the hospital. This category includes infections that are acquired and occur during the period of staying in hospital, and those that are acquired in the hospital but occur after discharge. It does not include infections acquired before admission to the hospital and existing upon admission. In addition, infections of health care workers in the hospital are also considered to be hospital infections. All of these types of infection represent an important source of avoidable morbidity and mortality, and their prevention and control consumes substantial medical and public health resources.

医院感染（HI）又称院内感染（NI）或医院获得性感染（HAD），是指患者或医务人员在医院环境内发生的感染，包括住院期间发生的感染和在医院内获得但在出院后发生的感染，不包括入院前获得或入院时已存在的感染。医院感染作为发病和死亡的重要来源是可防可控的，其防控消耗了大量的医疗和公共卫生资源。

9.13.2 Based on source of pathogen

9.13.2 根据病原体来源分类

1.Exogenous nosocomial infection

Exogenous nosocomial infection or "cross infection", refers to patients infected by pathogens from other patients, health care workers, accompanying personnel, contaminated environments or medical appliances while they stay in hospital.

1.外源性医院感染

外源性医院感染包括"交叉感染"、环境感染、医源性感染，是指被其他病人、医护人员、陪同人员、被污染的环境或医疗器具的病原体感染，即各种原因导致患者在医院内遭受非自身体内病原体侵袭而发生的感染。

2.Endogenous nosocomial infection

Endogenous nosocomial infection or "autogenous nosocomial infection" refers to patients infected by

2.内源性医院感染

内源性医院感染又称为"自身医院感染"，是指患者在住院期间被自身病原体感染。病原体一

pathogens coming from themselves while they stay in hospital; these pathogens are part of the normal microbial flora in the body.

3.Mother-infant infection

Mother-infant infection refers to infants infected by pathogens acquired through the placenta or birth canal in the process of delivery.

9.13.3　Based on the traits of pathogens

Hospital infection may be characterized, according to the traits of pathogens, as caused by: common pathogenic microorganisms, conditional pathogenic organisms, chance pathogenic microorganisms, or bacteria that are resistant to multiple drugs.

9.13.4　Based on infection location

Hospital infection is classed into twelve categories according to the location of infection: respiratory system, cardiovascular system, blood system, digestive system, central nervous system, urinary system, operation location, skin and soft tissue, skeletal and joint, reproductive system, oral, and other location.

9.14　Measures of Prevention and Control of Hospital Infection

9.14.1　Strengthening organizational management

According to the "Management Regulations for Hospital Infection" of the National Health Ministry of China, all hospitals at different levels shall have a department dedicated to managing hospital infection or have special personnel who are responsible for hospital infection, all reporting to the dean or deputy dean

般为寄居体内的正常菌群。

3.母婴感染

母婴感染是指婴儿在母亲分娩过程中通过胎盘或产道获得病原体感染。

9.13.3　根据病原体特点分类

根据病原体的特征，医院感染可分为常见病原体感染、条件致病菌感染、病原微生物感染、机会致病菌感染或耐药菌感染。

9.13.4　根据感染部位分类

根据感染的部位，医院感染分为12类：呼吸系统、心血管系统、血液系统、消化系统、中枢神经系统、泌尿系统、手术部位、皮肤和软组织、骨骼和关节、生殖系统、口腔和其他部位感染。

9.14　医院感染的防制措施

9.14.1　加强组织管理

根据国家原卫生部《医院感染管理条例》，各级医院应设立专门的医院感染管理部门或专人负责医院感染工作，均直接向院长或副院长报告。医院感染预防和控制部门的人员数量取决于医院的床位数量。医院感染管理部门主要负责预防和控制医院感染，护理部门主要指导护士在其职责

of hospital. The number of personnel in the department of hospital infection prevention and control is dependent on the number of beds in the hospital. The department of health care is primarily responsible for preventing and controlling hospital infection and the department of nursing mainly directs nurses to deal with hospital infection problems within the range of their duties.

9.14.2　Surveillance of hospital infection

Hospital infection surveillance refers to a long-term, continuous and systematic process of observation, collection, and analysis of the occurrence, distribution and determinates of hospital infection A good program disseminates data and provides scientific evidence for prevention and control of hospital infection.

An effective hospital surveillance system must include the following four aspects:① Well-trained doctors for infection control; ②Nurse specialists in infection control; ③ A reporting system for hospital infection; ④ Organizational capacity for conducting infection monitoring and control.

Hospital infection surveillance covers three tasks: ① Closely monitor the hospital infection situation and provide evidence for the committee of infection to set up effective prevention and control strategies and measures; ②Quickly investigate the reasons for hospital infections and swiftly take special measures to controlling their spread; ③Assess the effectiveness of currently used measures for preventing hospital infection.

范围内处理医院感染问题。

9.14.2　医院感染监测

医院感染监测是指对医院感染的发生、分布和决定因素进行长期、连续、系统的观察、收集和分析的过程。医院感染监测信息的反馈为医院感染的防控提供科学依据。

一个有效的医院感染监测系统必须包括以下四个方面：①训练有素的感染防制医生；②有感染防制的护理专家；③医院有感染报告系统；④有感染监测和防制的组织能力。

医院感染监测包括三项任务：①密切监测医院感染情况，为感染委员会制定有效的防控策略和措施提供依据；② 迅速调查医院感染的原因，采取特殊措施控制其传播；③ 评估目前预防医院感染措施的有效性。

9.14.3 Routine management of hospital infection

1.Reinforcing management of hospital regulations

Standard and qualified wards for communicable diseases must be set up in hospitals, and they are specially used to receive patients with communicable disease. Hospitals must avoid placing communicable disease patients and non - communicable disease patients in the same ward. Once a patient with a non-communicable disease acquires an infection or carries pathogenic bacteria, he or she must be isolated promptly from other patients. Likewise, patients with a high risk of being infected, such as those with hematological malignancies, lymphatic system diseases, organ transplantation and major burns, must be isolated. When visiting inpatients, visitors must avoid carrying pathogenic bacteria from the outside into the hospital or from the hospital to the outside. The rules for visiting are especially important and must be strictly adhered to when visiting patients with communicable diseases or weak immune functions.

2. Enhancing management of disinfection and sterilization

Medical appliances that are used to enter body tissues or organs in aseptic procedures entail a high risk of infection and must be sterilized; those used in contact with skin or mucosa present a medium risk and must be disinfected; and those with low risk are cleaned using regular methods. Quality control of disinfection and sterilization must be rigorous, and managers should regularly check the concentrations of disinfectants and monitor whether bacterial contamina-

9.14.3 医院感染的常规管理

1. 加强医院规章制度管理

医院必须设立标准、合格的传染病病房，专门用于接收传染病患者。医院必须避免将传染病患者和非传染病患者放在同一病房。一旦非传染病患者感染或携带致病菌，必须立即将其与其他患者隔离。同样，必须隔离具有高感染风险的患者，如血液系统恶性肿瘤、淋巴系统疾病、器官移植和严重烧伤患者。探访住院患者时，探访者必须避免将病原菌从外部带入医院或从医院带到外部。探访规则尤其重要，在探访患有传染性疾病或免疫功能低下的患者时，必须严格遵守。

2. 加强消毒灭菌管理

在无菌操作中，进入人体组织或器官的医疗器械具有较高的感染风险，必须消毒；与皮肤或黏膜接触的器械具有中等风险，必须消毒；对风险较低的器具采用常规方法清洗。消毒和灭菌的质量控制必须严格，管理人员应定期检查消毒剂的浓度，监测其中的细菌污染是否超标。对其他消毒方式，如紫外线，也应定期测试，评估其强度是否符合标准要求。

tion in them is over criteria. Other disinfection modalities, such as ultraviolet light, should also be tested at regular intervals to assess whether their intensity meets standard requirements.

3. Reinforcing management of rational use of drug and medical treatment

Hospitals should strengthen education on the rational use of antibiotics and medical treatments, make guidelines for them, strictly supervise and monitoring their use, seriously control overuse, and prevent deficiencies of dosage and other types of misuse.

4. Motivation and education

Motivation and education to encourage prevention and control of hospital infection should be provided for health care workers, patients and accompanying persons. In this way, health care workers' knowledge of prevention and control of hospital infection can be improved, and they may actively use more measures to decrease the occurrence of hospital infection.

5. Strengthening monitoring and management of latrogenic transmitting factors

Liquids for diagnosis and treatment should be periodically tested for bacteria, and infected liquid discarded. Blood and its products, as well as donors of blood, must be screened for bacterial infection, hepatitis A virus, and HIV.

6. Strengthening management for buying and using disposable aseptic medical supplies

The quality of disposable aseptic medical devices should be strictly monitored to prevent unqualified items from being introduced into clinical care services. At the same time, used items should be disinfected and/or destroyed so as to prevent them from causing serious public health problems in the community.

3. 加强合理用药和医疗救治的管理

医院应加强合理使用抗生素和医疗手段的教育，制定使用指南，严格监督和监测，认真控制过度使用，防止剂量不足和其他类型的滥用。

4. 激励和教育

应为医护人员、患者和陪同人员提供激励和教育，以鼓励预防和控制医院感染。这样可以增加医护人员关于医院感染的预防和控制的知识，从而积极采取更多措施减少医院感染的发生。

5. 加强潜伏性传播因素的监测和管理

应定期对诊断和治疗用液体进行细菌检测，并丢弃感染液体。对血液及其制品和献血者必须进行细菌、甲型肝炎病毒和艾滋病毒感染检测。

6. 加强对一次性无菌医疗用品的购买和使用管理

严格监控一次性无菌医疗用品的质量，防止不合格用品进入临床医疗服务。同时，应对用过的物品进行消毒或销毁，防止在社区引起严重的公共卫生问题。

9.14.4 Management of hospital infection

Immediately after a hospital infection is recognized, persons responsible for hospital infection control should collect samples to detect the pathogen(s) causing the infection and should conduct an epidemiological investigation to explore relevant features of the infection. Meanwhile, the following measures should be carried out:

1.Isolate patients

After recognition of a hospital infection, the infected patients should be isolated until no pathogenic agent is detected on several consecutive laboratory tests and risk of further infection no longer exists.

2.Field quarantine

Terminal disinfection should be performed in wards and departments in which hospital infection has occurred and new patient should not be received in these wards until after a time interval that is at least as long as the longest incubation period of this disease. Contacts should remain under close medical observation.

3.Detect carriers

If the source of hospital infection cannot be found through an epidemiological survey, a search for possible carriers should be considered and may include health care workers, patients, accompanying persons and visitors.

9.14.4　医院感染的处理

在确认医院感染后，负责医院感染控制的人员应立即采样，检测导致感染的病原体，并应进行流行病学调查，探析感染的相关特征。同时，采取以下措施：

1.隔离患者

在确认医院感染后，应隔离受感染的患者，直到在连续几次的实验室检测中未检测到病原体，确定不存在进一步感染的风险。

2.现场检疫

在发生医院感染的病房和科室进行终末消毒，经过至少一个最长潜伏期后，才可接收新患者。对接触者应保持密切的医学观察。

3.筛检携带者

如果通过流行病学调查无法找到医院感染源，应考虑寻找可能的携带者，包括医护人员、患者、陪同人员和访客。

Problem-set and answer

Distribution of Disease

1. Which of the following measures is used frequently as a denominator to calculate the incidence rate of a disease?　（　）

　　a. Number of cases observed

　　b. Number of new cases observed

　　c. Number of asymptomatic case

　　d. Person-years of observation

　　e. Persons lost to follow-up

2. In a study of the effectiveness of pertussis vaccine in preventing pertussis (whooping cough), the following data were collected by studying siblings of children who had the disease.

Immunization status of sibling contact	Number of siblings exposed to case	Number of cases among siblings
Complete	4 000	400
None	1 000	400

What was the secondary attack rate of pertusis in fully immunized household contacts?　（　）

　　a. 0%

　　b. 10%

　　c. 25%

　　d. 40%

　　e. 75%

Answer: 1. d ; 2. b

习题及答案

疾病的分布

1. 下面哪一项是疾病发病率计算公式的分母?

　　　　　　　　　　　　　　　（　）

　　a. 观察到的病例数

　　b. 观察到的新发病例数

　　c. 无症状病例数

　　d. 观察人年数

　　e. 失访人数

2. 在一项关于百日咳疫苗预防百日咳效果的研究中，研究人员通过研究患病儿童的兄弟姐妹，收集了表1所示的数据。

表1

同胞接触者的免疫状况	同胞中接触病例的人数	同胞中患病人数
有	4 000	400
无	1 000	400

完全有免疫力的家庭中百日咳的续发率是

　　　　　　　　　　　　　　　（　）

　　a. 0%

　　b. 10%

　　c. 25%

　　d. 40%

　　e. 75%

答案：1. d ;　2. b

Descriptive Studies

1. A research team wishes to investigate a possible association between smokeless tobacco and oral lesions among professional baseball players. At spring training camp, they ask each baseball player about current and past use of smokeless tobacco, cigarettes, and alcohol, and a dentist notes the type and extent of the lesions in the mouth.What type of study in this?

( )

    a. Case-control

    b. Cross-sectional

    c. Prospective trial

    d. Clinical trial

    e. Retrospective cohort

2. After the players have been questioned about use of smokeless tobacco and examined for lesions of the mouth, the data on the 146 player are tabulated as follows:

	Mouth lesion	No lesion	Total
User	80	30	110
Nonuser	2	34	36
Total	82	64	146

In this study, which measure of disease occurrence can be calculated? ( )

    a. Incidence rate

    b. Cumulative incidence rate

    c. Incidence density

    d. Prevalence

    e. Relative risk

3. Which of the following statements in true?

( )

    a. the odds ratio is equal to $(80/110) \times (2/36) =$

13.1

描述性研究

1.一个研究小组欲调查在职业棒球运动员中无烟烟草与口腔病变的关系。在春季训练营，调查员询问所有棒球运动员目前和过去使用无烟烟草、香烟和酒精的情况，牙医记录了这些运动员口腔病变的类型及程度。这项研究属于什么类型的研究？ ( )

    a.病例对照研究

    b.横断面研究

    c.前瞻性试验

    d.临床试验

    e.回顾性队列

2.在询问了球员使用无烟烟草的情况并检查了口腔的病变后，该研究小组将146名球员的数据列表如下（表2）：

表2

	口腔病变	无病变	总数
使用烟草	80	30	110
未使用烟草	2	34	36
总数	82	64	146

本研究中，可以计算下列什么指标？ ( )

    a.发病率

    b.累积发病率

    c.发病密度

    d.患病率

    e.相对危险度

3.下列哪项陈述是正确的？ ( )

    a.优势比＝$(80/110) \times 2/36 = 13.1$

b. A temporal association between smokeless tobacco use and oral lesions can be established

c. The statistical association can be calculated using the chi-square test

d. Selection bias could overestimate the result

e. There should be an equal number of exposed and nonexposed subjects

Answer: 1. b; 2. d; 3. c

Case-Control Studies

As an epidemiologist, you are asked to recommend the type of study appropriate to the needs of researchers who would like to study the causes of a rare form of sarcoma. They have discovered a registry of this form of cancer and have access to the largest database of patients with this form of cancer, which, unfortunately, is only a few years old. They have funding for only one year from the National Institutes of Health and note the budge will be tight. What type of study design do you recommend?　（　　）

a. Prospective cohort

b. Retrospective cohort

c. Cross-sectional

d. Experimental

e. Case-control

Answer: e

Cohort Studies

1. The association between low birth weight and maternal smoking during pregnancy can be studied by obtaining smoking histories from women at the time of the first prenatal visit and then subsequently assessing and assigning birth weight at delivery according to smoking histories. What type of study is this?　（　　）

a. Clinical trial

b.无烟烟草使用与口腔病变之间的时间关联可以确定

c.可以使用卡方检验计算统计关联

d.选择偏倚可能会高估结果

e.暴露和未暴露的人数应相等

答案：1. b；2. d；3. c

病例对照研究

某研究团队想研究一种罕见肉瘤的病因。研究者已经发现了关于这种肉瘤的登记册，并且已经获得了患者的大量数据，但只有几年的数据。该项目获得美国国立卫生研究院一年的资金支持，经费紧张。作为流行病学专家，你推荐该项目使用下列哪种研究方法？　（　　）

a.前瞻性队列

b.回顾性队列

c.横断面研究

d.实验性研究

e.病例对照研究

答案：e

队列研究

1.要研究低出生体重与母亲在孕期吸烟的关系，研究者在孕母第一次产检时获取其吸烟信息，然后在其分娩时根据其吸烟信息收集和分析婴儿体重。这是什么研究类型？　（　　）

a.临床试验

b. Cross-sectional

c. Prospective cohort

d. Case-control

e. Retrospective cohort

2. The results of a study of the incidence of pulmonary tuberculosis in a village in India are given in the Table 3. All persons in the village are examined during two surveys made two year apart, and the number of new cases was used to determine the incidence rate.

Table 3

Category of Household at First Survey	Number of Persons	Number of New Cases
With culture-positive case	500	10
Without culture-positive case	10 000	10

2.1 What is the incidence of new cases per 1 000 person-years in house-holds that had a culture-positive case during the first survey? （ ）

a. 0.02

b. 0.01

c. 1.0

d. 10

e. 20

2.2 What is the incidence of new cases per 1 000 person-years in households that did not have a culture-positive case during the first survey? （ ）

a. 0.001

b. 0.1

c. 0.5

d. 1.0

e. 5.0

2.3 What is the relative risk of acquiring tuberculosis in households with a culture-positive case compared with households without culture-positive case? （ ）

---

b.横断面

c.前瞻性队列

d.病例对照

e.回顾性队列

2.一项在印度农村开展的研究，利用相隔2年的2次调查的数据计算发病率，其中肺结核发病率数据见表3。

表3

首次调查的住户类别	人数	新增病例数
有肺结核病例	500	10
无肺结核病例	10 000	10

2.1 在第一次调查期间，有肺结核病例的家庭中，每1 000人年的新病例发生率是多少？ （ ）

a. 0.02

b. 0.01

c. 1.0

d. 10

e. 20

2.2 在第一次调查期间，没有肺结核病例的家庭中，每1 000人年肺结核的发病率是多少？ （ ）

a. 0.001

b. 0.1

c. 0.5

d. 1.0

e. 5.0

2.3 与无肺结核病例的家庭相比，有肺结核病例的家庭感染结核病的相对风险是多少？ （ ）

a. 0.05

b. 0.5

c. 2.0

d. 10

e. 20

3. The incidence rate of lung cancer is 120/100 000 person-years for smoker and 10/100 000 person-years for nonsmokers. The prevalence of smoking is 20% in the community.

3.1 What is the relative risk of developing lung cancer for smokers compares with nonsmokers? (　　)

a. 5

b. 12

c. 50

d. 100

e. 120

3.2 What percentage of lung cancer can be attributed to smoking?　　　　　　　　(　　)

a. 52%

b. 78%

c. 80%

d. 92%

e. 99%

3.3 If the prevalence of smoking in the community was decreased to 10%, the excess incidence rate of lung cancer that could be averted in that community would be?　　　　　　　　(　　)

a. 11/100 000

b. 22/100 000

c. 50/100 000

d. 60/100 000

e. 110/100 000

Answer: 1. c; 2.1 e; 2.2 d; 2.3 e; 3.1 b; 3.2 d; 3.3 a

a. 0.05

b. 0.5

c. 2.0

d. 10

e. 20

3.肺癌的发病率在吸烟人群中是120/10万人年，在不吸烟人群中为10/10万人年。社区人群吸烟率为20%。

3.1 与不吸烟人群相比，吸烟人群发展为肺癌的相对危险度是多少？　　　　　　(　　)

a. 5

b. 12

c. 50

d. 100

e. 120

3.2 肺癌归因于吸烟的归因危险度百分比为多少？　　　　　　　　　　　　(　　)

a. 52%

b. 78%

c. 80%

d. 92%

e. 99%

3.3 如果社区人群吸烟率降低至10%，那么社区人群的肺癌超额发病率将降低多少？　(　　)

a. 11/100 000

b. 22/100 000

c. 50/100 000

d. 60/100 000

e. 110/100 000

答案：1. c；2.1 e；2.2 d；2.3 e；3.1 b；3.2 d；3.3 a

Experimental epidemiology

1. In the study of the cause of a disease, the essential difference between an experimental study and an observational study is that in the experimental investigation （ ）

a. The study is prospective

b. The study is retrospective

c. The study and control groups are of equal size

d. The study and control groups are selected on the basis of history exposure to the suspected causal factor

e. The investigators determine who is and who is not exposed to the suspected causal factor

2. An investigator is designing a randomized, double - blind, placebo - controlled clinical trial to see whether vitamin E will prevent lung cancer. Which technique is likely to maximize compliance with the allocated regimen? （ ）

a. Using the placebo

b. Performing a run-in phase

c. Using intent-to-treat analysis

d. Double blinding the study

e. Limiting the number of subjects enrolled

3. Which is most likely to affect the validity (source of bias) of the study? （ ）

a. Loss to follow-up

b. Incidence of lung cancer

c. Prevalence of smoking in the source population

d. α error

e. β error

4. A randomized trial shows that a new thrombolytic agent reduces total mortality by 30% in the first 30 days after a suspected myocardial infarction compared with a placebo （P=0.002）. Which of the following

实验流行病学

1.病因研究中，实验性研究和观察性研究最基本的不同是，在实验性研究中 （ ）

a.这项研究是前瞻性的

b.这项研究是回顾性的

c.研究组和对照组的人数相同

d.研究组和对照组是根据疑似原因的历史暴露情况选择的

e.调查人员确定哪些人没有接触到可疑的因果因素

2.想要设计一个随机、双盲、安慰剂对照的临床试验，以研究维生素 E 是否可以预防肺癌。下列哪种技术可以最大化地遵守分配方案？

（ ）

a.使用安慰剂

b.使用导入期

c.利用意向性分析策略

d.双盲研究

e.限制登记的受试者人数

3.下面那一项最有可能影响研究的真实性（偏倚来源）？ （ ）

a.失访

b.肺癌发病率

c.源人群中的吸烟率

d.α错误

e.β错误

4.一项随机试验研究显示：一种新的溶栓剂与安慰剂相比，在疑似心肌梗死致死后的前30天内，总死亡率降低30%（P=0.002）。那么下列哪一个问题是最需要回答的？ （ ）

questions would be the most important to have answered? ( )

a. Was the trail blinded ?

b. What was the power of the study?

c. What happened to surviving patients in the next year?

d. What percentage of patients in each group actually had a myocardial infarction?

e. What was the effect on mortality from coronary heart disease?

Answer: 1. e;2. b;3. a;4. c

a.该试验使用盲法了吗?

b.这项研究的效力是多少?

c.在接下来的一年里,幸存的患者发生了什么?

d.每组患者中有多少比例的人患有心肌梗死?

e.对冠心病致死率的影响是什么?

答案: 1. e; 2. b; 3. a; 4. c